Health
Communication

Communication and Careers

SERIES EDITORS
Thomas W. Bohn, *Ithaca College*
Joseph R. Millichap, *University of Tulsa*

HEALTH COMMUNICATION
Theory and Practice

Gary L. Kreps
Rutgers University

Barbara C. Thornton
University of Nevada, Reno

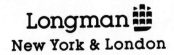

Longman

New York & London

Health Communication

Longman Inc., 95 Church Street, White Plains, N.Y. 10601

Associated companies, branches, and representatives throughout the world.

Developmental Editor: Gordon T. Anderson
Editorial and Design Supervisor: Frances A. Althaus
Production Supervisor: Ferne Y. Kawahara
Manufacturing Supervisor: Marion Hess

Library of Congress Cataloging in Publication Data

Kreps, Gary L.
  Health communication.

  (Communication and careers)
  Bibliography: p.
  Includes indexes.
  1. Communication in medicine—Case studies.
I. Thornton, Barbara C., 1936–   . II. Title.
III. Series. [DNLM: 1. Delivery of health care.
W 84.1 K92h]
R118.K73 1984   610'.141   83–958
ISBN 0–582–28410–4
ISBN 0–582–28411–2 (pbk.)

Manufactured in the United States of America

Printing: 9 8 7 6 5 4 3   Year: 92 91 90 89 88 87 86 85

CONTENTS

PREFACE

Doctors, dentists, pharmacists, nurses, and other health professionals depend on their ability to communicate effectively with colleagues and patients in the performance of their health care duties. For example, the doctor who interviews a new client to establish an accurate medical history, the dentist who probes a client's mouth to discover the source of a toothache, or the pharmacist who describes and explains the correct use of a prescribed drug to a client are all depending on their ability to communicate effectively. All too often, training for health care professionals has failed to stress the importance of human communication in health care delivery and as a consequence many health professionals are ill prepared to fulfill the communicative demands of their jobs. Communication training for these health professionals can provide the impetus necessary to facilitate development of effective health communication skills.

Health Communication: Theory and Practice is intended to guide the training of health professionals and consumers in developing effective knowledge and skills in health communication. Undergraduate and graduate students in preprofessional health care programs of study as well as practicing health care professionals seeking in-service training in communication will find this text useful. We take a pragmatic perspective on communication in health care, relating communication research and theory to realistic health care situations. A wide variety of research on health and communication is integrated and applied to the many problems facing the modern health care professional in the delivery of high quality health care services. Although the book avoids simplistic "cookie cutter" solutions to complex human problems, it does offer insights and strategies the health professional can use to analyze and cope with difficult health communication situations.

It is our strong contention that in order to solve health communication problems the study of communication ideally should be interdisciplinary. That is, members of the various health professions should study communication together so that each profession can become aware of the communication problems common among related disciplines. Since it is not always possible to study together, we have designed this textbook to fill many interdisciplinary needs and to function as a bridge between health professionals.

The text is divided into eight major chapters, each beginning with a case history and ending with selected readings by noted health communication researchers, scholars, and practitioners. The cases were written to help introduce and apply the concepts of the chapters for the reader. The readings were chosen to supplement the content areas developed in each chapter, and are excellent discussion starters for classes and training groups, allowing both students and professionals to integrate and expand upon health communication concepts of particular interest to them.

An extensive thirteen-section bibliography of communication in health care follows the last chapter, covering such topic areas as verbal and nonverbal communication in health care, health care interviewing, therapeutic communication, group communication in health care, conflict in health care, intercultural communication in health care, communication with the terminally ill, ethics in health care, and media in health care. We feel that the text, supplemented by the epilogue, case histories, readings, and extensive bibliographies will provide the reader with a broad understanding of the role of communication in health care practice.

In writing this book we have paid special attention to using language clearly and sensitively. We have attempted to demystify complex social psychological jargon by providing explanations and examples to flesh out and illustrate new and often complex concepts. We have chosen to include both the male and female pronoun when describing health practitioners and clients to avoid sexist language usage and sexist stereotypes. On the advice of some of our students, we have decided to limit our use of the connotatively passive term "patients" to describe health care consumers, opting for the more assertive term "clients" throughout the text. Throughout the book we attempt to encourage consumer participation in the health care process, and using the term client rather than patient is one way to help empower health care consumers.

Several people have been of great service to us in writing this book. Our special thanks to Tren Anderson, Executive Editor at Longman Inc., for his professional insight and cooperation. Tom Bohn has done much as our editorial advisor to encourage our creativity in developing the raw material of this book into a finished text. We appreciate the excellent critiques and suggestions our reviewers offered, many of which we adopted in the book. Our sincere thanks to Janet Morgan, who did most of the typing of the manuscript. Our colleagues in our universities and the Health Communication Division of the International Communication Association continued to encourage our work on this project. Our students provided insightful feedback on earlier versions of the book. Most of all, we sincerely appreciate our family members, who helped us maintain our sanity while writing, were patient with us when we neglected them, and were understanding when we went through crises and revisions in the evolution of the book. To Stephanie Kreps and Bill, Bret and Dan Thornton, we thank you. Special thanks to Rhoda Cohen-Kreps (who epitomizes therapeutic communication) and Margery Cavanaugh.

Health
Communication

1.

INTRODUCTION TO HEALTH COMMUNICATION

The young woman needed four wisdom teeth extracted. The procedure was a routine one that could be performed in the dentist's office. Nitrous oxide was administered as an anesthetic. The woman's mother accompanied her but was directed to sit in the waiting room, with the promise that she would be called if needed. During the course of the treatment, the woman had a drug reaction. She began to experience terror and wanted her mother. She felt her mother could help her feel secure enough to relax, and perhaps even enjoy the novel drug experience. The client tried to ask for her mother, only to find that she was unable to talk. Feeling helpless only increased her terror.

At no time during the one-hour dental procedure did either the dentist or the dental assistant inquire into the client's comfort. After the procedure, the client had several psychological reactions, including nightmares which persisted for several months. Today, almost a year later, she continues to feel aversion toward dentists. The dentist and his assistants, questioned by the parent as to why they had not inquired into the client's comfort, explained that they typically become so involved in the procedure that they often do not inquire; also they felt at a loss as to how they should approach the client during a procedure.

Many similar stories can be recounted of inadequate communication with clients who are experiencing pain or fright. However, health professionals (with rare exceptions) perceive themselves to be helpful and altruistically motivated persons. How does the communication disparity between "intent" and "execution" occur?

1

THE COMMUNICATIVE DEMANDS OF HEALTH CARE PRACTICE

Health communication is an area of study concerned with human interaction in the health care process. It is our contention that human communication is the singularly most important tool health professionals have in providing health care to their clients. Not only do health providers offer their services to consumers through communication contact, but they also gather pertinent information from their clients, explain procedures and regimens to clients, and elicit cooperation among members of their health care team through their ability to communicate.

Health care professionals depend on their abilities to communicate effectively with their colleagues, clients, and often the families of their clients to competently perform their health care responsibilities. The clarity, timeliness, and sensitivity of human communication in health care is often critical to the physical and emotional well being of health care clients.[1] In compiling a client's case history the practitioner must be able to evoke clear, accurate, and detailed information from the client in order to competently diagnose the client's current state of health, identify relevant health experiences he or she has had, and develop effective strategies for health care intervention and maintenance.

Regardless of the health care professional's level of health science expertise, if he or she does not communicate effectively in establishing the client's history there will be insufficient information available to the practitioner to direct the client's treatment. In the course of health care treatment the practitioner must utilize communication skills to gather information from the client, answer the client's questions, give the client directions for self care and establish a therapeutic relationship with the client. Human communication is the primary tool the health care professional has in delivering health care services to the public. Additionally, communication is also pragmatically important to the physician and other health professionals. One physician writer reports evidence that developing good client/practitioner relationships can lessen the number and costs of malpractice suits.[2]

Though a natural ability to communicate effectively with people is certainly advantageous to a health care professional, to function as a "professional" demands a more disciplined awareness of the manner in which human interaction occurs. The practitioner needs to develop increased awareness of the ways in which his or her own communication behaviors affect the meanings created and behaviors taken by others. The effective health care practitioner should react perceptively to the wide range of verbal and nonverbal messages clients and co-workers transmit in health care situations. Development of these human communication skills will allow the health care provider to respond appropriately and effectively to clients and co-workers. For example, in the case history at the beginning of this chapter, if the dentist and the dental assistants had been aware that their client was showing nonverbal cues of discomfort they would have realized how terrified she was of the treatment, and could have helped dispel her fears. Because these health professionals were not alert to their client's communication, they failed to react appropriately, and actually aggravated her anxiety.

Effective human communication skills and competencies do not just happen; people are not born with effective communication skills, nor do they necessarily develop naturally. Skills and competencies are learned behaviors that have to be examined and practiced in order to be mastered. This book is designed to direct your examination, practice, and mastery of effective human communication knowledge and skills to be used in the delivery of health care services.

HEALTH COMMUNICATION IS FOR THE ENTIRE HEALTH CARE TEAM

The need for knowledge and skills in human communication for health care delivery is not limited just to the physician, but it is equally important for the nurse, pharmacist, therapist, aide, health care administrator, social worker, and health care client to be thoughtful and effective communicators. Each member of the health care team must work interdependently with other team members as well as with clients in accomplishing health care tasks. Each individual performs an integral role in the complex and multi-faceted health care delivery system.

The health care delivery system is like a wagon wheel with many different spokes (see Figure 1.1). The hub of the wheel is the client's role. The entire health care system should revolve around the health care needs of consumers. Each of the spokes of the wheel represents one of the health care professional roles. Each of these roles performs important functions for the consumer in the delivery of health care. The client is the point where each of these professional roles meet. The combination of the specific health care skills of each of these professional areas provides the client with health care services. The quality of treatment provided to the client often depends on the effectiveness of human communication between the different parts of the health care delivery wheel.

The active and accurate communication between interdependent health professionals, as well as between clients and practitioners, enables coordination within the health care system. A breakdown in com-

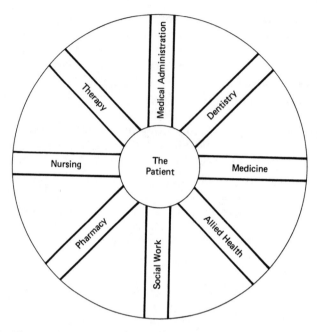

Figure 1.1   The Health-Care Delivery System Wheel.

munication between any of the spokes of the wheel or between any spoke and the hub of the wheel can jeopardize the effectiveness of the entire health care system by weakening the strength of the wheel. Together, all parts of the wheel add strength to the health care system. Effective communication keeps the parts of the health care delivery system working in concert and enhances the quality of health care.

PROBLEMS AND ISSUES IN THE DELIVERY OF HEALTH CARE

Evidence in recent years has revealed mounting inadequacies in the quality of human communication between people in health care settings. Practitioners are often unaware of the ways in which their messages to clients may frighten or confuse these clients. Clients often fail to recognize how important it is for them to explain their symptoms clearly and fully to their health care providers in order to receive appropriate treatment. Both clients and practitioners report frustration and dissatisfaction in their health care encounters with others. Korsch and Negrete concluded, in their 1972 *Scientific American* article, "the quality of medical care depends in the last analysis on the interaction of the patient and the doctor, and there is abundant evidence that in current practice this interaction all too often is disappointing to both parties."[3] While more emphasis has been placed on communication in health care since that article was written, there is no evidence to indicate that health care communication is much improved.

Client Cooperation with Health Care

An often identified problem area in health care is poor compliance with prescribed health care programs. The compliance literature addresses such issues as clients' failures to (1) comply with keeping health care appointments, (2) follow health care regimens, (3) use prescribed drugs correctly, or (4) abide by the rules of the health care institution.[4]

Poor consumer compliance in health care is generally recognized as a major problem impeding the delivery of high quality health care services.

The identification of this problem area as "patient compliance" indicates a one-way practitioner orientation. The responsibility for poor "compliance" is directed towards the client. In this book we prefer to speak about compliance in terms of cooperation between the client and the practitioner, where responsibility for health care outcomes are shared jointly by the client and the practitioner. By examining the communication between health care providers and their clients we can identify the development of cooperation.

Cooperation is not a naturally occurring part of human endeavor but rather the outcome of relationship development. Instead of viewing client noncompliance as a maladaptive client characteristic, it is more productive to view the problem as one of cooperation, due to the kind of communication relationship established between the client and the practitioner. Health care providers can evoke client cooperation with their medical regimens, directions, appointments, and procedures through the development of effective communication relationships. In chapter 2 we will discuss the relationship development process and suggest strategies for developing effective client–practitioner communication relationships.

Miscommunication in Health Care

Another rampant problem in the delivery of health care is the misinterpretation of communication between people. This is known as *miscommunication*. Miscommunication does not mean that communication has not occurred. *It means that often the meanings that communicators create in response to messages sent to them are very different from the meanings that were intended.* Miscommunications happen often in health care situations for a number of reasons. Some of these reasons include the complexity of health care information, the widespread use of medical jargon, and the extreme urgency and emotionality of many health care situations.

Miscommunications are not indigenous solely to health care interaction. Misunderstandings occur regularly between people in all kinds of social, business, and educational situations. The reason miscommunication in health care is of such vital importance is the crucial need for accurate and timely information in client diagnosis, treatment, and long-term care—miscommunication can actually be a matter of life or death. For example, if a hospital lab technician reports the results of a client's blood test to the client's attending physician over the telephone (as sometimes is the case in busy hospitals), there is a good opportunity for miscommunication to occur. An inaccuracy of even 1 decimal point in reporting these blood test results can strongly affect the physician's diagnosis of the client and the regimen prescribed. An incorrect diagnosis and prescription would undoubtedly complicate the original health problem confronting the client, with the ultimate potential of endangering the client's life.

Misunderstandings between clients and their health care providers can be a cause of noncompliance. It is difficult for a client to follow a health care regimen that he or she does not understand. Part of establishing an effective practitioner–client relationship is being able to communicate clearly, honestly, and accurately. In the following chapter we will discuss the use of verbal and nonverbal messages in communicating meaningfully with others, as well as the utilization of feedback in human communication to counteract the problem of miscommunication.

Unrealistic Expectations in Health Care

Another source of problems in the delivery of health care are unrealistic expectations held by both clients and professionals concerning each other's performance and the outcomes of health care treatment. Studies have indicated that health professionals and clients tend to stereotype one another.[5] These stereotypes are often unrealistic generalizations of the attitudes, inclinations, and abilities of people in health care situations.

Consumers may enter the health care situation expecting the health professional to perform minor miracles—eradicating their ailments and making them better than they were before they encountered their health care complaint. The doctor is often seen as a cultural hero by the public, able to solve any and all problems.[6] Media doctors on "Mash" and "St. Elsewhere" may be able to solve all of their clients' problems, but it is impossible for real-life doctors to do the same. These unrealistic stereotypes put the health professional in an untenable situation in which they can never meet clients' expectations.

Health care professionals also stereotype their clients. Research has indicated that health professionals prefer certain clients over others.[7] Depending on age, illness-type, sex, status, or level of attractiveness a client may be stereotyped in different ways by the health professional, because different stereotypes receive differing styles of treatment. Health care providers also often underestimate their clients' level of understanding of their health care treatments and problems.[8] These unrealistic evaluations of clients can inhibit high quality health care delivery. In Chapter 2 we will examine the perceptual process and discuss strategies for minimizing the ill effects of stereotypes in health care.

Lack of Sensitivity in Health Care

A final problem in the delivery of health care that we will identify here is insensitive communication between health providers and their clients. Insensitivity may be the greatest source of dissatisfaction people feel about the health care system. Due to heavy workloads, high stress, and constant contact with human suffering, the health professional may become callous to the feelings of others. Practitioners can become "burnt-out" after extended tours of duty on busy hospital wards, making them less responsive to the needs of their clients.[9]

Clients also have been known to be insensitive toward the needs and feelings of their health care providers. They often see their own problems as being preeminent over the problems of other clients or health practitioners. Clients may demand immediate attention to their problems and can become belligerent when the practitioner cannot instantly leave whatever he or she is doing and rush to the client's side. Certainly, upon reflection, the client's sense of urgency is understandable. Clients can become apprehensive and fearful about their health condition, and because of their fear can see only their own problems. Nonetheless, the self-centered perspective taken by many clients is a major impetus to insensitivity in health care.

We certainly do not intend to infer that all health care practitioners and consumers communicate insensitively. There are many extremely sensitive individuals in health care. Yet, the people who do behave in an unfeeling way to others in health care cause many other health care problems. A major tenet of this book is that effective health care is delivered through the establishment of effective communication relationships, and insensitivity is a giant block to such development. The previous health care problems we have identified (cooperation, miscommunication, and unrealistic expectations), are strongly related to insensitive communication. Throughout the rest of this book we will identify strategies available to health communicators to help them develop healthy relationships with clients and practitioners in delivering high quality health care.

Dissatisfaction with Health Care Services

The health care problems of lack of cooperation, miscommunication, unrealistic expectations, and insensitivity between people involved in health care have caused widespread dissatisfaction with health care practice by both consumers and practitioners.[10] This dissatisfaction, in turn, can cause people who may be in need of health care treatment to avoid seeking professional help. Clients who are receiving health care services are not always satisfied with the benefits of their treatment, which may relate to the increase in health care malpractice suits. Health care professionals who are dissatisfied with their roles and outcomes in health care practice are more likely to become disenchanted with the health care system, eventually leading to burnout and turnover of health care staff.

Human communication is strongly related to each of the health care problem areas we have identified. We have linked client cooperation to the establishment of effective communication relationships. Miscommunications are caused by ineffective use of messages and feedback in health care. Unrealistic expectations of health care are based on overgeneralized perceptions and stereotypes of the people involved in the health care system. Lack of sensitivity in health care causes people to communicate callously with one another, and precipitates the breakdown of health care relationships. All of these problems lead to dissatisfaction with health care and loss of effectiveness in the health care delivery system. Improvement in human communication in health care will certainly not solve all of the problems that are part of the complex health care system, but it can help improve the levels of satisfaction people have with their health care relationships.

NOTES

1. Thornton, Page, and Dangott, 1982, Section E.
2. Herlicky, 1970, Section A.

3. Korsch and Negrete, 1972, Section A.

4. Alpert, 1964, Section A; Blackwell, 1973, Section A; Caron, 1968, Section A; Davis, M., 1971, Section A; Davis, M., 1968a, Section A; Davis, M., 1968, Section A; Davis, M., 1968c, Section A; Davis, M., 1967, Section A; Davis, M., 1966, Section A; Davis, M., and Eichorn, 1963, Section A; Gillon and Barsky, 1974, Section A; Harper, 1971, Section A; Hertz and Stamps, 1977, Section A; Hulka, et al., 1975b, Section A; Jonas, 1971, Section A; Komaroff, 1976, Section A.

5. Blackwell, 1967, Section A; Enelow and Adler, 1972, Section H; Johnson, J., 1972, Section A; Mechanic, 1972a, Section H; Myerhoff and Larson, 1965, Section H; Nelson, 1973, Section A; Pollack, 1965, Section H; Seward, 1969, Section F; Spiegel, 1954, Section E; Tagliacozzo and Mauksch, 1972, Section H.

6. Myerhoff and Larson, 1965, Section H.

7. Nelson, 1973, Section A; Nguyen, 1975, Section B.

8. Kane and Deuschle, 1967, Section A.

9. Bates and Moore, 1975, Section G.

10. Anonymous, 1976, Section A; Ben-Sira, 1976, Section E; Corea, 1977, Section H; Crown, 1971, Section A; Dichter, 1954, Section A; Dodge, 1961, Section H; Ehrlich and Bauer, 1967, Section E; Fuchs, 1974, Section A; Gruen, 1970, Section A; Hulka, 1971, Section H; Illich, 1976, Section J; Kaiser and Kaiser, 1974, Section H; Kane and Deuschle, 1967, Section A; Knowles, 1973, Section J; Lambert, 1978, Section A; Mendelsohn, 1979, Section A; Nelson, 1973, Section A; Pellegrino, 1966, Section A; Scoggins, 1976, Section A; Slocum, 1972, Section F; Tagliacozzo and Mauksch, 1972, Section H; Walker, 1973, Section A.

READING

PREVIEW OF READING

The article in this chapter's reading section is written by an anonymous client about experiences as a consumer in a hospital. "A Consumer Speaks Out About Hospital Care," is an angry, critical perspective on the current health care delivery system. It is useful because it allows the health professional to see health care as it might look to the client. The author points out several problems experienced in the hospital, the most glaring of which seems to be a lack of sensitivity to the client's needs and feelings. This perspective on health care is probably not representative of health care in general, but does illustrate problem areas in health care delivery and the need for improved communication in the health care system.

A CONSUMER SPEAKS OUT ABOUT HOSPITAL CARE

Anonymous

Hospital employees talk too much and they talk too little. They ask patients questions that are none of their business; they fail to ask patients questions that they should. On occasion they give more of themselves than we might expect; on occasion they fail to act even remotely humane. They decline to communicate information about the patient's condition to the patient; they volunteer information to the patient which is no patient's business.

To protect the guilty, I choose to remain anonymous, but my identity is known to the editor. I'm past middle age, a professional person but not a physician or a nurse, have extraordinarily acute hearing but must wear trifocals, and have almost total recall, a photographic memory for faces and for illustrations in the PDR, and a working knowledge of biochemistry and physiology. My sex is irrelevant to this article.

When the surgeon recommended elective surgery for late spring, 1975, I marked off two weeks on my calendar.

An admitting clerk telephoned for preliminary information, observing that I would be called "on Monday before eleven" with definite word about a bed being ready. At one Monday afternoon, I called admitting, where a clerk insisted I had already been admitted.

"Funny thing . . . I haven't signed any papers and no one has taken any blood from me and I'm still sitting here at home."

"Well, I don't know . . . I must have you confused with someone else. C'mon down right now and I'll find you a room somewhere."

By four o'clock I was in a semi-private room, at $130 per day. At six, a tray was brought, with apologies: "This is the dinner the patient before you ordered before the heart collapse. They took the body out just before you came, you know. If you don't want this, I'll find something else." Assuming that the previous occupant of my bed had not died of botulism, I ate the meal.

At ten o'clock an unidentified nurse appeared: "Your medication." I said none had been prescribed. She was adamant. I asked her to read the orders again.

"Aren't you X?"

"No—I'm Y."

"Wow!" she blurted, "Wrong room again!" and disappeared.

The next two days were spent in minor "tests." These, before the malpractice crisis, would have been done in a quarter of the time and on an outpatient basis. [The five-minute perfunctory examination by the consulting internist was one exception. For $60, he advised my surgeon to perform the operation for which I had been hospitalized.] On each night following the "tests," attempts were made to give me medication not intended for me. Had I been the normal docile patient, I might have swallowed it.

My operation was scheduled for nine o'clock on the third morning, and the expected NPO sign went up on the doorway at bedtime. At midnight an orderly awakened me to announce that he was removing my water carafe because of the pending surgery. Luckily, I sleep easily and am not nervous.

At six I was rolled onto a cart and wheeled to a "holding ward." Without glasses, paper or pencil, and expecting a long wait, I began focusing on the conversations going on around me, and on the staff's actions. Some of the aged patients were so frightened they were shaking. Some of the blacks were screaming about discrimination, saying that they had been kept waiting too long.

An aide asked the RN at the desk for instructions about one of the shouters. "Do as you think best," said the RN.

"But *you're* in charge. I don't have any authority."

"Listen, G," said the RN. "You *know* this is only my second day on this job and you've been here a month. *I* just don't know. Why the hell can't you handle the situation?" Shrugging her shoulders, the aide did what she thought best—nothing.

Shortly afterward, an anesthesiologist in a green scrub suit sauntered over to the RN, now injecting something into the hip of a pre-op patient. Putting one hand over her eyes and wrapping an arm around her waist, the doctor said, "Guess who, honey." The statistical probabilities of the nurse bending or breaking the needle would make an interesting study. Fortunately for the patient, she did not.

"My God, my God, please take me *now* instead of after the operation" was the next cry I heard. Fear spread quickly to the woman on the adjacent cart, who began sobbing that "they" wouldn't let her keep her rosary.

"Anyone for coffee?" came a cheerful query from an off-duty aide passing through.

And so it went, on and on. If TV sitcom writers climbed into hospital gowns and, tape recorders at the ready, spent a morning in a holding ward, they could collect enough material for a full season.

Nine o'clock and unconsciousness really came too soon for this observer. About an hour later I woke up, not in a recovery room but in a "post-anesthesia room" that looked like an auto-repair shop: 40 carts with 40 patients, each with IV apparatus on high, parked parallel. At each cart station were four jets: air, water, oxygen, and God-knows-what. At each station, emergency tools lay atop spanking-white towels, above each station, a cabinet held tape, hemostats, scalpels, bandages, and all the miscellaneous "just in case" paraphernalia. When I was billed $25 for "use of PAR," I knew the auto-repair shop analogy had been correct.

Three nights later, well after eleven, an orderly woke me, insisted I was being operated on in the morning and that he was, therefore, removing my water carafe.

While I had an uneventful recovery, not a day went by without someone trying to give me medication meant for someone else. One midnight, however, a nurse appeared with medication I knew was intended for me. She asked my name and then, with a flashlight—thus showing compassion for my roommate by not flooding us with overhead illumination—checked my name and patient number on the wrist identification band. "We seem to make *so* many mistakes," she explained. "I like to be sure, because I'm not always on this floor."

A young lady with a badge identifying her as a "prenursing student volunteer" came in one afternoon, unaccompanied, called me by name, and said she had to take my blood pressure. While I knew this was a teaching hospital, I had not been aware that it was a self-teaching institution. Stating that she was still in high school, the girl fumbled with the cuff. When, after five unsuccessful attempts, she confessed, "I just can't seem to find the artery," I adjusted the position of the stethoscope and gave her a standard reading. She went happily on to another victim.

Daily, some staff member offered to give me a bath; others proffered back rubs. On one of the 14 days of my stay, the "Bookmobile" was trundled through the hall on its much-advertised "daily" rounds. An underdeprived and overfed matron from suburbia suggested I might enjoy a magazine or book "and there's no charge," but she didn't have a list of what was available, didn't know "for sure" what she had, and didn't wheel the cart to my bedside. At the moment,

I was absorbed in the current issue of *Science*, so my reply probably spoiled her day, as she had spoiled my concentration.

After visiting hours, nightly, nurses would come in to inspect the shelf of books I had brought with me and would casually relate the peccadilloes of the nursing staff, the idiosyncrasies of the medical staff, the brash advances allegedly made by some resident physicians, and the disdain with which most nurses regarded medical students. I learned of the practical jokes played on the more pompous surgeons, of the substitution of specimens for new members of the tissue committee, and of general adolescent behavior by all but a few prune-faced ancients.

Would the staff have told me what they did if they had known that my surgeon was my cousin and that many of the RN's had been to nursing school with my daughters and nieces? Or were they so open *because* they knew of my relationships and hoped I would repeat their tales? Whatever the answer, nothing can change the facts that for 14 consecutive days I was offered the wrong medication and that only one nurse positively identified me before giving me a drug.

Would the horseplay outside the operating room have continued if the staff had been aware that a keen ear was listening, albeit coupled with spectacle-less, unfocusing eyes? Would the RN in the holding ward have told the aide to do as she thought best if the nurse knew she was being overheard by, say, a newspaper reporter or a plaintiff's lawyer in a malpractice suit? Would an aide have asked me a few days later, in hushed tones of confidentiality, whether urology had anything to so with urine, if she had had an understanding supervisor?

And what can one say of the staff member who, confusing two people with similar surnames, administered mineral oil to my roommate—sedated and in traction—and then vanished for four hours? During that time, the oil proved it was fresh, viscous, and efficacious, but the poor patient's signaling to the nursing station brought no response whatsoever.

If ever I must be hospitalized again, I will still choose the institution where all these gaffes occurred, but I will again insist that my surgeon write on the order sheet: IDENTIFY ALL MEDICATION TO PATIENT.

2.

COMMUNICATION PROCESSES AND THEORIES

Rhonda and David Coleman had been married for nine years but had not been able to have the children they very much wanted. When a new obstetrician-gynecologist moved to their area they were delighted to hear that he was a fertility expert. They began treatment with Dr. Dolan and after six months, Rhonda became pregnant. The couple was delighted and chose to continue with Dolan. Rhonda did have some reservations about this decision as she had found communication with him difficult but his obvious technical and medical skills attracted both of the Colemans.

The Colemans' delight at the pregnancy turned into a nightmare during the following nine months. Rhonda had many concerns because of her history. Dolan was brusque and noncommunicative when he was examining her and the examinations were efficient but brief. After one examination, appearing overworked and exasperated, he suggested that she go to the local bookstore and buy some books on pregnancy that would make her a more informed patient so that she wouldn't have so many questions. Rhonda came home in tears but the couple was afraid to change doctors at that point in the pregnancy.

Rhonda called a friend who was a nurse. She was helpful in answering many questions and alleviating some of Rhonda and David's concerns. At the end of nine months Rhonda went into labor. The long labor was difficult partly because of her intense animosity and distrust toward Dr. Dolan.

After giving birth to a healthy baby, the Colemans found Dr. Allard, a pediatrician whom they liked and admired. One of their criteria at that point was communication, and the

pediatrician they chose took time to reassure families and
answer questions. When the Colemans told of their ordeal with
the obstetrician-gynecologist, Dr. Allard agreed to talk to
Dr. Dolan, who was a friend as well as a colleague. Dolan was
terribly distressed at hearing the Colemans' complaints. He had
assumed they were simply grateful to have a healthy baby. After
further talks with Dr. Allard he did admit that he had had other
complaints about his communication ability. He finally agreed
that he must do something about this problem. What should he
do? How could he learn to understand and improve his
communication?

THE NATURE OF HUMAN COMMUNICATION

Perhaps the greatest problem with human communication in health care
is the assumption that communication is an easy thing to do well. This
assumption is only half true. It is easy to communicate, but it is difficult
to communicate well, as Dr. Dolan found out in the previous case. Even
though we have been communicating with others all of our lives we are
not always effective communicators. In this chapter we will discuss the
nature of human communication, examining the major aspects of the
communication process and identifying strategies for communicating
effectively in health care.

*Human communication occurs when a person responds to a message and
assigns meaning to it.* The two key parts to this definition of human communication are the *message* and the *meaning*. Messages are anything that
people attend to and create meanings for in the communication process.
Messages can take many different forms. They can be spoken words,
written words, facial expressions, environmental cues, temperatures,
thoughts, or feelings. Basically, there are two groups of messages: *internal messages*, those we send to ourselves, and *external messages*, those we
react to from our environment (including other people). Meanings are
mental images we create to develop a sense of understanding. People
respond to messages (emanating both internally and externally) and create meanings for these messages when communicating.

Human communication occurs at various levels. The most basic
level of human communication is *intrapersonal communication*. Intrapersonal communication occurs when we communicate with ourselves.
People constantly have an ongoing dialogue of thoughts within themselves. For example, health care practitioners constantly use intrapersonal communication to make choices about client care, to interpret

messages from clients and co-workers, and to decide how to explain health concepts and treatments to their clients. The intrapersonal process for creating messages is known as *encoding*, and the intrapersonal process of interpreting messages is known as *decoding*.

Both encoding and decoding are translation processes people use to link the two most crucial elements of communication together, meanings and messages. In the encoding process the health practitioner translates the meanings he or she has about a given situation into the most appropriate messages available for use in communicating with others. Decoding is the translation of messages into meanings. Intrapersonal communication is the most basic form of human communication because the processes of encoding and decoding enable people to send and receive messages, which in turn make it possible for them to communicate on interpersonal, small group, and organizational levels.

Interpersonal communication is communication between two people (a dyad), usually face-to-face, although people can use communication media (such as the telephone) to communicate interpersonally without being in each other's immediate presence. Interpersonal communication builds upon intrapersonal communication because each member of the interpersonal dyad must communicate with him or her self to communicate effectively with each other. Intrapersonal and interpersonal levels of communication occur simultaneously when one person speaks with another person. The interpersonal communicator uses intrapersonal communication to decode the messages of the other person with whom he or she is communicating and to encode messages he or she intends to send to the other person.

One of the most important outcomes of interpersonal communication is the development of human relationships. As we discussed in the first chapter, people depend on their interpersonal relationships to elicit cooperation from others. In the fifth chapter we will discuss in more depth the importance of establishing effective client–practitioner relationships in the delivery of health care. As in intrapersonal communication, the interpersonal level of communication enables people to communicate at the next higher level of human communication—the small group.

Small group communication occurs between three or more people interacting with one another in an attempt to adapt to their environment and achieve commonly recognized goals. As in interpersonal communication, small group communication usually occurs face to face but may also develop through use of communication media (for example, teleconferencing). The total number of small group communicators is generally limited to the number of people who can actively participate together in a group conversation.

Small group communicaton is more complex than interpersonal communication because group interaction is composed of many different interpersonal communication relationships. As the number of communicators within the small group is increased, the complexity of the communication situation is increased geometrically due to the rapid increase in the number of potential message exchanges that can occur between group members. For example, Bostrom (1970) has calculated that a group of eight people has a possibility of 1,056 interactions.[1]

Another aspect of group communication that differs from interpersonal communication is the dimension of *group dynamics*. Group dynamics is the potential for the development of sub-groups and opposing coalitions within the group membership. The development of these coalitions complicates group communication and the relationships between group members. The different ways group dynamics can develop within a group can have a strong impact on the output of the group.

The small group is an important work unit in health care. Small group communication occurs in health care teams, therapy groups, consumer education classes, and decision making committees within health care organizations. These groups perform important functions in the health care system by providing information, support, and problem solving abilities that individuals couldn't possibly provide independently. In chapter 6 we will discuss in more detail the functions and processes of small group communication in health care, emphasizing the development and operation of effective health care teams.

The fourth and most complex level of human communication to be addressed in this chapter is *organizational communication*. An organization is a social system composed of interdependent groups of people sharing the performance of commonly recognized goals. Organizational communication refers to human communication between organization members during the performance of their organizational tasks. Organizational communication encompasses the prior levels of communication—intrapersonal, interpersonal, and small group.

Organizational communication is integral to the functioning of health care institutions because it is the means by which health care practitioners (from all aspects of the health care system) coordinate their activities to accomplish the goals of the organization. Because of the great size and complexity of many modern health care organizations it is virtually impossible to have face-to-face communication between all members of the organization. To cope with the complexity of organizational communication, organizations must develop formal channels of communication between different parts and members of the organization. We will discuss in much greater depth some current communication problems and coping mechanisms for health care organizations in Chapter 7.

In summary, there are four levels of human communication that build upon one another and increase in complexity from intrapersonal communication to interpersonal communication to small group communication to organizational communication. Figure 2.1 illustrates the hierarchical nature of the four basic levels of human communication.

As you can see in Figure 2.1, intrapersonal communication is the largest and most basic form of human communication. It is at the intrapersonal level that we think and process information. Interpersonal communication builds upon the intrapersonal level, adding another person to the communication situation and introducing the dyadic relationship. Small group communication, in turn, builds upon interpersonal interaction, utilizing several communicators and adding the new dimensions of group dynamics and multiple interpersonal relationships to the communication situation. Organizational communication exists through the combination of the three previous levels of communication in coordinating large numbers of people in the shared accomplishment of complex goals. It is important to recognize how each of the higher levels of communication is dependent upon the effectiveness of its lower levels of communication. Effective communication at each level is developed through effective communication at preceding levels.

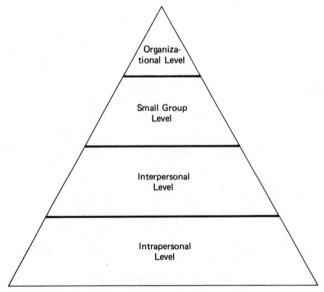

Figure 2.1   Hierarchical Levels of Human Communication.

In addition to these four basic levels of human communication, there are also two special forms of communication that do not fit neatly in our hierarchy but utilize elements from each of the levels: *public communication* and *mass communication*. Public communication is when a small number of people (usually only one person) addresses a larger group of people. Although the speaker takes the major responsibility for the public communication and sends the preponderance of verbal messages, that person is not the only person engaging in communication. The audience also sends messages to the speaker, primarily through nonverbal channels. Speeches, lectures, oral reports, and dramatic performances are all forms of public communication.

Mass communication occurs when a small number of people send messages to a large, anonymous, and usually heterogeneous audience through the use of some specialized communication media. Mass communication uses such diverse media as film, television, radio, newspapers, books, and magazines. Mass communication is similar to public communication in that the source of the message takes primary responsibility for the communication. However, mass communication has the potential for reaching larger audiences than face-to-face public communication, and has less opportunity for audience participation.

Both public communication and mass communication have the advantage of being able to reach large audiences, thereby communicating with many people in a short amount of time. On the other hand, both forms of communication also have the disadvantage of limited shared communication with the audience. The reactions an audience has to communication is known as *feedback*, and, as we will discuss later in this chapter, feedback is an important part of communication by both clarifying and humanizing human interaction. To maximize the advantages of public and mass communication, while minimizing their disadvantages it is useful to utilize already existing intrapersonal, interpersonal, small group, and organizational levels of communication. By utilizing all of these forms of communication the health provider can at once reach a large number of people, in a clear and personal manner. Throughout the rest of this book we will examine the ways in which health care professionals can utilize all of these levels of human communication.

COMMUNICATION AS PROCESS

Human communication is a *dynamic, ongoing process—communication does not start and stop*. People are constantly involved in communicating with themselves and with other people. We are immersed in a sea of messages and meanings. *Human beings cannot not communicate*. As long as you are alive, you are involved in some means of communication.

It is easy to oversimplify the human communication process. Many early models of human communication assumed that one person (a source, or sender) sent a message to another person (a receiver) in communication. This is an oversimplification. No one individual is only a sender or a receiver in human communication. *In human communication we simultaneously send and receive many messages on many different levels*. We are constantly encoding and decoding. These early linear models of human communication fail to recognize the continuously developing nature of the communication phenomenon.

By seeing communication as an ongoing process you must recognize that human *communication is irreversible*. Human *communication is bound to the context in which it occurs*. Context refers to the time and space surrounding human communication. When communication occurs and how people feel about the timing of the communication has a major impact. For example, it is a far different communication situation depending on whether a friend phones you at 8 P.M. or at 3 A.M.! Time also refers to the day of the week and month of the year, and so forth. The setting where communication occurs also has great impact on the interaction. You certainly communicate differently with people in a class, at a party, in a clinic, or on a hospital ward. Even if you say exactly the same thing in several different situations to the same people, the changes in context will inevitably alter the communication that takes place.

Once you have communicated something to someone you cannot retract it. The communication event that transpired became permanent the moment it occurred. By restating or changing the messages sent you do not remove previous messages, you merely add on to them. For example, a nurse tells a hospitalized client to prepare for surgery, and later finds out the client is not scheduled for surgery until the next day. No matter how many times the nurse explains the mistake the impact the communication has had on the client remains. It is similar to a judge in a courtroom murder trial telling the jury to disregard an outburst from a courtroom spectator who yells that the defendant is a killer. No matter how the judge implores the jury to be impartial the communication has had its effect. The irreversible nature of human communication underscores the importance of careful communication in health care, for whatever the health professional says, it is in some way always remembered.

Human communication is a deceptively complex process. There are many different aspects of communication that interrelate in the communication phenomenon. In this book we will take a *transactional* perspective on human communication. Transactionality implies that communication is a process composed of a myriad of different components, interacting simultaneously to produce communication. Some of these key components include the messages to which people react, the meanings people actively create, the time and place of the communication (context), the relationships established between communicators, the past experiences of the communicators, the personalities and dispositions of the communicators, the purposes people have for communicating, and the effects of human communication on people and situations. Throughout this book we will be examining communication in health care from a transactional perspective, identifying the crucial parts of the communication process and determining the effects of human communication on the delivery of health care services.

COMMUNICATION AND THE CREATION OF MEANING

Human beings have an insatiable appetite for creating meanings. We strive to know what is going on around us, to understand the people we interact with, and to get a handle on the different situations in which we find ourselves. Human communication is the primary tool available to us to help develop a sense of understanding people and situations. We gather information from the messages available to us and interpret these messages to create satisfying meanings to help us cope effectively with the world around us.

The creation of meaning is a very personal process. *All people are unique and their perceptions of reality and creations of meaning are unique*. We have the cognitive ability to create very rich meanings of great depth at many different levels. Because the creation of meaning is a personal process we each create meanings in different ways, often interpreting the same situation in very different ways. The creation of meaning is not a mechanical process, it is part of a learned psychological process.

Meanings are in people, not in words, objects, or things. People actively create meanings in response to the world around them. No object or word has inherent meaning. Human beings create meanings for words and objects to develop a sense of understanding for them.

Selective Perception

Human perception is a process by which people become aware of internal and external messages and interpret these messages into meanings. Human beings perceive the world around them through the use of their sensory mechanisms. These sensory mechanisms include sight, hearing, touch, taste, smell, balance, awareness of heat, cold, pain, pleasure, and pressure. In addition to perceiving *external messages* through use of our senses, we also perceive internally generated messages. *Internal messages* are both physiologically oriented (as in feelings of hunger, fatigue, or nervousness) and mentally oriented (as in thinking, daydreaming, and choice-making).

An important internal channel of mentally oriented messages is something we label "channel Z" or the ability to imagine and create rich fantasies. Channel Z is a mental mechanism people create to transport themselves from their physical environment to a convivial fantasy land of their own making. Humans' ability to enter channel Z can be very therapeutic for them if they use their imaginations in appropriate situations. Use of channel Z can be a refreshing and rejuvenating experience, helping people cope with stressful situations by providing them with an important repose from reality. Some people are unable to control their use of channel Z, daydreaming and fantasizing in inappropriate situations, when they should be focusing their attention on externally generated messages. The ability to control perceptual processes is an important communication skill.

A major problem in controlling human perception is the overwhelming number of potential messages available to the perceiver. People cannot possibly perceive everything there is in any given situation, even if they are able to block out their own internally generated messages, because of the wide range of external messages available to them. People have limitations to the amount of *cognitive space* available to them for processing information. If we attempted to perceive all of the messages available to us we would suffer from *information overload*—our inability to process all of the messages bombarding us causes such overload and would leave us disoriented and confused.

To complicate the perceptual process even more, people don't have the ability to perceive everything around them due to their *sensory limitations*. There are limitations on our hearing, sight, smell, and so on. We cannot hear all of the sounds around us or see all of the light waves bombarding us.

Human beings have developed the cognitive process of *selective perception* to maximize the effectiveness of the messages they do perceive and minimize the perceptual problems caused by cognitive and sensory limitations. Selective perception is a process by which people select the most important messages out of the total pool of potentially perceivable messages, and use those selected messages to make sense out of their current situation. There are three interrelated parts to the selective perception process. They are:

1. *Selective Attention*: focusing in on the key messages in any situation;
2. *Habituation*: focusing out of consciousness extraneous or unimportant messages in any situation;
3. *Closure*: putting together the messages collected through selective attention and arranging them into a meaningful configuration.

The messages people select through selective attention are chosen due to the unique past experiences and predispositions of each individual. Not only do people select the most important messages around them through selective attention, but they also prioritize the messages they attend to. The most important messages are given the most cognitive space (attention), and the less important messages are afforded less cognitive space. Every split second people update the selective attention choices they have made and reprioritize the messages they have selected.

Selective attention and habituation work hand in hand, and operate simultaneously. In order to give full attention to any set of messages an individual must be able to block out competing messages. This is why habituation is so important. To habituate effectively people must be able to block out both external messages and internal messages. External messages that compete for attention might be noises or distracting visual cues while competing internal messages might be fatigue or daydreams. People develop their ability to habituate well through continued practice.

The individual must then provide closure: make sense out of the situation based on limited information gathered from the messages attended to. This is done by filling in the blank spaces between messages through educated assumptions based on the perceiver's past experiences and sense of logic. The better individuals are at creating closure the more likely they are to develop a strong sense of understanding for the perceptual situation.

Since each person develops their own method of perceiving the world around them through their own version of selective perception it is likely that different people will select different messages on which to focus. Additionally, they will block out different messages, and put the messages they have attended to together in different ways. These individual differences in the selective perception process are the primary reasons for divergent creations of meaning by different people. There is no objective reality, only subjective realities created by different people based on individual perceptions of the world around them. The major implication derived from perceptual differences between people is the need for interpersonal communication to check and clarify the meanings people create. *People cannot exchange meanings: they can exchange messages*. The more effective the messages they send to one another, the more likely it is that communicators will be able to create overlapping (similar) meanings, thereby developing communicative understanding for one another.

CONTENT AND RELATIONSHIP LEVELS OF COMMUNICATION

Messages people send one another have both a *content* and *relationship* dimension. The content aspect of human communication refers to the basic information being presented in the message. The primary topic, theme, and data of what is being said is contained within the content level of communication. The relationship level of communication, on the other hand, refers to the feelings communicators express for each other through their communication. Expressions of respect/disrespect, like/dislike, powerfulness/powerlessness, love/hate, or comfort/discomfort are all parts of the relationship dimension of human communication.

The content and relationship aspects of human communication are expressed simultaneously in every message sent and received in inter-personal communication. Since interpersonal communicators send and receive a multitude of messages all the time, content and relationship levels of messages have a major impact on interpersonal communica-tion. It is important to recognize that every time you tell someone some-thing you are not merely expressing information about the topic but you are also defining the relationship you are in the process of establishing with your communication partner.

Even the most common statement such as, "How's it going buddy?", has content and relationship communication aspects. On a content level the statement expresses an inquiry into the status of the receiver's mental, physical, and social condition at that given moment, as well as expressing a greeting from one person to another. On a rela-tionship level the statement might imply concern for the receiver's well-being, interpersonal attraction between the sender and the receiver of the message, empathy for the receiver's current situation, or merely an expression of friendship.

The content level of communication provides people with infor-mation about the world around them. As we discussed in the perception part of this chapter, people have an insatiable appetite for knowing about the people they relate to and the environment in which they live. The world is a complex and confusing place. Information helps people understand the world around them by reducing the uncertainty they have about other people and things.

Every situation people find themselves in has a certain level of uncertainty. We never know everything there is to know about any given person, place, or situation. Every bit of information we gather through content communication provides us with more knowledge about the world around us. The content level of human communication helps us to understand the world we live in and to cope with uncertainty.

The relationship level of human communication provides people with information about the relationships they are developing with others. We are in constant need of human companionship. Human beings are social creatures and depend on their relationships with others to provide mutual emotional support for one another, solve difficult problems, and coordinate complex activities.

Every time a message is sent between people at least one aspect of that message communicates something about the relationship being established between communicators. Relationships develop due to the communication established between people. Every time you communicate with someone you are affecting in some way your relationship with that person. Communication can increase or break down the effectiveness of human relationships, depending on the relative degree of personal or object communication inherent in the messages being communicated.

The relationship aspect of interpersonal messages can be placed on a continuum between *personal and object communication*. Personal communication shows respect for the other person. A communicator sending messages on the personal end of the continuum (see Figure 2.2) communicates with the other person as an equal, allows the other person's perspective to affect the messages sent, and generally communicates in an honest and trustworthy manner. Object communication, on the other hand, is insensitive and demonstrates lack of respect for the other person. It tells the person what to do without seeking his or her input on the matter and treats the other person as an unintelligent and unimportant being.

Personal communication tends to be a humanizing form of human interaction, while object communication tends to be a dehumanizing form of human interaction as Figure 2.2 illustrates. Personal communication makes us feel good about ourselves. It bolsters our self-image,

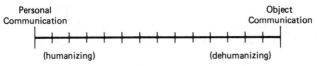

Figure 2.2   Continuum of Personal and Object Communication.

by communicating the relational message that who we are and what we have to say is important. Conversely, object communication tears down our self-image, it makes us question our worth and we become angry at the person treating us an object rather than as a person.

Since personal and object communication are parts of the relational aspect of communication it is possible to communicate the same general content information in very different relational ways using either personal or object level messages. For example, a dentist can ask a client to cooperate with a dental regimen in either a personal or object manner. On the object level, "If you don't brush your teeth regularly it won't be much longer until you have no teeth," or on a more personal level, "I'd appreciate it if you'd consider brushing your teeth every day because it will counteract the buildup of tooth decay and make your teeth last longer." The object approach to client communication treats the client as though he or she had to be bullied into complying with the dental regimen, while in the personal approach the client is treated as a responsible individual who will cooperate with the dentist if given good reasons. Which manner of communication would you prefer? More than likely, you would rather be communicated with as a person rather than as an object.

Personal communication can be beneficial to the establishment of effective client–practitioner relationships. Object communication, on the other hand, can be detrimental to effective client–practitioner relationships. It takes no more time to communicate personally with people than it does to communicate in an object manner. It does take respect, honesty, and a genuine concern for yourself and the other person. Throughout the rest of the book we will consider the perils of communicating on an object level with clients and co-workers, as well as explore strategies for utilizing personal communication in client-practitioner relationships, health care teams, health care organizations, and in developing therapeutic communication.

COMMUNICATION AND FEEDBACK

As we discussed earlier in this chapter, *feedback* is a communicated response to another individual's communication. It functions by providing communicators with information about how they are being perceived by others. With this feedback communicators can adjust their message strategies to communicate more effectively. Because feedback guides people in adjusting the messages they send to one another it helps to clarify human communication.

Effective communicators constantly seek feedback from the people with whom they are communicating to determine how these people are reacting to the communication situation. Intrapersonally, you send yourself feedback about your thoughts or actions when you review your ideas and behaviors. Interpersonally, feedback helps you determine what effects your communications are having upon your dyadic partners and how they feel about you. In small groups feedback is used to determine the ideas and reactions of group members about problems and their solutions. In organizations feedback determines the adequacy of member information and effectiveness of organizational policies. In public communication feedback allows the speaker to gauge the responses of the audience to his or her presentation. Even in mass communication, where feedback works most slowly, feedback is needed to evaluate the effectiveness of a mass communicated event or program.

Seeking feedback from people in communication situations is a way of humanizing the interpersonal interaction. It is important for health providers to do, not only because it gives them information about the level of information the client possesses, but also because on a relational level it communicates to the client that the health professional is interested in his or her perspective on the health care situation.

Metacommunication is a specialized form of feedback about the manner in which people communicate. Metacommunication is communication about communication, where the communicator is given feedback about the way he or she is communicating. *Metacommunication is a primary tool in socialization, because rules of interaction are learned from metacommunicative processes.*

Every human relationship, group, organization, and culture develops rules for the ways in which people are supposed to communicate. Later on in this book we will discuss these communication rules in more depth, identifying them as norms. Some of these rules include the accepted manner of address people have for one another, the type of dress codes that exist, the use of specialized language (jargon, slang, or foreign languages), and the ways in which people are allowed to touch each other in different situations. The primary function of metacommunication is in teaching people the correct rules for communicating.

When you were a child you were probably given many metacommunication messages to teach you how to act correctly in different situations. For example, children are often taught how to speak politely with metacommunicative messages like, "Always say thank you when you are given a present, even if you don't like the present." As people grow older the metacommunicative messages they receive become more subtle. Usually adults teach other adults communication rules by using less obvious nonverbal metacommunicative messages. When a person breaks a communication rule his or her contemporaries will usually indicate nonverbally through a frown, a harsh look, or laughter that what that person has said or done is not acceptable.

Some people are less perceptive about metacommunicative messages than others, and therefore are slow to learn the correct rules for communication in different situations. These people are often shunned by others because they don't act in accordance with social rules. To be effective in any communication situation, whether it be interpersonal, group, or organizational, you must be able to recognize metacommunication messages and learn the rules for appropriate communication behaviors. We will discuss metacommunication again in relation to learning group and cultural norms.

VERBAL AND NONVERBAL MESSAGE SYSTEMS

Messages are the tools people use to communicate with one another. As we discussed earlier in this chapter, in human communication people exchange messages to evoke each other's creation of meaning. We identified two kinds of messages, internally generated messages (thoughts), and externally generated messages. Human beings use these external messages to communicate with one another. There are two kinds of external messages, verbal and nonverbal.

Verbal message systems include the use of words and language, both spoken and written, while *nonverbal message systems* include the wide range of messages people perceive and assign meaning to that are in addition to the use of words. Nonverbal communication contains many different kinds of message systems, ranging from body movements to environmental cues.

Verbal and nonverbal communication often work closely together. In fact, there is no way to use verbal communication (words) without using some form of nonverbal communication. Nonverbal messages always surround and influence the verbal messages people send because the medium used for sending verbal messages is always nonverbal (as in vocal or visual cues). Later on in this chapter we will discuss in more depth the relationships between verbal and nonverbal communication.

Verbal communication is a *digital* form of communication, in that words represent objects or things. Digital communication is based on the use of an arbitrary symbol system designed to name some phenomenon. Words are not the things they name. They are symbols that are used to signify some experience. There is nothing about the words "tree" or "house" that directly describe either a tree or a house. Language is a synthetic means of communication because people designate which word will stand for which experience. This is one of the main reasons we stated earlier in this chapter that meanings are in people, not in the words people use.

Nonverbal communication is generally an *analogic* form of communication, in that nonverbal messages actually describe the phenomenon they are communicating. Analogic communication is based on the use of symbols that have a likeness to the objects they are representing. Nonverbal messages like facial expressions, postures, gestures, or vocal cues directly represent the feelings and emotional states of the communicator expressing them.

There are some significant differences between analogic and digital modes of communication. Analogic communication is primarily used to communicate emotionally-oriented information, while digital communication is used for communicating data-oriented, technical information. To take this one step further, nonverbal communication (primarily analogic) is most effective at conveying relationship information, and verbal communication (primarily digital) is most effective at conveying content information. It is difficult to convey very technical, complex information nonverbally, and it is equally difficult to express an intense emotional feeling to someone with words (unless these words are surrounded by powerful nonverbal messages such a vocal volume, touch, or eye-contact). Watzlawich et al. (1967) go as far as to write, "Indeed, wherever relationship is the central issue of communication, we find that digital language is almost meaningless."[2]

The implications of the relationships between verbal communication, digital modes, and content information indicate that words are effective at expressing complex technical topics. The relationships between nonverbal communication, analogic modes, and relationship information imply that emotionally charged information is best suited to nonverbal messages, and that nonverbal communication has a strong effect on defining and developing interpersonal relationships.

Language as a transmitter of complex information has performed an important *timebinding* function for humanity. Timebinding is the storing of human knowledge and experiences and conveying of this knowledge over time. Written language has provided humankind with a relatively permanent, stable, and widespread source of information. The development of computer languages and advanced technologies will allow present and future generations to timebind information and process complex messages more effectively than ever before.

Verbal communication is usually thought of only in the spoken mode, but written language is also an important part of verbal communication. The spoken word allows people to communicate about information in a personal and dynamic manner. Yet, it is common for people to forget or misinterpret information that was spoken. The spoken word is very transitory, the words fly past us so quickly at times that it may be difficult to understand all of the messages being sent. In written communication, however, you can usually read at your own rate, as well as carefully review difficult parts of the text. The transitory nature of spoken communication underscores the importance of actively using feedback when speaking with others. Written communication, although less dramatic than spoken interaction, has the advantage of stability, permanence, and formality. To derive the benefits of both spoken and written communication it is wise to use one to augment the other when you want to make an impact on the person you are communicating with and you also want a formal record of your messages.

There are four interrelated perspectives on the study of verbal communication:

1. *Phoenemics*: Examination of the performance of spoken language focusing on the sounds and pronunciations of words.
2. *Syntactics*: Examination of the structural aspects of language usage, emphasizing the grammar of verbal communication.
3. *Semantics*: Examination of the meanings associated with words, developing such tools as dictionaries and thesauri.
4. *Pragmatics*: Examination of the behavioral functions of language use by people in different situations.

In this book we will be most concerned with the semantic and pragmatic aspects of language.

As we discussed earlier in this chapter, meaning is a very rich mental process, and the study of semantics recognizes the depth of human meanings for words by separating meanings into two major types, *denotations* and *connotations*. Denotations are the generally accepted public meanings words have assigned to them. Definitions that you might find in a dictionary are the denotative meanings of language. Connotations are more personal, subjective meanings people create and assign to words. While the denotative meanings associated with words are usually limited to less than ten, the connotative meanings any word might evoke are limitless. These many different denotative and connotative meanings assigned to language indicates one of the primary reasons people interpret verbal messages differently, and once again implies the importance of seeking feedback to check people's perceptions of words and meanings.

The pragmatic perspective in language examines the ways in which language is used in different situations by different people. An important area of pragmatic language use in health care is the use (and sometimes over-use) of *jargon*. Jargon is a secretive linguistic code used by different groups of people. Sometimes jargon is technical in nature, while at other times jargon is used to communicate social information. Jargon serves a variety of functions for its users including:

1. *Expedites interaction* by combining complex concepts and terms into a single word or phrase that can be recognized by other group members. Examples of this expediting function might include use of abbreviations to communicate lengthy health care concepts such as: Ob-Gyn, CPR, or MCI, as well as short terms in place of more complex ones such as coding, prepping, or detox.

2. *Establishes group membership* by identifying individuals with access to specialized vocabulary and information. If you can use the jargon of a specialized group of people such as occupational therapists, medical administrators, orthodontists, or neurosurgeons, you are far more likely to evoke cooperation from these individuals when speaking to them about their specialized area because you can identify yourself as being knowledgeable in that specific topic. On the other hand, if you use health care jargon incorrectly you will immediately identify yourself as a novice!

3. *Creates status* for users over nonusers of the specialized linguistic vocabulary. People sometimes use jargon to impress or intimidate the uninitiated by making those who do not understand the jargon feel confused and foolish. In health care, as in all organizational systems, information is powerful. Jargon users can attempt to establish power over nonusers by intimating through their word choices that they possess specialized knowledge and information about health care that the other person does not. Establishing power, however, may not be such a good strategy in health care practice because it can deteriorate the relationship and interfere with cooperation between the communicators. Moreover, use of specialized jargon with nonusers will most certainly block the communication of information because the nonusers have no denotative meanings for the jargon terms and phrases. Dr. Kenneth Walker discussed this use of jargon, calling it the "me God, you moron" system of communication utilized by many of his physician colleagues. Walker sees this as a way physicians can put themselves on a pedestal and not communicate because they basically do not want to do so.[3]

4. *Insulates* users of jargon from nonusers. Jargon use can be used to protect the group of jargon users from infiltration by outside groups of people who do not understand the specialized language. This func-

tion of jargon can be useful when a health professional needs to communicate specialized information that for reasons of confidentiality should not be known by others. The health provider can use jargon to explain the situation to a peer without risking loss of confidentiality if nongroup members happen to overhear the communication exchange. On the other hand, this insulating aspect of jargon can frustrate others who would like to know what the health professional is talking about and believe they have a legitimate right to possess the health care information.

As you can see, jargon can be used in many different ways in health care practice. Some of the uses of jargon are extremely beneficial to the health care delivery system, while other uses of jargon may be detrimental to high quality health care. Improper use of jargon in health care can alienate users of jargon from nonusers, because the unnecessary use of jargon with nonusers can be a form of object communication and cause the nonusers to feel dehumanized. The decision whether or not to use jargon in different health care situations is an ethical decision health care practitioners have to make. In chapter 8 we will discuss in more depth the nature of health care ethics and how it affects the communication that occurs in health care situations.

Human language is a tool that is used for different groups of people. Languages change as the needs of the people who use them change. Because language is constantly changing and evolving to fulfill the needs of its speakers human language is an *emergent phenomenon*. To be an effective user of language you must be able to keep up on the changes and developments in language use. Not only are new words developed and introduced into the language, but existing words also develop new usages. Because information and knowledge are stored and transmitted through language it is important for language to be in constant flux and development to keep up with our growth in human knowledge. Nowhere has human knowledge expanded more rapidly than in the medical and health care sciences, so it is important for health care professionals to learn current linguistic additions so that they can keep up with this growth in knowledge. This can be done by reading current literature and talking to other professionals.

As indicated earlier in this chapter, nonverbal communication refers to the wide variety of message sources people perceive and assign meaning to that are in addition to verbal communication. In essence, this is saying that nonverbal communication is every possible message source people respond to besides words. Moreover, as we discussed earlier, nonverbal communication surrounds and influences all verbal communication.

There are many different types of nonverbal messages, and to lump them all together under the extremely general rubric of "nonverbal communication" would be simplistic and confusing. Rather, we will identify seven different, but interrelated, nonverbal systems. These systems work together, usually simultaneously, in human communication. They are:

1. *Artifactics*: People's personal appearances, body shapes, sizes, smells, skin colors, hair styles, bodily hair, makeup, perfumes, clothing styles, as well as objects they carry around with them (such as briefcases, books, jewelery, pens, combs, watches), and the objects people choose to decorate their environment with (clocks, paintings, furniture styles and colors, books, etc.). These artifactic messages have a strong influence on the initial perceptions and first impressions people have about others.

Traditionally, health care practitioners have identified themselves through the use of easily recognizable artifactic cues, such as uniforms, equipment, and patient files. Health care uniforms are usually white (or light in color), symbolic of cleanliness and disinfection. Artifactic cues that you use can have a profound effect on the judgments clients make about your competence and cleanliness. Attention to your personal appearance, such as neatness and cleanliness of your uniform and grooming, tasteful (moderate) use of jewelry, makeup, and perfumes can be important in convincing clients you are a health care professional with all the knowledge and skills necessary to give them effective treatment.

2. *Kinesics* include the way people move their bodies and position themselves, including postures, gestures, head nods, and leg movements. There are three basic types of gestures: *emblems*, which are gestures that have direct verbal translations such as nodding the head for yes and shaking the head for no, or waving the hand for hello; *illustrators*, which are gestures that accompany speech and accentuate what is being said, such as banging of hands on a table when the person speaking is angry; and *adaptors*, which are unconscious nervous gestures such as cracking the knuckles, scratching, or tapping the foot. Kinesic messages often indicate the level of someone's involvement in a given situation, as well as whether they are reacting positively or negatively to those around them.

Health practitioners must be aware of their client's gestures simply for the fact that clients during treatment are often unable to express themselves through the use of words. Various emblem gestures are used to convey answers to questions by the practitioner such as, "Does this hurt?," "Are you comfortable?" Client adaptor gestures can often indicate their fear and tenseness to you (such as gripping the arms of the chair, or wringing their hands). You can use the information derived from these kinesic cues to better direct your responses to the client during treatment.

3. *Occulesics* consist of facial expressions and eye behaviors. The face is the primary emotional message sending center of the human organism. Moreover, people monitor the facial expressions of others closely, as well as keeping close track of their own facial expressions to determine the emotions the face is expressing. Eye behavior includes eye-contact, gaze (direction, intensity, and duration), as well as blinking behaviors. Occulesic messages can tell us about the person's emotional state and level of interest in a situation or person.

Your face is a major source of emotional information for the client. You must constantly be aware of the expressions you present to the client, because they are often watching you while you are working on them. If your face communicates feelings of fear, surprise, anger, disgust, or contempt, you may be causing the client to become unnecessarily nervous and fearful. As much as possible try to smile and show support and interest to the client with your face. By doing so you can often alleviate many of their tensions. Eye-contact is also an important part of occulesics in establishing rapport with the client. Maintaining eye-contact with client's, and smiling pleasantly can communicate your interest, respect, and caring for the person. Thoughtful and considerate use of occulesics can help clients feel more at ease in health settings.

4. *Paralinguistics* are vocal cues accompanying speech, as well as environmental sounds. Vocal cues include the volume, pitch, tone, rate, and expression in someone's voice. Environmental sounds include music, wind, heavy machinery, train whistles, and so on. The vocal aspect of paralinguistics is the form of nonverbal communication that is most closely tied to verbal communication. Research has indicated that the tone of voice a health professional uses with a client has a significant affect on the client's level of compliance.[4] The sounds surrounding us in our environment also affect the disposition and feelings of people.

Clients can often determine your level of sincerity and caring for them more from the way you speak to them than from what you actually say with words. Loud, rapid, forcefully spoken words can intimidate clients and communicate aggressiveness and even contempt. Soft, slow, expressionless speech may communicate disinterest in the client. It is usually best to attempt to speak clearly (loudly enough for clients to hear all your words, but not loudly enough to frighten them), and expressively to hold patient interest and attention. Environmental sounds can either add or detract from establishing a relaxed communication climate for clients.

5. *Tactilics* are touching behaviors, including self-touching, touching others, and the touching of objects. Skin to skin touching (*haptics*) is the most intimate form of touch. Research has indicated that human touch fulfills physiological and sociological needs for people.[5] An important need fulfilled by human touch that is related to health care practice is the expression of caring and empathy.

Health communication research has shown that touching behaviors in health care are not adequately meeting client needs.[6] Watson (1975) reported in a study of touch initiated by health care staff working in a geriatric facility, that severely impaired clients were touched less often then those who were only mildly impaired, although those who were most ill were probably in great need of sensitive touch by health professionals.[7] Moreover, this study showed that when practitioners did touch clients, they did so significantly more often for instrumental (job-related) purposes than for expressive (emotional) reasons.[8] These research findings suggest that the health care practitioners' use of touch in this health care facility was not generally directed toward expressing empathy and caring for clients, which, it should be noted, can limit the effectiveness of health communication. In health care practice it is important to be able to touch clients in a sensitive and supportive way if they are in need of emotional support. You must, however, be careful to touch only clients who give you cues that they are willing to accept your touch, or otherwise a client may feel as though his or her privacy has been invaded.

6. *Proxemics* is the study of the distance between people and objects, including the distances established in interpersonal relationships, group meetings, and environmental design. Interpersonally, each person maintains an expandable spatial bubble around themselves as an interpersonal buffer between themselves and others. This is referred to as *personal space*. We desire less personal space in social situations with people with whom we are comfortable and more personal space in social situations in which we are uncomfortable. Personal space is a relational process. In a dyad both communicators make personal space decisions and attempt to maintain "acceptable" boundaries of personal space. Sometimes your personal space expectations and the expectations of others conflict, and the result is *spatial invasion*. Spatial invasion makes people very uncomfortable and precipitates a communicative reaction of either fight or flight. Obviously neither reaction is useful for the maintenance of healthy relationships, so in health care practice one must be careful to recognize and abide by the personal space expectations of others.

Another aspect of proxemics dealing with the objects and space claimed and protected by people is territoriality. Territoriality differs from personal space in that it usually does not expand and contract in response to different situations and does not have to surround the person. People are territorial about their "possessions" or objects for which they claim ownership. These objects can range from smaller ones like clothing and books to major possessions such as homes and automobiles. People will generally protect their territory vigorously and will become quite angry if their territory is limited or their possessions are taken from them. In medical organizations, like hospitals, where institutionalized clients are denied many of their belongings such as clothing or jewelery, these clients may become upset and angry. The health practitioner should be careful in such cases to explain to clients why they cannot have these possessions and exactly how the institution is holding them in safe-keeping. Possessions should not be removed unless absolutely necessary.

Still another part of the proxemic system of nonverbal communication is *small group ecology*, or the spatial arrangement of group members at meetings. Different spatial arrangements can have strong impact on the group communication that occurs at meetings. For example, it is easier to have a participative group discussion when members sit around a table or in a circle than it is if they sit in rows or are bunched haphazardly. Additionally, different group positions around a table tend to evoke different communication roles. For example, people who sit at the heads of the table are most likely to become group leaders, while people who flank the leaders (on either side) are likely to form coalitions with and support the leaders. People sitting towards the middle of the table are likely to participate less in the group discussion. People will communicate more actively with one another if they are positioned face to face (*sociopetal orientation*), than if they are positioned away from one another (*sociofugal orientation*).

Architectural design and environmental planning also have a major impact on human communication. Open offices with glass windows through which people can see are more conducive for active communication than closed offices with walled in barriers to communication. Some modern health care organizations have designed facilities with movable walls and partitions (*semi-fixed space*) to elicit increased communication between members of health care teams who would have previously been separated from one another by unmovable walls and doors (*fixed space*). Moreover, the amount of space available to us in our immediate environment can affect our moods and attitudes. Small offices with low ceilings and no windows can cause people to feel boxed in and make them sullen and depressed, while cathedral ceilings and picture windows looking out on gardens and open spaces evoke feelings of peacefulness and contentment.

7. *Chronemics* deals with how time affects communication, including

communication behaviors patterned over time, appointment keeping, and length of time communicating with others. Time is, perhaps, the form of nonverbal communication that people are least aware of, yet time has a major impact on human interaction. Human beings develop cyclical behavior patterns based on time of day, week, month, year, and so on. We depend on schedules and appointments to organize our lives. The more time you spend communicating with others, regardless of the topic of conversation, the more you are telling them you believe they are important individuals. Conversely, the more time you keep people waiting to interact with you, the more you are implying they are insignificant to you. Health practitioners often keep clients waiting without recognizing how the waiting time can work against the establishment of effective practitioner–client relationships. To counteract this chronemic problem the health professional should avoid keeping clients waiting, or if a waiting period is inevitable, the practitioner should show respect for the client by explaining why the waiting period was necessary and expressing an apology.

Nonverbal communication is a very large and important part of the total human communication process. Each of the seven nonverbal systems includes a wide range of message types that affect innumerable communication situations. Yet none of these nonverbal systems operate in isolation from other nonverbal systems, and nonverbal communication in general operates in concert with verbal communication. Knapp (1978) suggests, "Verbal and nonverbal communication should be treated as a total and inseparable unit." He describes six ways that nonverbal messages affect verbal messages in the total communication process, "Nonverbal behavior can repeat, contradict, substitute for, compliment, accent, or regulate verbal behavior."[9] By developing sensitivity to the verbal and nonverbal messages human beings constantly encode and decode the health care practitioner can learn both how to send the most appropriate messages to others and to interpret the variety of messages expressed consciously and unconsciously by patients and co-workers in health care situations.

SUMMARY

In this chapter we have explored the human communication process, identifying the major theories and principles of human communication that relate to the development of effective health communication skills. In an attempt to organize and summarize all of the information presented here, the most important propositions about the nature of human communication are listed below:

1. Human communication occurs when a person responds to a message and assigns meaning to it.
2. Human communication is a dynamic ongoing process.
3. Human beings cannot not communicate.
4. In human communication we simultaneously send and receive many messages on many different levels.
5. Human communication is bound to context and is irreversible.
6. Human communication is a transactional process.
7. Human communication is the primary tool people use to develop a sense of understanding about other people and situations.
8. All people are unique and their perceptions of reality and creations of meaning are unique.
9. Meanings are in people, not in words, objects or things.
10. Every message people send one another has both a content and a relationship dimension.
11. Personal communication shows respect for the person and tends to be a humanizing form of interaction.
12. Object communication shows disrespect and tends to be a dehumanizing form of interaction.
13. Feedback helps to clarify communication between people.
14. Rules of interaction are learned through metacommunication.
15. Verbal communication is a digital form of communication, and is most effective at communicating content information.
16. Nonverbal communication is an analogic form of communication, and is most effective at communicating relationship information.
17. Language is an emergent phenomenon.
18. Verbal and nonverbal communication work together as a total inseparable unit.

NOTES

1. Bostrom, 1970, Section N.
2. Watzlawick et al., 1967, p. 57, Section A.
3. Woods, 1975, Section A.
4. Milmoe et al., 1967, Section B.
5. Montagu, 1971, Section C.
6. Aguilera, 1967, Section B; Barnett, 1972a, Section C; Day, 1973, Section C; and Watson, 1975, Section B.
7. Watson, 1975, Section B.
8. *Ibid.*
9. Knapp, 1978, p. 21, Section C.

READING

PREVIEW OF READING

In "The Mystification of Meaning: Doctor–Patient Encounters," Barnlund describes the symbolic aspects of human illness and relates it to medical practice. He argues that effective medical practice demands sensitive and effective communication by physicians, illustrating how traditional medical education often fails to train the physician to perform the communicative aspects of medical care. Barnlund explores the subjective aspects of meaning, demonstrating the unique ways that people create meanings for their illnesses and their medical treatment. Moreover, he identifies several basic reasons why doctors and patients perceive reality very differently and suggests strategies physicians can use to demystify health care by improving doctor–patient communication.

THE MYSTIFICATION OF MEANING: DOCTOR–PATIENT ENCOUNTERS

Dean C. Barnlund

The words "mystique" and "mystify" have a curious affinity in language and life. "Mystique" refers to the magical aura that surrounds objects or persons which endows them with talismanic and magical influence. To "mystify" is to confuse, perplex, or make obsure or difficult to understand. They go together. Mystification is simply the means by which persons are endowed with mystique. While professional mystique seems to be an elusive idea, the process of communication that creates it is capable of systematic analysis.

Reprinted by permission from the author and *Journal of Medical Education* 51 (1976): 716–25.

Dr. Barnlund is a professor, Department of Speech Communication, School of Humanities, San Francisco State University.

Examining communicative relationships within the medical profession requires some broad appreciation of the communicative process itself. A good starting point might be this: every person from birth until death is engaged endlessly in a search for meaning. To survive physically and psychically, people must inhabit a world that is fairly stable, relatively free of ambiguity, and reasonably predictable. Though people tolerate occasional doubts, few can accept continuing meaninglessness.

To aid in coping with a chaos of fleeting sensations—what William James called this "blooming, buzzing confusion"—we seek to give events some structure that will render them intelligible. Repeated success in interpreting events contributes to an accumulating set of assumptions on which all future acts depend. These assumptions, as George Kelly once noted, provide templates or guides which every person fits over the realities of life.[1] Gradually people within a culture and within a profession acquire specialized frames of reference which, though they speed the process of judgment, often induce a certain blindness. What is "information" to the specialist may be only "noise" to the lay-person; what the physician regards as "noise," his patient often treats as "information." To the patient excessive thirst may be only an inconvenience, but to the doctor it is a symptom of diabetes; to the examining physician the color of the patient's chart may seem irrelevant, but to the patient it is an ominous sign.

All knowledge of the world is inescapably subjective. In effect, each person stands at the center of his or her own universe of meaning, transforming the flow of sensations into organized and intelligible events. Each of us views the world selectively and fits it to our own past experience and changing purposes. Each notes some details and overlooks others; each finds plausible some relationships and rejects others. Since every interpretation of events rests on fallible senses and personal motives, what is known is always incomplete and always subject to error.

It is tempting in the daily clash of words to forget that it is the perceived world—not the real world—that we talk about, argue about, laugh about, cry about. It is not scalpels and crosses and bedpans that regulate human affairs, but how people construe them that determines what they will think, how they will feel, and what they will do about them. Meanings do not come from the world but are assigned to it by every interpreter, and it is he who is the final arbiter of events.

SYMBOLS AND MEANING

Language plays a critical role in the construction of the frames of reference through which we view events. It is the most elaborate and most flexible system humans have devised for transforming shapes and sounds into meaningful events. There is wide recognition that the single species-distinguishing attribute of humanity is the capacity to transform experience into symbols. As Langer[2] has emphasized, the brain works as naturally as the kidneys, carrying on a constant process of ideation, even when we are asleep. It follows its own internal law of translating sensory data into symbols to feed our insatiable appetite for meaning.

Life is so permeated with symbolism that it is difficult to imagine any human experience that is not mediated by language. Language tells us what to look for and what to disregard. It suggests causality here and denies it there. It can paralyze us or rouse us to act. It triggers fear and moments later transforms that fear into hope. It is the slender thread by which we overcome our isolation from each other. Yet if words sometimes clarify, they may also distort. If they induce trust, they may also arouse suspicion. If they contribute to insight, they can also lead into error.

SYMBOLIC DIMENSIONS

Symbolic mediation, the intervention of words between people and their experiences, would seem to be an especially sensitive problem in the treatment of human beings. A physical mechanism, a clock or computer, may break down; but any damage to the mechanism is easily identified and repaired without complications. To an animal, injury or disease is simply another physical state. Any suffering is tied directly to disturbances of normal function. Diagnosis has no influence upon the course of the disease, nor does the prognosis complicate recovery.

This is not the case with human beings. Human illness is not only a physical condition but a symbolic one as well. No animal talks itself into becoming sick, suppresses its symptoms because it fears a diagnosis, prolongs recovery because of the symbolic payoff it receives, or spontaneously recovers because it has redefined its situation.

Yet humans do all of these things. They avoid critical examinations that might save their lives. They seek unnecessary treatments and disregard essential ones. They often suffer more from the name of their illness than the physical pain it produces. They suppress some symptoms and invent others. They convert discomfort into excruciating pain and transform extreme suffering into tolerable discomfort. They can go into shock without physical justification and accept a painful death with serenity.

In short, every medical problem is in part a symbolic one. One cannot damage the physical self without injuring the symbolic self, nor can one inflict insult repeatedly on the symbolic self without damaging the physical self. Research on "experimenter influence" and the "placebo effect" convincingly demonstrates that neither physicians nor patients are free of the influence of the way they define their situation. Diagnosis and treatment are in large part symbolic problems, and to ignore this fact may distort or defeat their aims. There is little doubt that how people think about themselves can alter their blood pressure, oxygen needs, and blood chemistry.

The notion that there are a limited number of "psychosomatic" illnesses has gradually given way to the idea that every illness has some psychosomatic reverberations. The broken leg of a young skier may mean a minor inconvenience amply compensated for by increased attention, a flood of sympathetic concern from acquaintances, and special privileges at home and at school. To an older person the same fracture may signal a loss of physical coordination, a sign of aging, or an omen of approaching dependence.

It was once thought that pain was directly proportional to the amount of physical tissue damaged. According to Melzack,[3] this can no longer be assumed, for pain itself depends on the meaning attributed to physical incapacity. This meaning in turn reflects the past experiences and future expectations of the patient. Higher brain functions are capable of modifying or even suppressing signals that accompany physical distress. If every experience of the organism is invested with symbolic significance, it is naive to assume that the most dramatic of life experiences—those involving physical survival itself—are immune to such effects.

To put this another way, for the patient there is no distinction between perceived pain and real pain and between perceived health and real health. This is a dichotomy implied by language but one without counterpart in human experience. It is perceived malfunctions that bring patients to seek care. It is the persistence of such perceptions that keep them in treatment. It is a change in these perceptions that causes them to terminate treatment.

Similarly for the medical profession, it is a perceived disturbance of normal function that mobilizes the physician. He, in turn, acts upon this perception. Through elaborate procedures there is a search to confirm this perception. Investigation may modify or strengthen an initial interpretation. Ultimately it may be shared in part or in full with the patient. Eventually both share a perception of recovery. But all who are involved in the treatment process will base every question, every inference, every recommendation upon meanings assigned to their impressions through the symbols they impose on them. As Friedson has remarked,[4] "illness is a meaning assigned to behavior" and "illness behavior is ordered by that meaning."

One is forced to conclude that there is no patient who does not present the medical profession with, at least in part, a symbolic problem. No illness lacks its semantic dimension. The professional who feels involved exclusively in the maintenance of a physical mechanism and who dismisses the communicative aspect of this work operates on a simplistic and even dangerous premise. Human beings are not merely symbol users; every moment of life is permeated with symbolism.

OBSTACLES TO COMMUNICATION

The study of communication is concerned with the process by which people attribute meaning to their experience and with their efforts to share such meanings. It focuses upon factors that undermine or facilitate the achievement of common meanings through an exchange of messages. The complexity of medical communication may be intimated by examining some of the more common and more serious barriers to interpersonal understanding in medical settings.

Ego involvement. Less complete communication is likely whenever the topic of conversation is highly ego-involving, such as when one or both parties are fearful of the matter under discussion. Few subjects would appear to arouse as intense feelings as adequacy of the physical or symbolic self. Recent cross-cultural research suggests that the least talked about of all topics are those relating to physical inadequacy, illness, and disease.[5] The anxiety associated with such matters triggers a number of defensive maneuvers, most of which interfere with a clear exchange of meaning. Some people flee and others attack, some refuse to listen and others refuse to talk, some exaggerate and others minimize. But rarely do people comprehend clearly when they are emotionally upset.

Differences in knowledge. Another factor complicating communication resides in the respective power of the communicants. We are beginning to appreciate that information is power. Where knowledge is unequal, where some people have access to the facts and others do not, equality of human relationships is impossible. It is not suprising, therefore, that incomplete and distorted communication surrounds so many encounters between specialists and lay people. To be uninformed is to be communicatively impotent, and this dependent state is not one mature people tolerate gracefully. Rarely is this condition absent between doctors and patients.

Social status. Difficulties are likely, also, when the social distance separating two communicants is great. The greater the disparity in education, income, and social standing, the less people are capable of hearing or of hearing what was said as it was intended. The presence of higher status figures—parents, teachers, supervisors, police—provokes fear quite apart from whatever they may happen to say. White[6] found his cardiac patients manifesting significantly different levels of tension when he discussed their cases with them in status-aggravating or status-minimizing settings. When status distinctions are emphasized, people avoid contact with each other, withhold information, and distort the meanings intended by the words of others.

Communicative purposes. Status differences are complicated further by differences in point of view arising in part from differences in position and authority. Rarely do communicative purposes overlap completely. Because of distinctive motives, student and teacher do not argue about the "same" grade; nor do husband and wife discuss the "same" child; nor for that matter do physician and patient talk about the "same" X-rays, the "same" disease, the "same" operation, or the "same" fee. Messages acquire much of their meaning from the perspective from which they are uttered. Unless people are sensitive to such differences in purpose or unless these are explicitly discussed, meanings will not coincide since they are anchored in discrepant motives.

Emotional distance. Through conversation people seek some similarity of thought, some congruence of feeling. Words like "rapport," "intimacy," "empathy," and "closeness" are used to describe satisfying encounters with others. But any such meeting of minds is difficult unless both communicants are willing to be "present," not merely available intellectually but totally present as persons. In the interaction of roles, in the encounter of facades, there is no commitment to communication. To give patients the feeling that they are a problem, a disease, or an intriguing curiosity rather than a human being is to undermine the process of sharing meanings. No one has put this point as cogently as Martin Buber.[7] The "I-It" relation, he argues, is demeaning and frustrating for it rests on perceptions of the other as no more than an object. It is only when people confront each other in an "I-Thou" relation that they meet as human beings with respect and mutual concern. When people cultivate emotional distance, they not only prevent any deep sharing of meaning but also arouse animosity and even hatred.

One-way communication. Once communication was regarded as a linear process. Someone, a sender or speaker, transmitted messages to a receiver or listener. Meanings obtained by the receiver were due to the skill of the sender. The sender did the work and the receiver merely paid attention. Any idea could be deposited in the nervous system of another person if one only chose the right words. Now we know better. No one deposits any meaning in the mind of others. Receivers do not passively absorb the intentions of others but creatively interpret what they hear in the light of their own perspectives, their own needs, their own expectations. Reaching any degree of interpersonal understanding requires a process of mutual accommodation. Each person must provide the other with clues to his or her meanings via words and actions. Each must attend to the clues of the other. And each must be prepared to clarify and elaborate his meaning from the viewpoint of the other. This process succeeds to the extent that both parties assume equal responsibility for achieving common meanings.

Yet the prevailing style of interaction from the clinic to the classroom is one-way rather than two-way. And, unfortunately, such channel restrictions impoverish the process and leave receivers confused and impotent. Labortory studies supply dramatic evidence of the seriousness of this phenomenon; where communication flows in only one direction. The simplest instructions are misinterpreted, errors are compounded rather than corrected and morale and human relationships deteriorate. It is easy to appreciate the source of such distortion and friction. Nothing is more demoralizing than to be placed in critical situations and then be prevented from clarifying obscure and confusing messages.

Verbal manipulation. Many efforts to communicate are prompted not by the desire to share or create new meanings but to maneuver the other person into a predetermined decision. Whatever the form of such efforts, from verbal seduction to verbal coercion, they derive from an assumption of moral superiority on the part of one communicant. They also involve disrespect for the integrity of other persons and appropriation of their right to determine their own destiny. Enlarging the communicative responsibility of one person requires some surrender of responsibility by the other. And while such dependency is tolerated by children, adults often find it demeaning and insulting. In a highly manipulative society it is not surprising that most people become adept at recognizing their manipulators. They become suspicious and verbally devious themselves. Thus, communication is often subverted and people antagonized when the authority of their own experience is denied equal weight in the process of making decisions affecting their own survival.

Ambiguity of language. Language itself may introduce barriers to mutual understanding. Through a system of symbols with culturally sanctioned definitions, people seek to share their experience and establish grounds for cooperative action. Yet every communicative code forces the infinity of events into a limited set of categories and fixes appropriate labels to them. "Illness" has perhaps a hundred meanings. "Surgery" may have several dozen. "Fracture" is imprecise. "Cancer" is inexact. If so many words are vague in their reference, messages composed of such ambiguous elements will be even less precise. Nearly every statement can support many legitmate and even contradictory interpretations. In some respects the vocabulary of illness constitutes a special case. Anyone who has attempted to describe a sickness knows the frustration of searching for words to convey the subtle inner disturbances called symptoms. As the great English novelist, Virginia Woolf, once said, "let a sufferer try to describe a pain in his head to a doctor and language at once runs dry." Most people have experienced the communicative paralysis induced by a poverty of words for inner states combined with innocent insistence upon clarity from the doctor.

Language by itself solves nothing. Words can confuse as easily as they clarify. As we have seen, communication is not accomplished by mere listening; it requires a persistent and sensitive effort to solve a mystery whose major clues are provided by words. Common meaning is achieved only through repeated and mutual checking of interpretations. Where people have little appreciation of the ambiguity of words, they remain unaware of the extent to which their remarks can be misunderstood. And they are unlikely to adapt their communicative style to this fact of life.

Role of jargon. Language isolates in another way. Not only do Chinese and Russians speak different languages but also so do males and females, young and old, soldiers and civilians. Every subculture, every trade, and every profession cultivates a dialect of its own. Lawyers, engineers, scientists, accountants and physicians foster their private jargons. These are neither ornament not luxury; they serve genuine needs; they increase the efficiency of communication within the group; they cultivate rapport among members; they provide a sense of common identity. While contributing to communication within a group, these same dialects when turned outward confuse, frighten, stupefy, alienate. And the more sensitive the topic of conversation, the more such private languages undermine the function for which language was designed. If medical personnel are occasionally puzzled or irritated by the words of economists, lawyers, insurance agents, or musicologists, they might consider the extent to which these same people may be mystified by the diagnostic remarks of physicians.

Pressures of time. Compounding these difficulties is the factor of time. In some ways our humanity seems threatened more by the pace of our lives than by any other single factor. There is no human relationship, no communicative act, that is enriched or improved by speeding it up. It takes time to explain, time to listen, time to dissipate fears, time to assimilate frightening facts, time to prepare for crises, time to enter the experiential world of another person. The urge to hurry must be overcome if people are really serious about preserving the human community.

Significance for Treatment

The factors that complicate the process of sharing meanings are nearly all present in doctor–patient encounters. And most are found here in their most extreme and destructive form. It is here that emotionally disturbing matters, sometimes of life and death, are discussed. It is here that the immense authority and power of one communicant faces the ignorance and impotence of the other. It is here that the need for rapport is largest, yet the emotional distance is likely to be greatest. It is here, too, that critical choice must be made with information which is clothed in an esoteric jargon that obscures and mystifies. And it is here that words are uttered rapidly, even unintelligibly, with little time to clarify or assimilate their meaning. Some of these obstacles to understanding are inherent in illness itself; some derive from the historical roles of physician and patient; others result from the personal communicative style of the physician or are a matter of cultivation by the medical profession.

Yet if people are really serious about improving medical communication, they must resist the appeal of conspiratorial approaches. It is always easier to take sides than to understand—to align ourselves simplistically with child against parent, worker against management, student against teacher, patient against physician. The temptation to search for demons is an addiction the human race has not overcome even in this sophisticated age. The number of villains in the world is probably overestimated, and they are by no means the exclusive property of the medical profession.

Human acts nearly always make sense. They arise from some compromise between private impulse and social expectation. If human behavior is to change, it may be less because we substitute virtue for vice than because we deepen the awareness of people to the total context from which they derive their meanings and motives. The communicative manner of medical specialists may spring less from any malevolent effort to claim omniscience and prestige than from an accident of the role in which medical professionals have cast themselves and been cast by society and from the process by which people are selected and prepared to assume medical responsibilities.

The doctor, as well as the patient, must cope with anxieties surrounding treatment. The doctor may be aware of the seriousness of the case and may know the real limitations of medical knowledge and skill. He may be sensitive to past errors and the possibility of committing further mistakes. There is the danger of making the wrong choice among alternative treatments. There is risk of patient criticism and peer disapproval. If medical personnel sometimes emphasize their authority and status, assert opinions as if they were unassailable, manipulate patients, maintain emotional distance, and discourage patient collaboration, are these not some of the same tactics most people use when threatened and unaware of viable alternatives? Mystification may seem the only constructive way of protecting the patient from undue anxiety in view of the limited assistance that medicine and surgery can provide. It may be used in the hope that mystique can accomplish what science cannot. Mystification permits physicians as well as patients some escape from anxiety, embarrassment, and frustration. This does not justify it, but it may identify its source in the human psyche.

MEDICAL EDUCATION

Consider acculturation into the medical profession. How much of this process is designed to promote respect for or insight into human personality? There appears to be minimal effort to assess candidates on their capacity to sustain extensive or intensive human relationships. Yet no profession has daily contact with so wide a spectrum of subcultures, and none exerts influence over such sensitive matters. How many courses are concerned with exploring the ways illness threatens the symbolic as well as physical self? How many class periods focus upon the communicative strategies patients use to cope with imminent threats to their survival? How much time is spent exploring the physician's own communicative style, the assumptions on which it rests, the impulses it reflects, the consequences for those he or she treats?

Throughout training the future physician is preoccupied with the physical properties of the body. Medical training is concerned with anatomy, chemical processes, manifestations of dysfunction, and the consequences of medical and surgical techniques. A vast array of instruments and technologies must be mastered. Is it surprising if later when faced with patients the physician should prefer to deal with physical their rather than psychic symptoms? Will medical specialists not be likely to feel more comfortable and competent handling X-rays, blood samples, printouts, and pathology reports than coping with frightened and distraught personalities? In some offices one gets the impression the physician would prefer never to meet or know the person being treated. If only somehow one could avoid dealing with the human being at all. It is understandable that few patients can effect so neat a surgery between illness and self.

A person's communicative manner derives from his view of human beings. Values are not elusive abstractions; they are manifest in every word. It is difficult to respect the integrity of others and the validity of their experience and at the same time manipulate them—as difficult as it is to see others as mindless children and still collaborate with them as equals. But commitment to humane values is rarely enough, any more than the simple desire to relieve suffering automatically confers diagnostic or surgical talent. Skill must be acquired to translate respect for patients as persons into capacity to engage them communicatively as equals. Communicative skills must be cultivated that respect patients' intelligence, acknowledge their needs, accept their feelings, value their opinions, and promote collaboration in decision-making. To acheive this sort of mature relationship demands some recognition of what often occurs under the guise of medical communication and of alternatives for building more effective encounters between physicians and patients.

RESEARCH

When one turns to ask what is currently known about communication between medical personnel and patients, the answer is itself mystifying. A phrase will suffice—very little. Here is a profession founded on science, dedicated to truth, committed to inquiry, concerned with the relief of suffering, yet either oblivious to or unwilling to examine its own communicative behavior. Is this simply a mote in an otherwise scientific eye? Or is it a defensive assertion of the medical mystique and the preference to do as one pleases?

If the suffering caused by communicative negligence were a result of some physical disorder, the response would be predictable: organize medical research, underwrite exploratory studies, encourage testing of alternative treatments, and counter the disorder. But when the suffering is a consequence of symbolic disorder—when it arises from the failure to listen, the failure to comprehend, the failure to respect and collaborate—even when such failures result, as they sometimes do, in suffering or death, should there not be an equally vigorous effort to remedy it? It is unfortunate that we have no clear idea of the precise extent of injury to the human personality—or for that matter to the body itself—by the unsought diagnosis, the unasked question, the unreported symptom, the uncomprehended explanation, the disregarded treatment, the incorrectly followed medication. We have only the horror stories so many tell, offset by occasional reports of sensitive and empathic collaboration. While we have some conception of the suffering imposed by broken bones and diseased tissue, we have only the vaguest notion of the damage done through communicative negligence.

This is an area of medicine where the questions far outrun the answers. And the reason there are so few answers is that so few within the field of medicine have raised questions about medical communication. Nearly everyone inside and outside the medical profession affirms that communication with patients deserves study, but few institutions have offered to support such research. To know little about something as complex as interactions between physicians and patients is nothing to apologize for. But to know little and to choose to remain ignorant about it is tragic for the patient and demeaning for the profession.

What are some of the questions that press for answers? We need to know more of the various types of patients and the manner in which they present their condition. There is no reason to assume that high and low income groups, females and males, blacks and whites, educated and uneducated respond in the same way to illness. To claim to respect all patients is nonsense unless medical personnel are willing to meet them on their own communicative terms. There is little reason, also, to assume that all types of illness and injury provoke similar reactions and similar questions or demand similar kinds of involvement. What is a helpful remark in one context may be frightening in another. If patients' reactions bear little resemblance to what seems appropriate, physicians must remember that it is patient's perceptions, not their own, that are the focus of treatment.

We need to know what types of communicative defenses are triggered by illness. It has been suggested that patients tend to be "copers" or "deniers," with the former seeking information in order to assimilate it and the latter avoiding information to keep from being overwhelmed by it. There may be many more ways of handling threatening news than this simple dichotomy suggests. There are, finally, a host of questions concerning the dominant style of the physician. Should it be primarily investigative, informative, supportive, persuasive, collaborative, or therapeutic? At what point and with which patients might each of these contribute to recovery and self-esteem?

Some indication of the kind of investigative work that is possible and its potential is found in a simple exploratory study undertaken in 1970 by Thomas Lonner for a master's thesis at San Francisco State University. It focused on the preoperative and postoperative contacts between one physician and several patients undergoing surgery. The findings are suggestive rather than definitive. But they illustrate the possibilities of such studies.

What the investigator found was this: the physician was genuinely interested in his patients, earnestly tried to provide the care they needed, and attempted to be as clear and informative as possible. His motives were impeccable and his approach was constructive. But it was also clear, in spite of this, that he had only one approach to all patients; that he failed to recognize differences in their reactions to stress; that he was unable to predict their postoperative responses; that he made little effort to confer with them; that he did not adapt verbally, often using words that had no meaning for them; and that when he failed, he sought no explanation for his failure nor did he consider varying his behavior to adapt to this failure. Yet to unsophisticated observers, including some of his patients, he appeared to be an adequate example of the doctor communicating with his patient.

Medical educators, it would appear, must recognize the symbolic and semantic aspects of illness and injury. They must recognize, as well, that all treatment involves a communicative relationship with patients. It is important not only that more intensive efforts be made to investigate this critical relationship between persons seeking treatment and those providing it but also that part of medical training should be developing sensitivity and flexibility in human interaction.

If, as was once written, it is more important to know what manner of man has the disease than to know what disease he has, one might add that to know the manner of man is impossible without appreciating the way he symbolizes his situation. This is a communicative problem of no small dimensions but one for which the medical profession cannot escape some responsibility. It is meanings, not merely physical symptoms, that prompt people to seek or avoid examination, that cause them to withhold or describe their condition, that intensify or minimize their physical discomfort, that prompt them to report or distort reactions to treatment, that lead them to obey or contradict medical advice, that determine ultimately whether they assist or sabotage efforts to cure them. The entire process, from the onset of illness to recovery or death, is invested with symbolism, with meanings that are unique, to every person and to every physical condition. And these meanings, in turn, complicate the conditions that are the focus of treatment. If medical personnel are concerned with the relief of suffering, they can no longer disregard their communicative style with patients. Suffering and the relief of suffering are influenced by symbolic as well as physical acts. Medical personnel are inescapably involved in influencing meanings in some of the most traumatic moments of human existence. Mystification would appear to be a questionable substitute for communicative sensitivity.

REFERENCES

1. Kelly, G. *The Psychology of Personal Constructs*. New York: Norton, 1955.
2. Langer, S. *Philosophy in a New Key*.Cambridge, Mass.: Harvard University Press, 1957.
3. Melzack, R. The Perception of Pain. *Scientific American* 264 (February 1961): 41–49.
4. Friedson, E. *The Profession of Medicine*. New York: Dodd, Mead, 1972, p. 224.
5. Barnlund, D. *Public and Private Self in Japan and U.S.* Tokyo: Simul Press, 1975.
6. White, A. The Patient Sits Down. *Psycoso. Med.* 15 (1953): 256–57.
7. Buber, M. *I and Thou*. New York: Scribner's Sons, 1958.

3.

ORAL AND WRITTEN COMMUNICATION IN HEALTH CARE

Members of the State Pharmacists' Association were growing more and more concerned with the ability of pharmacists within the state to impact upon public attitudes about pharmacy and provide the public with accurate information about pharmaceutical products and services. More specifically, they were concerned about the poor public recognition of the pharmacist as a health professional and an integral member of the health care team, lack of public knowledge about important health care issues, low job-satisfaction and self-image of many pharmacists, as well as the misuse and abuse of medications within the state.

Ernie Floyd, the education director of the Pharmacists' Association decided, in consultation with the association administrator, that it might be a good idea for the association to develop a Pharmacists Speakers' Bureau. He composed a brief questionnaire to survey the reactions of the association membership about the speakers' bureau idea. Results of the survey showed that the vast majority of pharmacists who were members of the association had responded positively to the idea of a speakers' bureau and strongly agreed with the need for improved information exchange with the public. Paradoxically, very few pharmacists volunteered to be members of the speakers' bureau and make public presentations.

The membership's mixed reaction—they thought the speakers' bureau was a good idea but were not willing to actively participate in it—had Ernie confused. In the past the association membership was usually more than willing to give of their time to participate in activities they thought to be important. After several discussions with pharmacists Ernie discovered the primary reason association members were reluctant to participate in the program—their lack of confidence in their ability to speak well in public.

To help pharmacists develop as effective public speakers and improve their presentational skills Ernie arranged a workshop for association members on presentational speaking. He drafted a promotional pamphlet about the workshop and sent it out to the association membership. Local and national experts on public communication skills training were contacted and arrangements were made for these experts to lead the workshop. The workshop was divided into two sessions. The first session was devoted to examining the public communication process, including preparing the speech, presenting the speech, and answering audience questions. The second session was devoted to practicing delivering public presentations, using videotape to provide feedback about areas for improvement of presentational style. Additionally, Ernie put together a speaker handbook containing tips on public speaking, information on how to handle questions and answers, how to publicize presentations, how to find an audience, how to outline a speech, how to utilize audiovisual materials in presentations, where to find information for presentations, and how to critique one's own presentational style.

Attendance at the workshop was good and it was very successful at helping the pharmacists apply their expertise to effective presentational communication. The handbook was distributed to all workshop participants. After the workshop several pharmacists expressed their interest to Ernie in joining the Pharmacy Speakers' Bureau. The bureau has grown in the months following the workshop, and there are many requests for speakers by different public audiences, including schools, churches, senior citizens groups, and business organizations. The speakers' bureau helps to provide these groups with important health information about such varied topics as drug costs, drug abuse, pharmacist services, pharmacy careers, correct uses of medications, vitamins and nutrition, and alcoholism. The Pharmacy Speakers' Bureau is an important part of the State Pharmacists' Association that works to promote better health through health communication.[1]

CONVEYING INFORMATION THROUGH PUBLIC COMMUNICATION

Presenting Health Information to the Public

One of the most important aims of health care is to disseminate information which will accurately explain what is happening to the client's body or mind. Conveying information, particularly technical information, is difficult because of differences in language use and cultural systems (see Chapter 8). It becomes even more challenging to convey health related information to large groups through oral or written channels in public settings. The purpose of this chapter is to present information that will make it much easier for health and health care information to be shared publicly through the spoken and written word.

In the case history at the beginning of this chapter the State Pharmacists' Association used both written and oral communication to develop a Speakers' Bureau. The education director used written communication in preparing a questionnaire to survey the attitudes of pharmacists toward the speakers' bureau, in preparing a brochure promoting the presentational communication workshop, and in preparing the speaker handbook. The presentational communication workshop was presented to the pharmacists through oral communication, both when the public speaking experts spoke to the pharmacists about public speaking, as well as when the pharmacists practiced delivering public presentations. As this case history indicates oral and written presentational communication is an important form of health communication.

Public communication is much more structured than interpersonal communication. In public communication (be it oral or written) one person is designated as the presenter and the rest become the audience; the presenter does the majority of the talking. The same analogy can be made for writing. The goal of the public presentation, oral or written, is to inform, persuade, stimulate, and often, to entertain.

Public presentation takes many forms. Oral presentations can consist of anything from speeches to laypersons for health education purposes to speeches to colleagues where technical information is conveyed. Television appearances are becoming more frequent for the health professional as mass media representatives are becoming more and more concerned with presenting information on health topics to their viewers (see Chapter 4).

Audience Analysis

It is important to analyze the person or persons with whom you want to share information. The process of doing this is called audience analysis and it is an important one for the health professional to understand. Audience analysis should be done before doing any speaking or writing. You should ask questions such as the following: Who are you addressing? What are they like? How do you think they will react to your presentation? For example, are you designing information sheets for the diabetic patient or are you conveying the results of some new research to the county medical association where the relationship is more collegial and more technical language is appropriate? Whatever the case, you need to think about the persons receiving the information, for, whatever their number, from 1 to 100, they are your *audience*. The health professional should analyze the audience members as to demographic variables such as age, education, sex and socio-economic status, emotional maturity, and the desire to know or understand what is happening to their health, in order to determine their cultural orientations and potential attitudes toward you and your topic.

Oral Presentations

It is important to determine the attitude the audience will have toward you and the information you will be presenting them with. Are you trying to convey information and gain good will? Even though you may be an expert, do the persons you are addressing recognize your expertise, or is it necessary to convince them? All of these questions refer to your *credibility*. In the broadest sense, credibility refers to an audience's willingness to trust what a person says or does. Your manner and presentation will need to be tailored according to how credible you are recognized as being. Additional audience analysis questions that should be asked when making an oral presentation: How will the audience arrive at your presentation? Will they be tired from other activities? Will they be dreading this speech or anxious to hear it? Is the audience composed of laypersons or experts? Is it a mix? How many will attend?

Regardless of how you answer these and other audience analysis questions, there will be a measure of persuadability in what you try to do in your speech. Although speeches can be designed to inform, to stimulate, and to entertain, all have at least a minimal persuadability component. That is, the speaker is trying to influence the attitudes, feelings, or behaviors of the members of the audience. We will discuss persuasion in a later part of this chapter.

After you have analyzed the audience, you will want to look at *your own motives* for giving the speech. Do you have important information you want to share with this group to enhance the health of your listeners? Do you want to enhance your reputation as an expert? In answering this latter question, don't be modest. All of us like to share our knowledge in some way or another. We simply need to be honest about our motive.

Purposes of Oral Presentations

There are several different types and purposes of public presentations. There are *speeches to inform*, *speeches to persuade*, and *speeches to entertain*. Speeches to inform may include in-service lectures, patient demonstrations, and client health education talks. Speeches to persuade may include fund-raising talks, medical supplies and equipment sales pitches, as well as talks to health consumers and their families to promote compliance with health care regimens. Speeches to entertain may include after dinner presentations at banquets, awards ceremonies, and humorous roasts of colleagues.

Modern speech theorists recognize that most public presentations combine elements of all three of these speech types: information, persuasion, and entertainment. For example, in a good health education lecture, although the primary purpose of the speaker is to inform the audience about a particular health care topic, the speaker also wants to persuade and entertain the audience. The effective speaker attempts to persuade the audience to accept and adopt the point of view of the presentation and not merely hear the information presented. The effective speaker also wants to make the presentation entertaining and engaging enough to keep the audience's attention and leave them feeling good about the lecture. The best speakers, then, are those that can combine the abilities to present clear, relevant information to an audience, persuade and motivate the audience to respond, and keep the audience's interest.

Before making a speech you should analyze your purposes for making the presentation, and analyze the audience you are speaking to. This prior analysis will help you prepare your presentation because it will provide you with a clear understanding of what you want to do and who you want to address.

Content and Organization of Speeches

Once the general audience characteristics are known, and the motives and goals are established, the speech can be tailored to fit the needs of the group. We have found the phrase "C.O.D." to be helpful. The letters stand for the content, organization and delivery which are the major elements of either speeches or lectures.[2]

Usually a topic has been preassigned for most speeches. It is important that the speaker decide on either a narrow or general interpretation of that topic. For example, if the topic is death and dying, the presenter might want to focus on that topic in general or, more specifically, on death and dying in the hospital context. The decision should be made according to audience needs and time constraints. The topic will come into perspective during the presentation stages as notes are prepared and the speaker reflects on the message to be given.

Four standards Haakenson suggests:

1. Material should be relevant. It should amplify the point being made.
2. It should be accurate.
3. It should be of interest and capture the listeners' attention.
4. It should be adequate and not overlong.

Haakenson gives us a religious illustration to support that premise: A veteran pastor was asked by his new assistant, "How long should I preach when I give my first sermon next Sunday?" "That's up to you," came the reply, "but we feel we don't save any souls after twenty minutes."[3]

Once the main premises of the speech are developed, the speaker needs to develop illustrations for these premises—case histories, examples, statistics, humor, quotations and audiovisual aids are all examples of supporting data. These data can come from personal experience, research and reading, or information obtained from others.

Important information (key points) given to an audience, needs to be replicated, or reinforced, so that these points will be remembered. It has been suggested by some researchers that this replication of relevant facts should take place utilizing a different sensory modality.[4] For example, if the point is originally made orally to the listener, it should be reemphasized visually. If the purpose is to tell the audience how much damage is done to the lungs by smoking, a slide of a polluted lung might be used as a visual aid to reemphasize that information.

The actual speech itself should have a central idea with major supporting points. The points should be supported by examples. We have included a speech outline which can be adapted to different kinds of speechs (see Figure 3.1). In preparing a speech the writer should also remember that the organization can be based on chronological or time sequences. Additionally, it can be logically or topically organized.

Figure 3.1   Skeleton Outline for a Speech To Stimulate a Change in Behavior

Technical Plot	How To Stop Smoking
Introduction	I. Secure the attention of the audience and establish a friendly feeling between yourself and the audience; the most common type of beginning is to relate an incident that can be tied with the behavior you will advocate.
Body Statement of importance of behavior Motive Appeal: Pride	II. Taking the lead from the incident you used in the introduction, point out the desirability for and importance of the behavior change.
Examples	A. Using examples, create a vivid picture of what happens when you smoke. 1. Use personal experiences. 2. Use narration and historical cases. B. Reinforce the importance of non-smoking through the use of startling facts, quotation from prestige sources.
Anecdote Quotation Example Instance Instance	1. Keep interest and attention high by using stories and other materials that focus on the importance of this behavior change. 2. Show a *general acceptance* of the behavior and of its desirability in society in general and the kind of people in this audience. C. Adapt to this immediate audience by narrowing your examples and other supporting materials to show that the behavior is also important to them.
Example Story	1. Use examples involving people like those in the audience. 2. Touch the feelings and emotions of the members of this audience. 3. Make the appeal close to the audience; make certain that the behavior is of real significance to them.
Statement of Behavior	D. Make a transition to a specific statement of the behavior (nonsmoking) that the audience is to intensify, suggesting some specific procedure to quit smoking.
Slogan	1. Use some novel device, such as alliteration or a slogan, to express and to impress the plan on the minds of the audience.

Fig. 3.1 (*cont'd*)

Explanation	2. State what you would like the audience to do positively, without argument.
Conclusion	III. Picture life as it will be when the audience has adopted the behavior—nonsmoking—and heightened the desirability in their own minds of doing what you suggest. A. Here you can afford a bit of mild exaggeration, since everyone should be with you and some overstatement will seem natural.
Example	B. Avoid the abstract—be vivid, concrete—making the picture lively and realistic. C. Fill in the speech with imagery, illustration, and narration. D. Start with a rapid restatement of the behavior; add a quotation that vividly suggests a personal commitment on the part of the audience to do as you ask; end with a challenge to the audience to do as you ask.

This outline was adapted from *Instructional Supplement With A Handbook of Communication Exercises: Communication Probes*, B. Peterson and R.W. Pace, Chicago, Science Research Associates, Inc. 1977, p. 82.

As the major ideas are tied together in some kind of sequence, transitions become important. The transitions need to tie part-to-part and part-to-whole. Transitions can be made through enumeration ("Secondly, in assessing your smoking behavior you should keep a daily record) or through summarization. Occasional summaries are often an effective way to make the speech clearer to the audience.

As the speech is organized, persuasive devices should be included where appropriate, particularly if a different kind of health-behavior is to be encouraged. The motivational process can be briefly summarized. An effective speaker needs to:

1. secure attention.
2. state a problem or need.
3. offer a solution.
4. help the audience visualize the desirability of the solution.
5. invite definite action.

Part of the motivation process is, of course, to seek change. Since most people either desire or fear change, the speaker or lecturer needs to be aware of how the audience views the particular change. Strategy then needs to be designed, which meets the audience's particular needs for the change contemplated by the speaker.

1. Persuasion, part of motivation, is accomplished in many ways. Persuasion can be accomplished through the writer's or speaker's reputation. To enforce your reputation (particularly when you are first building one) you should be forceful and knowledgeable. Additionally, you should use supporting materials that are clear, relevant, and innovative.
2. Persuasion also takes place through emotion. People respond to certain words or ideas in a similar manner. The emotions of the audience can be appealed to by knowing the audience's attitudes.
3. Persuasion can also be accomplished through logic or reason. Using valid evidence and sound reasoning assists in this regard.

Audiovisual Aids

Useful tools for the speaker can sometimes be movie or overhead projectors, graphs and charts, tape or phonograph recordings, or an easel. Each aid utilized must meet certain criteria, however, or it should not be utilized. These criteria are:

1. *The aid should be important to the speech.* It should specifically amplify the point being made in the speech. It should not be distracting.
2. *The aid should be seen only as an assisting device.* The point being made should stand without an aid but be better because of it.
3. *Aids should be visible, audible, and in working order.*

The final aspect of the third criterion, "working order" causes major problems with the use of audiovisual aids. Can you even count the events you have attended where the projector broke down or didn't focus or the plug to the overhead didn't fit in the wall? Murphy's law of "whatever can go wrong, will go wrong," seems to apply to use of audiovisual aids. One invaluable rule is to check out the equipment *before you decide to use it* and once again *just before* the presentation. You should practice the speech with the aids in the very area in which the speech is to take place, whenever possible.

Aids should be simple and clear. Complicated displays can distract the audience from the major points being made. If the aid is not neat and clear, the audience will start worrying about the speaker's credibility.

The handout is often used as an aid in medically related presentations. While it can be invaluable in presenting detailed and complex
material or in summarizing the presentation, care should be taken in
handing it out before the speech. Often it will distract the audience.
One exception to this is an outline which, when given at the beginning
of a complex presentation, can simplify information for the listener.

Introduction, Body, and Conclusion

Generally, there should always be three discrete sections to every public
presentation, the introduction, the body, and the conclusion. Each of
these sections performs a different and important function in the oral
presentation.

The *introduction* is where the speaker identifies him or herself, and
sets the topics and goals of the presentation to the audience. Introduc-
tions are used to orient the audience to the presentation, as well as to
establish audience interest and attention. A good approach for establishing attention is to relate the topic of the presentation to the specific
goals or backgrounds of the audience members. Credibility can be established in the introduction section of the presentation by demonstrating
the source of your expertise, your trustworthiness (or pure motives for
the presentation), and your charisma.

The *body* of the presentation is where the data and evidence for your
topic is exhibited to the audience. Statistics, quotations, personal testi-
mony, stories, and examples are often used in the body of the presentation to illustrate the major points of the speech. The body of the
presentation should follow up on the goals set for the presentation in
the introduction, explicating fully the reasons for these goals and providing the audience with information supporting your primary topic. In
most speeches, the body is the longest part of the presentation.

The *conclusion* section of the presentation is used to summarize and
amplify the primary points of the presentation. The main topics should
be restated in the conclusion in a clear and dramatic manner, thus driving these points home to the audience. If you want the audience to act
upon any of the information you have provided them, you must forcefully identify specific actions the members of the audience can take. Be
sure to offer recommendations that the audience has the potential to
accomplish, explaining how and why they should do what you are asking of them. For example, if you are suggesting that each member of
your audience be on their guard against hypertension, it would behoove
you to explain why that is important and specify how and where
they can get their blood pressure checked. The more specific your con-

cluding suggestions are, the more likely it is that your audience will follow your advice.

The introduction, body, and conclusion sections of your presentation provide your speech with structure and direction. The introduction sets up the topic of your presentation for the audience. The body is used to explicate the main points of your speech, and provides the supporting evidence for your position. The conclusion is used to tie the main points of your presentation together, and leave the audience with a sense of closure and direction.

Delivery of Oral Presentations

Once the content of the speech is established and it is well-organized, the delivery aspects should be analyzed. This area includes the speaker's psychological set (happy, sad, or firm) the bodily expressions (nonverbal communication), voice, articulation, and language.

First and foremost, speeches need to be delivered with excitement, animation, and enthusiasm. Even topics that are highly technical can be made more interesting by the speaker's own interest in his or her presentation.

The nonverbal communication is also important. Gestures need to flow rather than be rigid. The speaker's stance (how she or he holds her or his body) has impact on the audience. One of the more common unconscious problems of many public speakers is the failure to keep both feet on the ground while speaking. Appearance is also part of the nonverbal communication and clothes should be chosen for the speech according to the image the speaker wants to convey. Eye contact and facial expression are factors. Make sure that you have eye contact with all members of the audience and that your face expresses your enthusiasm for your topic.

Speakers also need to think about their voice and how it affects the audience. Can they be heard in the back of the room? One trick is to always project the voice to the person in the furthermost corner. The pitch of the voice also needs to be considered. The voice should be neither too high or too low. Additionally, the speaker needs to change inflection once in a while during the speech for persuasive purposes.

Words need to be articulated carefully and at the right rate of speech. Fast speeches are ignored and slow speeches are boring. Additionally, the language of the speech should be appropriate and sometimes eloquent or dynamic. Words such as "uh" and "okay" should be avoided. Again, jargon or "medspeak," as health-related jargon is often called, should be avoided unless the audience will understand the jargon. If the audience consists of laypersons, the speaker should remember the international and national findings that patients do not interpret medical terminology in the same way professionals do and care should be taken to avoid such terms.[5]

Some additional delivery tips include the following:

1. A pause should take place after the speaker stands up. This pause allows organization of notes, a survey of the audience and a deep breath!
2. Humor can be part of the delivery only if such humor is comfortable for the speaker. Humor should not be forced.
3. The speaker should not apologize for coughing, for forgetting or for any part of the presentation. In fact, it is very important for him or her to convey an air of confidence about the whole performance.
4. The final movements of the speech or lecture should be effective, persuasive, and enthusiastic. As stated in the content section, a summary is important and the audience should be left thinking about the major points.
5. Speakers should watch other speakers in person and on television for good speaking tips as well as for problems to avoid.

Special Notes on Television Presentations

Television provides invaluable opportunities for health education. However, organization becomes of paramount concern as time is so limited. Often the health professional will be asked, for example, to give a full analysis of the pros and cons of eating dairy products in three minutes. Obviously, there is far more information about this topic than the three. minute limit will allow you to present. In preparing for any television performance, the speaker should think of no more than three major points to convey in a half-hour presentation and the rest of the time should be used in supporting those points. In preparing for talk show presentations (and the preparation takes place with the moderator for five minutes before the camera rolls) the speaker should emphasize the kind of issues he or she thinks will be important to the audience, for few talk show hosts or hostesses know the subject as well as the speaker. Often they have no idea of the questions to begin asking on technical subjects.

Some ideas for television presentations are:

1. Wear a dark suit or jacket with some contrast in a shirt or blouse. Make sure your clothes aren't too busy.

2. Look at the host or the other panelists. Don't stare into the camera!
3. Watch your feet. Place them firmly on the ground and sit with your back touching the back of your chair. Don't be too rigid or too relaxed.
4. Try to forget you are on television. Talk with the other participants as you would talk with colleagues or friends.
5. Be enthusiastic about your topic.
6. Don't be long winded. Answers to questions and comments should be forceful but short. Use examples or cases to support your points when possible.
7. Don't be late. Live TV shows can't wait for you. Additionally, make sure you know the studio location in advance. Most of them are hidden in remote areas.
8. Be sure and tell your family and friends to view your performance. If you want to assess your own performance, videotaping machines are ideal.

Notes on Lecturing and Teaching

The lecture is a very important communication tool in health care education. There has been much criticism recently of medical and nursing school teaching. The criticism focuses on such issues as boring lectures, lack of interest in students and little attention to feedback from the students. Once again, we want to stress that all oral presentations contain elements of speeches to inform, persuade, and entertain. This is especially true of the lecture. A good lecture should do more than merely present information to an audience. The lecture should be designed to present pertinent information, motivate the audience to accept and use the information, and keep the audience involved and interested in the lecture.

It should be noted that the roots of the word doctor derive from the Latin words "to teach." Teaching is an essential part of health care practice, as it is an essential part of both providing consumers with relevant health care information and training health care professionals about the latest health care methods. While efforts have been made to improve health-related teaching by adding "teachers of teachers" to several medical and nursing school faculties, recent cutbacks in the funding of these programs have eliminated some of these programs and thereby the focus on good teaching. In an attempt to facilitate increased recognition of the importance of oral communication in teaching, as well as the abilities to communicate effectively in teaching situations we suggest a few teaching tips.

The effective lecture will focus on informing, persuading, and entertaining the audience, in the same manner as a good speech. The lecture needs to contain interesting and stimulating material, be pertinent to the specific audience, and be well organized and well delivered. The use of humor, case studies and other devices can be effective in emphasizing important points. Handouts are often useful for presenting highly technical or complex material.

The major difference between the lecture and most public presentations is in the area of feedback from the audience. In most public presentations, there is a specific time period set aside for questions and answers. During a lecture, however, students generally need to ask questions, and at times engage in discussion, throughout the lecture period. Often these interchanges can divert the class and the teacher from the lecture topic. An effective lecturer needs to be flexible enough to deal with student concerns while tying class interaction in to the lecture topic and meeting the time demands of the class period. The lecturer should attempt to make transitions between the comments students make and the lecture topic being presented. In this way, the lecturer is able to answer the questions and respond to the audience's ideas while keeping the presentation on topic. Additionally, building in time for questions during or after the lecture can help the lecturer keep track of the topic and make the presentation within the given time limits.

Research on audience attention-span, as well as our personal experiences as educators suggests that lectures can reach a point of diminishing return for the speaker if they are too long. Generally, the lecturer should not speak to an audience on a complex topic for more than 45 minutes at a stretch if students are expected to retain material.[6] It is a good idea to break up long lectures with question and answer sessions, illustrations, exhibits, media, group exercises, or group discussions to keep your audience's attention.

An important technique for teachers (as well as for other speakers) is to seek feedback from students as well as to answer questions. In seeking feedback, the lecturer can find out if students are understanding the material, and if they think the lecturer is effective. Those of us who have taught, know how difficult it is to accept this feedback. However, if students are to learn we certainly need to ascertain the effectiveness of our teaching.

Lectures to one's colleagues follow much the same format as to students, however, they can be more technical. For special information on this topic Calnan and Barabas have designed a useful guide in their short book, *Speaking at Medical Meetings*; although this book is directed toward physicians, it is also useful for those in other health professions.[7]

Public communication often overlaps with group communication. In formal group situations the group leader, as well as selected group members, may find themselves in the position of addressing the group. These presentations to groups contain many of the same characteristics of speeches that have been discussed in this chapter. Chapter 6 will examine the topic of communication in groups, addressing the topics of health care teams, self-help and therapy groups, health education groups, and problem solving group discussion.

WRITTEN COMMUNICATION

Conveying Public Information

Both the oral and the written word are important to the health professional. As we have discussed, the setting, the audience, and the time are some of the factors that influence whether information should be shared on an oral or written basis. Speeches are usually more informal. Oral language must be understood immediately and it is more difficult to replicate information orally. The speaker has an opportunity to gain feedback, particularly in informal settings; it is much more difficult for the writer to achieve that dialogic component.

The reasons that writing is chosen over the speaking modality, however, are many. Sometimes writing is a reinforcement to speaking. For example, a physician might prescribe medication, giving the patient oral instructions, and then choose to replicate with the new written information sheets provided by the American Medical Association in its Patient Medication Instruction program. He or she might also choose to design their own information sheets. Writing is also important if the health professional wants to reach large numbers of people. Writing often reaches a larger audience because it is easier to disseminate written materials, and people can view these materials at their own leisure, in their own home environment. It is also considered academically and scientifically important that many health professionals "publish" at some time in their careers.[8] As we saw in the previous chapter, when discussing language, the written word is an important means of time-binding knowledge across generations. Writing is considered particularly credible for the researcher because the written document allows scrutiny by one's peers. Types of health or medically related writings are prescriptions, written patient instructions, technical-research papers, case reports, and patient records. The health professional might also choose to write poetry or publish both fiction and nonfictionalized accounts of health care.

One serious concern that faces the writer of information-sharing technical papers is the long period of time from the generation of a research idea to the date of publication of the results. Often painstaking research work becomes outdated before it is published. The prospective writer needs to be aware of the lengthy process of article submission, review, and actual publication. Publication sources should be chosen accordingly.

Anyone considering serious writing of any kind should be clear about their motives. Are they writing for professional advancement and/or recognition by their peers? Are they writing to share data with their colleagues that might assist patient care? Are they writing because they have a creative urge? Being clear on one's motives is important because it helps guide the direction of the written work.

The second important question is "What do you want to write?" After the first goal question is answered, the answer to this second question becomes clearer. For example, if you are writing for national recognition from colleagues, you might want to write a carefully structured and somewhat original article or letter to a national journal. Research might be presented in several ways: orally at a specific convention, and in written form to specific and more generalized audiences. Some professional associations have combined both goals by publishing oral presentations in written form in a proceedings format.

The third question, "What audience do you want to address in your writing?" ties into the other questions. By deciding what you want to write, you usually demarcate a possible audience. If you are a nurse practitioner wanting to share some carefully constructed case studies, you need to find the appropriate journal. If you are a pharmaceutical researcher, your audience will usually read pharmacy journals.

Content and Organization of Writing

In the early part of this chapter, we advocated the "Content-Organization-Delivery" method of speech organization. That method is equally applicable to writing. In this section we will apply that method to the writing of a research report. Case studies will also be mentioned.

The *title* is important as it indicates not only the subject material, but where the material will be filed in abstracts and indices. It is important that the title encapsulate the paper. Usually, the title is followed by an abstract which is a summary or overview of the entire research endeavor. The *abstract* gives the reader an opportunity to decide whether he or she wants to read the entire report and should be comprehensive and stimulating.

The *introduction* to the report gives justification for the research. It is this paragraph or paragraphs that are the most difficult to write. Rather than agonize over this first paragraph or sentence, we encourage the author to put anything down just to get started. In fact, this first paragraph can more easily be made consistent with the paper after the paper is complete. These first paragraphs should also incorporate the research goal, which, of course, should have been established before the research was started.

Failure to delineate the problem clearly in the introduction reflects on the research as well as the writer's ability to think clearly. However, once again, rather than agonize over the appropriate words at this stage of writing, a raw statement of the purpose can be temporarily put on paper so that the writer can move ahead to the body of the paper which is usually the easiest part of the paper to write. An example of a first paragraph follows:

The purpose of the study was to investigate correlations between human and animal infanticide. It was hypothesized that the instinctual drive that leads to baby-killing in animals may have a counterpart in humans which leads to child abuse and maltreatment.*

Related research is usually discussed at the beginning of the research report after the statement has been clearly presented. In this section of the report the author summarizes the relevant research of others and gives the citations of those research reports so that the reader can look them up if necessary. This is generally one of the easiest sections of the paper to write since it is simply a compilation of the data of others. It is important in this section of the report to summarize and quote accurately.

The *method and design* of the research is presented next. The writer needs to explain what method was used (experimental? historical? descriptive?) and how it was used. It is in this section of the report that a description of the subjects and the methods employed is pertinent. Ethical considerations and safeguards should also be noted.

In the *result* section of the report, the researcher sets forth the interpretations of the data. If the research utilized hypotheses, this is the time to state whether those hypotheses were rejected or accepted according to the data analysis.

The last part of the paper centers around a *discussion* of the research. A summary is included at this point and the resolution of the initial

* This was adapted from a news story on animal infanticide research. *Nevada State Journal*, October 26, 1982.

research problems is discussed. Conclusions are stated here as well as applicability to specific situations. Suggestions for future research based on the study can be discussed at this point. *Notes and references* follow the body of the paper. It is important that every quote be properly identified as well as all other material utilized directly from other sources.

Examples of research papers and technical reports which are medically oriented can be found by looking at major index sources (see Figure 3.2).

The Case Study Report

In recent years the case study report has often been deemphasized while laboratory studies have been more prominent in the medical journals.

Figure 3.2   Selected Health and Medicine Indexes

Abstracts of Health Care Management Studies: Includes articles on general health care. Abstracts are given.

Hospital Literature Index: This index offers material related to hospitals and health care in many types of facilities.

Index Medicus: This is probably the major index focusing on health related subjects. It includes subject and author sections. Journals indexed are found in the January issue. It does not abstract.

International Nursing Index: Has subject and author sections and each topic is indexed under at least three headings. Journals are in the January issue. The index also has publications of organizations and agencies as well as authors.

Medical Socioeconomic Resource Source: This is designed to integrate material from social science and the health care field. Economic and public health are two of the fields indexed. It does contain brief abstracts.

Newsbank: A newspaper clipping service not available in all libraries. Indexes articles from over 100 cities. Topics are included from socioeconomic, political, and scientific fields.

Hospital Literature Index: This index offers material related to hospitals and health care in many types of facilities.

Abstracts of Health Care Management Studies: Includes articles on general health care. Abstracts are given.

Medicine and health, however can often be better understood and health practice methods can be shared if the case study is utilized. It is also a good starting point for medical writers.[9] Case studies need to be presented carefully and be somewhat unusual so that the material will be useful to the reader. The writer of the case study report, in conjunction with any technical writer, needs to research his or her subject well to make sure that identical case presentations do not already exist in the literature, or that if they do exist, this new presentation brings new and thoughtful ideas. The writer also needs to find a suitable journal which encourages case studies. In other words, the writer needs to find the right audience. Once again, Figure 3.2 needs to be consulted for major health and medically related index sources. These sources list the major publications of the many health fields in addition to providing information on research reports in these journals. Another important advantage of the case study report is that it gives private practitioners a conduit to their academic colleagues. Harlen emphasizes the fact that private practioners are not part of the "in-group" that writes articles for medical journals although they have much to offer the practice of medicine. He suggests that writing cases is one way to improve communication between academicians and practitioners.[10] His ideas on this would apply to any health care field.

Delivery or Presentation of Written Communication

Though the term delivery is usually associated with public speaking, we argue that it needs to be considered as equally important to the written communication. The delivery or presentational aspects of the material often determine whether the document will be read or not. A paper, a book, or even an instruction sheet to a patient needs to be neat and pleasing to the eye. The typing or printing of the document should be done carefully with no errors. Headings should draw the reader's attention. Pages should be carefully numbered.

Additionally, the document should not be too lengthy. Unless it is full of highly important technical data which a specialized audience will read, major points and summaries should be stressed with citations included for anyone who wants to do further research. Put yourself in the place of one of your hoped for readers and ask if you would read the document you have prepared. This question, more than any other, will assist you in preparing your manuscript or document for delivery to a publisher or audience.

Turning Speeches into Written Papers

There is a desire common to many writers to turn oral presentations into written papers which can be submitted for publication. Unfortunately, this is not as easy as it sounds. Words that sound well during a speech, are often too informal to be committed to paper. While speech-making requires some color and warmth, technical papers require more formal and remote presentations. Points made in writing are longer and more complex. While the same formula can be used for either speeches or writing (content, organization, and delivery) the ways words are presented in the different speaking or writing contexts must be evaluated differently by the speaker-writer. Often reworking the speech with these considerations in mind can solve the problem. Sometimes, however, a new outline needs to be originated with more attention to examples suitable for writing as well as charts and visual aids more appropriate for a paper than a speech.

Instruction Sheets

The relatively recent finding that it is important to repeat information to patients is beginning to penetrate medicine and health care. The physician, or nurse, or other health educator is often called upon to take highly technical information and reduce it orally and in writing so that the patient can understand and follow a regime. The challenge becomes particularly acute in instruction sheets where the information needs to be condensed to one or two pages. Nowhere is content, organization, and delivery such a challenge. Avoiding "Medspeak" (the jargon health professionals, particularly physicians, use to share information) and asking clients to edit the material before it is printed are two important tips. In a study on communication with patients, it was found that 81 percent of the physicians underestimated their patient's capabilities of understanding explanations. The study found that patients actually were able to understand most problems if they were discussed in ordinary language.[11]

In writing instruction sheets, points can be underlined and enumerated (1, 2, 3, 4, etc.) to indicate their importance. Headings are also important on short documents.

Letters

Health practitioners who have little time but much to say are often found writing letters to editors. *The New England Journal of Medicine* is noted for the dialogue that takes place through letters on major health issues. The letter writing sections of journals provide a democratic forum for an exchange of ideas among colleagues as well as members of other professions.

Such communications should be written on standard business paper and should follow business form. They should follow some logic, be brief, and be to the point. Even if disagreement is being expressed, the letter is usually more effective if it relies on facts and logic rather than a passionate subjective opinion. Letters sometimes need to be written to colleagues and patients. Neatness, clarity, and a direct approach to the subject are the cornerstones of an effective business letter. The presentation and delivery are also of importance. Impressive printed stationary and no typographical errors are examples of the latter.

Seeking Reaction from Others

One of the most important steps in writing of any kind is to have your work reviewed and edited informally before it is submitted to official reviewers. This is not an easy thing to accomplish. Friends and family members are sometimes too complimentary or too critical. The person or persons who are seeking to informally review your work should be persons who have some knowledge of your subject, ideally, who will in some way represent the audience you are seeking through your writing. Present the copy of your material to them widely spaced and with plenty of room for margin writing. Ask them to change mispellings, to mark awkward sentences and to comment on the readability and accuracy of your writing. Be sure and indicate the time they have to do the criticism. Most importantly, put yourself in a state of mind where you will look forward to the criticism knowing that it will make a better final product. Don't be defensive with your informal review. Take all criticism given but decide for yourself what changes need to be made in your writing. At this point, put yourself in the place of your audience.

Some Last Comments

In this chapter, we have been more prescriptive than in many other parts of this book. Public presentations (both oral and written) lend themselves to the prescriptive format because of the lack of interaction that takes place. Nevertheless, the individual writer or speaker needs to put his or her own stamp of individuality on a presentation. Planning presentations through use of the COD method (content, organization, and delivery) will enable the speaker or writer to spend extra time in adding the small touches that will make the presentation unique. A joke or a thoughtful personal comment can be important in the oral presentation just as a thoughtful introduction can be important in a written document.

NOTES

1. This case history is based upon the activities of the Indiana Pharmacists' Association, 1981, and specifically upon the work of their director of education, Ernest Boyd, P.D.

2. Haakenson, 1977, Section N.

3. Ibid. p. 208.

4. Bandler and Grinder, 1975, Section A.

5. DiMatteo and Freidman, 1982, Section A.

6. Harlem, 1977, p. 70, Section A.

7. Calnan and Barabas, 1972, Section B.

8. Harlem, 1977, p. 73 Section A.

9. Ibid, p. 81.

10. Ibid, p. 80.

11. DiMatteo and Friedman, 1982, p. 89, Section A.

PREVIEW OF READING

In the article, "Doctors Down the Logorrhea," by Chriss, the overuses of medical jargon are examined in light of the work of the DeBakey sisters in combating the use of stilted medical language. Chriss stresses how important it is that physicians speak clearly and he generally describes the educational programs devised by the DeBakey sisters to teach effective language use in medical practice. Moreover, the article identifies some of the reasons why "medicalese" develops in the first place. Although Chriss is addressing the problem of medical jargon in the physician-patient relationship, the same considerations apply to speaking and writing which is why we have included the article in this chapter.

DOCTORS DOWN THE LOGORRHEA—
DeBakey Sisters Cure 'Medicalese'

Nicholas C. Chriss

Most people have heard of Dr. Michael E. DeBakey, the famous Houston surgeon who mends and replaces hearts. Not nearly so many have heard of Lois and Selma DeBakey, his sisters.

But inside the often anonymous world of medicine, the De Bakey sisters are almost as well known as their brother. Just as he has fought heart disease, they have spent their careers fighting a disorder that afflicts many medical doctors—logorrhea.

That is not a venereal disease. Logorrhea means excessive and stilted wordiness. If there is anything that Lois and Selma DeBakey dislike, it is the pompous, confusing, vague, monotonous and ambiguous medicalese that so often turns up in learned journals of medicine and in the conversations of physicians.

They combat it by giving seminars and symposiums around the country and abroad to doctors who would like to become more articulate.

Several decades ago the sisters made a startling discovery. Medical doctors, among the brightest and most highly educated of people, have difficulty speaking and writing simple, clear English. At the urging of their famous brother, they explained in an interview, they began to do something about it.

The sisters are professors of scientific communication at the Baylor College of Medicine here. They also are responsible for introducing a course on scientific communication at the medical school of Tulane University, and at the Ochsner Medical Foundation in New Orleans. In addition, their work has given many schools thoughts about instituting some humanities courses in medical school.

"By dissecting published scientific articles in class, and stripping them of their jargon, cliches, vogue words, pretentious diction, verbiage and imposing-looking statistics, our students have learned to expose the claptrap, bombast, empty thesis, flimsy or illogical argument and invalid conclusions," Lois DeBakey said.

The "cant and circumlocution" of medicalese is almost an obligatory acquisition during a doctor's medical school days, she added.

Early in medical school, Selma DeBakey said, students discover that scientific lingo is useful. "It helps the physician seem wise when he may be uninformed about a certain subject.

"The medical student becomes so accustomed to the medicalese that he recognizes no flaws in it; he may even consider it the exclusive property of the initiated who need communicate to no one else," she went on.

The sisters said that for years a medical student's reading is limited to medical publications that are "marred by vagueness, repetition, monotomy, ambiguity, confusion and actual misstatement."

The sisters also said that in medical schools, as in many other schools of higher education, true-false tests have replaced written essays and that poor English is often a problem for modern doctors.

An otherwise brilliant surgeon might state in a report that "the patient's pelvis was fractured by being thrown from an automobile," they said.

"The DeBakey sisters are the greatest thing that's come along in medicine for ages," said Dr. Irvine Page, a Cleveland physician, medical educator and editor of Modern Medicine.

Lois DeBakey said one indication that medical science has become ineffective in communicating health information is that patients increasingly turn to popular newspaper columnists for answers to medical and sex problems. "Sadly, columnists' answers are not always correct," she said.

Columnist Ann Landers recently admitted in a talk to physicians: "I feel as if I'm practicing medicine without a license."

Like many other lovelorn columnists, her mail is heavy with medical concerns. In a 1974 column she wrote: "Dear Doctor: Ann Landers has a problem. She receives almost 1,000 letters a day and in every mailbag, there are at least 100 letters that should have been sent to you."

The DeBakey sisters pull no punches in their talks to the medical men, telling them that doctors are getting further and further from the public by using scientific doublespeak. They say flatly that too many medical journals are filled with "claptrap."

A doctor may be a wizard in the operating room or the research laboratory, but completely inarticulate in describing the advances that have been made in medical science, they say.

Dr. Frank Ingelfinger, longtime editor of the New England Medical Journal, points out also that being able to communicate with the public and its lawmakers is becoming more important because laypersons are becoming more and more involved in medical decisions concerning such questions as abortion, smoking, the use of behavior-modifying drugs, research involving splitting genes, and similar fields.

In their seminars, Lois and Selma DeBakey also suggest something that medical doctors often agree with privately: "Physicians sometimes misuse language as a protective shield against the fears of anxiety they experience while attending their patients."

It is difficult for many of them, the sisters said, to talk realistically about terminal illnesses, sex problems, emotional sicknesses and so on.

For the doctor, Selma DeBakey said, "the cost of being misunderstood, especially by his patients, is exorbitant. More than a few patients express the need for an interpreter to translate the language of the physicians and some even switch physicians on this account.

"The resident psychiatrist who labels his patient as a narcissistic personality may be expressing his own feelings of inadequacy in the presence of the patient."

The sisters say their seminars and criticism of medicalese are well received by doctors. They are just as tough on medical advertisements that they believe mislead consumers.

"By mimicking the pseudo-scientific phraseology of medical journals, advertisers can seduce the public into drawing a propitious conclusion that the manufacturer would not dare state," the sisters said.

It is the sisters' attacks on medical doublespeak, however, that have attracted the most attention.

The medicalese that physicians use, the sisters say, can often result in a dehumanizing treatment of humans who become cases rather than patients.

"Many doctors end up concentrating on the organ, rather than the patient," said Ingelfinger of the New England Medical Journal.

Michael Crichton, the well known author and medical doctor, wrote not long ago in the same journal that "an eminent surgeon strides purposefully into the operating room each day—but to read his papers, you wonder how he finds the courage to get out of bed in the morning. His writing indicates he is unsure of everything, and has no particular convictions on any subject at all."

Crichton said it is traditional for physicians to conceal their knowledge from patients through the judicious use of language. He quoted the 13th-century surgeon Arnold of Villanova: "You may not find anything about the case. Then say he has an obstruction of the liver, and particularly use the word, obstruction, because they do not understand what it means, and it helps greatly that a term is not understood by the people."

The days when such distinguished scientists and physicians as Da Vinci, Galileo and Pasteur wrote simply, elegantly and accurately are gone, but Lois and Selma DeBakey would like to lead medical science back into the atmosphere of that time by helping physicians become articulate.

So, they often pass on to their students the words of the famed 18th-century writer and lexicographer, Dr. Samuel Johnson: "Read over your composition, and whenever you meet with a passage which you think particularly fine, strike it out."

4.

MEDIATED COMMUNICATION IN HEALTH CARE

St. Francis Hospital of Indianapolis was encountering an unexpected problem. A rather large number of patients at the hospital whose physicians had recommended a gastroscopy for them refused to sign the informed consent statement and would not undergo the procedure. Gastroscopies are a fairly routine procedure which involves the use of a gastroscope instrument to inspect the interior of the stomach. The gastroscope, which is a tube-like instrument with something similar to a light on its end, is inserted through the client's mouth, down the esophagus, and into the stomach. The procedure is invaluable in examining ulcers, discovering tumors of the stomach, and generally discovering stomach disease. Although the procedure sounds rather involved and uncomfortable, it is relatively simple and causes most clients very little discomfort. Lack of adequate information from the physician about what the client could expect before, during, and after the procedure was thought to be the problem. After reviewing the situation, including interviews with hospital staff and clients, it was decided that there should be a gastroscopy educational program developed. The hospital media department produced an informative videotape designed to describe the gastroscopy procedure and its uses. The videotape program included interviews with physicians, nurses, and those who were just recovering from the procedure. The videotape program was shown to each hospital client recommended for a gastroscopy. Client response to the media program was extremely positive. The informed consent turn-down rate was reduced by 35 percent for those who watched the brief videotape presentation.

MEDIA

A large percentage of health communication in the modern health care system involves the use of *media*. McLuhan describes media as the "extensions of man."[1] The use of media extends people's ability to communicate, to speak to others far away, hear messages and see images that would be unavailable to their perception without media. As extensions to human communication, media allow health care professionals to reach more people with health related messages in less time than through nonmediated communication channels. Media enable people who are geographically removed from health care organizations and personnel to access health care information without traveling long distances. Media have been used as a powerful educational tool, serving a wide range of audiences, such as students of the health sciences, practicing health care professionals, and health care consumers. The case history at the beginning of the chapter describes a real situation where videotape was used as an in-house tool in an urban hospital for providing health care consumers with relevant information. Media provide powerful tools for storing and transmitting important health care information. Modern health care services depend upon the use of media as communication tools, and these uses and applications of mediated communication in the delivery of health care will continue to expand in the future.

Media are tools that people use to communicate. A definition of media follows: *media are an intermediary communication delivery system using some form of technology*. By an intermediary system we mean media are used as a specialized channel of communication between communicators. Different kinds of media technologies have been developed to link communicators. These include print, audio, video, and computer technologies. Some of these media are designed to appeal to the general public. The public channels of mediated communication are known as *mass media*. Other forms of media are designed for use with selected groups of people, usually within the boundaries of organizations. These private channels of mediated communication are generally known as *in-house media*. In this chapter we will explore a wide range of applications and implications of mass media and in-house media on the delivery of health care.

In discussing mediated communication, we will distinguish among three broad types of media, each possessing various different specialized media tools. The three broad types of media are: *print media, audiovisual media*, and *interactive media*. Print media and audiovisual media are commonly used as both in-house and mass media channels of communication, while interactive media have primarily been used as in-house media tools. The use of interactive media with the public may change dramatically in the future because of the current development of the technological tools needed to present interactive media systems to mass communication audiences.

PRINT MEDIA

Print media are the oldest and most traditional of the three types of mediated communication. Print media rely on the use of the written word, incorporating photography and sophisticated graphics as well. Print media are broadly used both in-house (as employee newsletters, annual reports, letters, booklets, bulletin boards, posters, payroll inserts, handbooks, company magazines, and exhibits), and also as a mass communication channel (in the form of books, newspapers, magazines, and billboards). Print media have great potential for use as health communication tools in educating consumers about health care maintenance and different health care services available to them.

The broadest application and distribution of print media in the modern world is the newspaper. Most of us are exposed to the newspaper every day. Newspapers have a strong impact on the public's beliefs, attitudes, and behaviors. Cohen (1963) contends that the press has a powerful impact on setting audience agenda, and the newspaper, specifically, is an extremely powerful tool for influencing what its readers think about.[2] This claim about the power of the press to direct public agenda setting has been confirmed with research on political campaigns, but, unfortunately, has not been found to be as influential in setting agendas for the public in health related campaigns.[3] Part of the reason for the impotence of the press in influencing public attitudes about health issues might be the fact that health issues are not written about in newspapers as often as other news issues.[4] Additionally, more than half of most newspapers' content do not cover public issues, but are devoted to advertising.[5]

Although the press by itself has not been found to be an extremely powerful tool in persuading public attitudes about health care issues, it has been found to be an important source of information for people already interested in a specific health issue. Wright (1975) found in a study of the comparative use of newspapers, radio, magazines and television as sources of health information that newspapers and magazines were used most frequently by survey respondents and they found these printed media most useful as sources of information.[6] The press has great potential as a vehicle for presenting health related information to the public, and as such has the responsibility of providing accurate health care information.

All too often we've heard hospital representatives complain that "The only time the hospital is mentioned in the newspaper is when there is some problem or scandal brewing." If this is so, it is because the media often have little or no knowledge of the commendable activities occuring at the hospital. The press is eager to report positive newsworthy information, but they must have access to such information in order to present it to the public. The common phenomenon of an adversarial relationship developing between health care organizations and the press points out the importance of establishing cooperative relationships between health care organizations and the media. Hospitals and other health care organizations must be active in their relationships with the public media. Hospital administrators cannot just wait for the local newspaper to report the positive contributions of their institutions, but must have their public relations staffs provide the media with accurate and interesting information about their organization in the form of press releases and public service announcements. Once a good working relationship is established between health care institutions and the public media, there is far less chance for unfair media coverage to occur.

Books are another important and pervasive form of print media providing health information to health care providers and to the public. Text books, professional books, and self-help books are among the different types of publications that provide health information. This book, for example, is both a professional book designed for practicing health providers and a text book designed to instruct students about communication in health care practice. Health professionals depend upon books as ". . . repositories of medical wisdom and experience."[7] Books also provide important information to the public about how to maintain personal health and innovative methods of treatment available. Professional journals are another important source of information for health care practitioners and consumers, informing them of the results of recent health related research. Yet the rapid expansion of health related information has produced a nightmarish situation where there are more books and journals containing pertinent health science information than any individual could possibly read, let alone understand and incorporate in their lives. Harlem (1977), an M.D., reports about the situation facing doctors trying to keep up with relevant health science readings: "We are drowned in a flood of medical and scientific publications, journals, conference proceedings, textbooks, and handbooks ad infinitum. What can we do about it?"[8]

Additional forms of print media have been developed to help health care practitioners cope with the information overload of health literature. Abstracts of pertinent literature can provide interested individuals with information more quickly than the original texts, giving these individuals an opportunity to pick and choose the literature they want to read in full. Many professional journals and other publications are now encouraging the submission of review articles, summarizing and critiquing areas of research and designed to help consumers of health care information quickly examine vast amounts of literature in a short amount of time. For example, the International Communication Association, in its annual publication, *Communication Yearbook,* provides a publication format with a review article summarizing and evaluating previous research in the area of health communication and identifying important developments within the health communication field, as well as providing a similar review article format in other areas of communication research. Indexes also provide a useful means of coping with health science information overload. Later in this chapter we will discuss the use of computerized data bases to help people cope with the ever expanding volume of health science information.

Print media do not only affect the public, but are also used as important forms of in-house media in health care organizations. House organs, or newsletters, can provide useful information for members of health care organizations. Self-help groups, such as "Weight Watchers" or "Make Today Count" (a peer support group for terminally ill individuals and their families) often use newsletters to announce meetings, topics of interest to members, and news about the group's membership. The newsletter can serve as a means of sharing relevant information among members, encouraging involvement in the organization, and motivating a sense of identification and involvement among members of the organization. Newsletters are also powerful and pervasive communication tools in hospitals. Kreps (1982), in a research and development study of nurse retention at Wishard Memorial Hospital of Indianapolis, directed the introduction of a nursing newsletter. The newsletter entitled "Dialogue," served as a means of keeping nursing staff informed about changes and developments at the hospital, ideas and progress of the newly instituted nurse retention program at the hospital, and personal information about members of the nursing staff.[9] Additionally, members of the nursing staff were encouraged to air their gripes and frustrations to the hospital administration via the newsletter. In this manner this nursing newsletter was used to facilitate upward, downward and horizontal channels of communication within the organization. Newsletters are potentially useful forms of organizational communication.

Another important form of in-house print media is bulletin boards. Bulletin boards are often taken for granted in many organizations, but can be a very useful means of communication. "They have the advantage of being relatively inexpensive and easy to maintain and have an immediacy that attracts attention. They do not have the problems of credibility often associated with other methods of controlled communication; employees and others tend to regard them as straightforward public notices of vital events."[10] In hospitals, bulletin boards can be used to announce and publicize in-service educational programs of interest to staff members, patient education programs of interest to clients, and job openings that hospital employees might be interested in applying for. In addition, bulletin boards can be useful media for honoring members of the organization who have achieved special accomplishments, or have offered outstanding service to the organization. Such employee recognition programs can be useful to the organization as a means of motivating employee involvement.

Other forms of print media that are of use in health care organizations include pamphlets, posters, handbooks, and letters. Pamphlets and posters are often used in patient education. Pamphlets are useful tools for explaining health care regimens and helping to ease clients' apprehensions about health problems by providing them with answers to commonly asked questions. In many hospitals pamphlets are used to explain serious illnesses to clients and their families. For example, people recovering from heart attacks, strokes, or other health problems are often given pamphlets explaining the causes, implications, and approaches for rectifying these health risk situations. Posters are useful for graphically presenting information about specific procedures and exercises prescribed for clients. Posters are also used to promote health campaigns, such as exercise for health, good nutrition, and giving up cigarette smoking. Exhibits often serve the same functions as posters in graphically representing information in organizations.

Letters are a pervasive aspect of all business and professional communication systems and are an important form of communication in health care organizations. They enable communication between individuals across distances, in a generally inexpensive and permanent, although sometimes time-consuming, manner. Letters to a hospital's public (consumers of health care services, providers of human and material resources, government agencies, etc.) are important public relations tools for health care institutions. If the written document is professional and personal it will create a positive image for the organization, but if it is written insensitively or carelessly it can damage the institution's image. In the previous chapter on writing in health care we presented specific guidelines for effective writing. Later in this chapter, we will examine the use of letters as a form of interactive media, as well as the use of the telephone in health care organizations as a useful adjunct to letters and other print media.

AUDIOVISUAL MEDIA

The second general type of mediated communication to be discussed in this chapter is audiovisual communication. Audiovisuals are one of the fastest growing areas of media, with many different forms of audiovisual communication now available. Audiovisual media involve mechanized technology which present sounds and sights to audiences in such forms as overhead transparencies, slide presentations, filmstrips, movies, recordings, videotapes, commercial radio and television programming, and closed circuit television (which we will also discuss later in this chapter as a form of interactive media). Audiovisual communication tools are widely used as both mass media and in-house media.

Perhaps the most widespread and pervasive tools of audiovisual communication are the mass media channels of television, radio, and film. These media are important molders of public image, but they do not always present an accurate image of the health care system. McLaughlin, in a study about the portrayal of medicine on televised doctor shows, demonstrates that these shows do not accurately represent the realities of health care practice and tend to idealize the role of the doctor; he reports, "The role of the medical doctor on television is therefore that of a powerful, almost omnipotent healer who performs his duties above and beyond normally expected capacities."[11] This televised portrayal of medical doctors can foster the development of unrealistic stereotypes about medical practice on the part of the public, who, based upon the information gleaned from television shows, may expect a doctor to solve all problems, physical or emotional, with a wave of his or her arm. After all, Hawkeye on "Mash" or Marcus Welby can solve all the problems their clients face! Doctors also might develop stereotypes about their health care abilities and the reactions their clients will have towards them, based upon the media portrayal of the health care system. What's more, this inaccurate portrayal of health care practice undoubtedly adds impetus to the health communication problem of unrealistic expectations about health care held by both practitioners and consumers that we talked about in the first chapter of this book.

Although early popular films of the 1930s and 1940s, such as "Young Doctor Kildare" (starring Lou Ayres and Lionel Barrymore, 1938) portrayed health care personnel and the health care system in an extremely positive manner, recent films unlike commercial television have often not presented stereotypically idealistic portrayals of health care practice. In fact, several films such as "Hospital" (1970, starring George C. Scott) and "Whose Life Is It Anyway?" (1981, starring Richard Dreyfuss) show the seamier side of the health care system, portraying health professionals in an extremely unfavorable light. In "Hospital" several hospital clients are killed by the negligence of the health care staff. In the film, a man entering a large, prestigious hospital, for minor treatment is mistakenly taken into surgery and dies as a result of an operation meant for another client. In "Whose Life Is It Anyway?" a young man who suddenly becomes a quadrapalegic due to a car accident, has to take the hospital to court to gain legal control over his own life. The movie "Hospital" portrays health professionals as being inept, while "Whose Life Is It Anyway?" portrays health professionals as being overly paternalistic and insensitive. Both of these films have exaggerated the negative aspects of the health care system, in much the same way many prime-time television shows have exaggerated the positive aspects. Neither portrayal of the health care system helps to develop a realistic, positive image for health care personnel and delivery systems.

Perhaps the most effective mass media presentation of health care can be seen in the growth and development of health educational programming in commercial television in recent years. Many nationally and locally televised news programs have introduced "health reporters" to their news staffs to present health issues and health education segments on their daily and nightly news telecasts. Often these reports outline new medical, dental, pharmacological, etc., discoveries and treatments and describe different types of health care services available to the public. Several nationally televised "news magazine" format shows in the United States, such as "60 Minutes," "20–20," and "Hour Magazine," generally present health-related entertainment and education features. Discussion oriented shows, such as "Donahue," regularly examine the pros and cons of various topical health issues, and provide communication time for proponents of different perspectives on these issues. Physical fitness shows, which have a long history in commercial television, are reemerging as of late, such as the "Richard Simmons Show," with strong emphasis on presenting the public with methods of preventive health care, and the development of positive health habits in such areas as exercise and nutrition. Several radio programs also focus on health-related issues.

The growing emphasis on health issues in audiovisual mass media has promising potential to become a powerful public medium for health education. Public health information and behavior change campaigns utilizing any one audiovisual communication medium have generally not been highly effective in changing public attitudes and reducing health risks.[12] Presentation of health campaign information through multiple media channels, however, has had some success in influencing the public's health behaviors. This is especially true when the media used in the campaign have been coupled with a detailed strategy to meet the characteristics of the target audience, guided by applied theories of mass communication, education, and audience motivation.[13] Future strategic uses of mass communication media can have great impact on public health behaviors.

Audiovisual media are also commonly used in health care institutions as important organizational communication tools. "The most common audiovisual media are videotape, film, and sound/slide."[14] Additional audiovisual communication tools used in health care organizations include audio cassettes (with many hospitals developing cassette libraries for their staff's in-house education), filmstrips, and multimedia productions. These in-house media are used for staff education, patient education, internal organizational communication, reports between shifts, documents of health care procedures (often for legal purposes), hospital initiated persuasive health campaigns, and hospital public relations projects.

Videotape is a powerful audiovisual communication medium that has found extensive use in health care organizations. Many hospitals use small-format videotape systems for ". . . recording first shift instructions for playback to the second and third shift . . . to document medical and surgical procedures," and to provide programs for ". . . patient information and education," as well as for developing materials for ". . . staff development."[15] In the case history at the beginning of this chapter the hospital described had its own in-house media production department that developed health education programs.[16]

Videotape has also been successfully used as an in-house educational tool for instructing health providers about interviewing and other health communication skills in health care organizations and educational institutions. Cassata and Clements describe a physician education program they developed and conducted using videotape as a feedback mechanism in teaching interviewing skills.[17] They report that the impact of videotape technology for providing students with direct feedback about their communication skills in medical interview situations is dramatic and suggest future applications of videotape technology in medical education.

Films are also used as in-house media in many health care organizations. Rarely do these organizations produce their own films, as they often do with videotape programs, but rent or buy films that have been produced by private companies. There are many films produced each year on health related topics that are used in both staff education and consumer education programs. Film provides an entertaining medium for presenting complex topics to many different health care audiences.

Slide/sound shows have developed in recent years as an increasingly popular form of audiovisual media in health care organizations. Although these programs do not lend themselves to visual movement and action in the way film and videotape media do, the expanded use of multi-image, stereo slide/sound programs has enhanced the attractiveness of this medium as an exciting and entertaining communication tool. Many of the topics presented with film and videotape programs can be presented through slide/sound media at significantly reduced production expense. Moreover, slide/sound media lend themselves to easy updating and re-editing, while film and videotape programs are difficult and costly to change once they are produced. Slide/sound shows have been used similarly to film and videotape media to present staff and consumer education programs, persuasive health campaign programs, and public relations programs. Kreps and his associates are presently developing a multi-image slide/sound program promoting positive health habits for school children, to be introduced into the Indianapolis Public School System elementary school health curricula.[18] This audiovisual media program will be used to foster the school children's development of increased self-esteem, personal responsibility, and the ability to make high quality health decisions.

Many hospitals have their own media development and production departments who work with house staff to produce audiovisual media for in-house use. Additionally, these departments often administer media libraries where clients and staff can view different health related media presentations. The use of audiovisual media in health care organizations has grown to become an important form of health communication, and will continue to grow as its uses expand in the future.

INTERACTIVE MEDIA

One of the most interesting and exciting applications of media in health care is the use of interactive media. Interactive media range from somewhat limited communication tools such as the telephone (although telephone technologies have expanded the medium's uses in recent years) to new and innovative computerized education and diagnostic media. Interactive media are communication tools that allow people to send and receive information through the use of technology. There are *reflective* interactive media tools that recreate the messages media users send (as in traditional uses of the telephone, mail, and closed circuit television), and there are *intelligent* interactive media tools that can interpret user initiated information and respond with appropriate internally generated information.

Interactive technologies are commonly used as in-house media, but rarely as mass communication tools. (Recall that mass media present information to the general public, while in-house media present information to selected, although sometimes large, audiences). Reflective communication media have been used in health care organizations with technical tools such as closed circuit television, two-way radios, and the omnipresent telephone. Intelligent media have been primarily used in health care organizations through the use of computer technology.

The telephone is a powerful communication tool that allows people all over the world the potential to interact with one another. Although the audience for the telephone is very large, it is considered to be an in-house and not a mass media tool, because information communicated over the phone is directed specifically at selected individuals and not to the general public. Even the use of conference calls is an in-house technology because, once again, the communication is limited to a specific group of individuals who have been selected as recipients of the interaction and not to the public.

As an in-house medium for communication, the telephone provides many benefits for business and professional organizations. Goodman (1982) presents the telephone as an ideal time-management medium.[19] His argument is that the telephone provides people with a vehicle for communicating over long distances without spending all of the time and money that might be necessary in traveling to interact face-to-face with someone. The benefits of using the telephone are not only its cost-effectiveness, but also the speed of reaching people. The pervasiveness of telephone use in the modern world makes the phone an important communication technology.

Technical advancements in telephone design have provided users with the ability to conference with several individuals simultaneously over the telephone. Automatic answering, call-back and call-out systems make the telephone more convenient to use and more effective as a communication mechanism. Additionally, the telephone is an effective communication tool when used together with other media, such as print. Initial contact with individuals might be made with print, and the telephone can be used to follow up the communication, as in follow-up calls from a dentist's office to remind a client of an appointment scheduled during the last visit, and following up a written reminder. The telephone can also be used to establish contact with individuals, with written media being used as follow-up. For example, health organizations' solicitations of donations often use this communication strategy. The telephone is a more personal initial contact for solicitations, while the letter can be used to obtain specific data and funds. Later in this chapter we will discuss the use of the telephone as an adjunct to interactive computers.

Some of the difficulties inherent in the use of the telephone as a mediated form of communication involve the limitations of the technical channel to hold information, and the tendency toward distortion and loss of information between communicators over the telephone. These two problems are closely tied to one another. The obvious limitation of the telephone as a channel of information, as compared to face-to-face interpersonal communication, is the loss of visual, tactile, olfactory, kinesic, proxemic, and artifactic information. The standard telephone used by the public is generally limited to providing users with verbal, paralinguistic, and chronemic information. As we discussed in Chapter 2, people use the various different channels of verbal and nonverbal communication messages to confirm and clarify the overall message being sent. They examine the range of messages available them and decipher the content of the communication situation through a process of comparison and contrast. In Chapter 2 we suggested that effective communicators are aware of the range of different messages they send, and strive to be perceptive of the various verbal and nonverbal messages others send to them. The telephone limits the range of messages communicators have available to send and receive. This constraint on the number of messages available to communicators increases the opportunities for message distortion in telephone communication situations.

The implications of these limitations on telephone communication serve to introduce several potentially troublesome situations for health communicators. One significant problem posed is the probability of sending and receiving misconstrued messages. The effectiveness of communication in health care often depends on the accuracy of message reception. For example, if a physician misconstrues a lab technician's telephoned report of the results of a lab test by just one decimal point, the resulting incorrect diagnosis or treatment plan enacted can have dangerous repercussions for the client. A second, related, potential problem in telephone communication is the use of the medium for purposeful deception. It is more difficult to detect deception over the telephone than in face-to-face communication, due to the limited range of messages the receiver has to interpret. For example, a caller may disguise his or her voice over the phone, without any fear of being recognized by a visual cue. To improve the accuracy of communication over the telephone and limit the occurrence of unintentionally misconstrued or purposefully deceptive messages, communicators must pay close attention to the verbal, paralinguistic, and chronemic messages available to them. Moreover, telephone communicators should utilize feedback to clarify messages sent and received. (See Chapter 2 for a discussion of how best to use feedback.) The introduction of telephones with the technical capability of transmitting both audio and video signals (the picture-phone) will increase the message sending capacity of the telephone, although it still will not approach the message capacity of face-to-face communication.

Closed circuit television is another interactive communication medium used in health care that is similar to the telephone, yet has the potential for providing users with more message information than the conventional telephone. Interactive television can provide users with both visual and audio message information. This can be essential in health care situations where a health care provider may have to see as well as hear a description of the consumer to effectively diagnose and treat an ailment. Park and Bashshur (1975) have described the use of two-way closed circuit television as "telemedicine," explaining its use as a communication tool for ". . . remote diagnosis, consultation, counseling, psychotherapy, and teaching."[20] They identify several interactive media programs that are being used to provide health care information and services to people via two-way television technology. The consequences of telemedicine for health care providers and health care practice suggest that health care services formerly unavailable to individuals in remote locations can now be offered via specialized media. Satellites have been developed to provide health communication information via two-way radio and television to remote geographic areas, affording people living in rural areas like "bush" Alaska with the benefits of modern health care information and services.[21]

Computer technology can be used with telephones and closed circuit television media to provide health care organizations with exciting interactive communication capabilities. Computers are powerful cybernetic communication tools that can process information and respond to different user requests. The computer is an intelligent interactive communication technology. When used as an adjunct to the telephone or the closed circuit television system, the computer can be used to rapidly evaluate and analyze incoming off-site information, search distant information banks for solutions to problems, and direct user behavior in accordance with precedents established in external health care facilities. The computer can be used to evaluate the likelihood of success of a given health maintenance procedure, analyze the data produced from many complicated lab tests, or search for related research and evidence upon which to base a health care decision, all in a highly time-efficient and cost-efficient manner.

A major problem encountered in computer use is the impersonality of many computers and computer programs. The computer is unable to interact on a "human" analogic level, is unable to understand emotions such as fear, anger, frustration, love, and so on, and is seen as being a cold, unfeeling machine by many users. Moreover, most of the programs designed for computers make the computer a very unforgiving communication tool. With these programs a user has to be able to send an absolutely correct entry message to the computer, using the computer's language or code, or the computer will not provide the user with the information or services requested. Minor message inadequacies, like a misplaced punctuation mark, or a lower case letter where a capital letter was needed, would be enough to jam up communication between the user and the computer.

Modern programmers have done their best to rectify the impersonality and rigidity of the computer by designing convivial programs for computer users. Convivial programs often use nontechnical computer languages modeled after human languages, and have personalized error messages that playfully identify any syntax problems a user may have presented to the computer. Older nonconvivial computer programs would merely reply to an incorrect user entry with a flashing "ERROR" statement, while newer convivial programs cue the computers to reply in a more friendly manner with a response such as, "Sorry, I think you made a mistake. Here is how to enter your request so I can read it. Thanks a lot!" Additionally, several computer games have been designed that are fun for users to play, and make the modern computer a much more enjoyable communication tool than older non-convivial computers. As computer programmers continue to develop convivial computer systems, and users become more sophisticated about computer methods and applications, the computer will continue to grow as an important form of interactive media in health care.

Computers have been used widely as a form of in-house interactive media. They are used to process both words and numbers for users. Computers have been found to be a handy and efficient means of storing data for future retrieval. Health care organizations depend on computers to store and process their financial data, medical records, personnel information, and inventory of supplies and equipment. Computer users communicate with the computer, using an accepted computer language or code, to access the information the computer has stored. New technologies have enabled computers to share information. That is, given the right access codes, one computer can obtain information stored in another computer, usually through a telephone interface. An organization with a computer and a telephone interface mechanism can access a wide range of information and information processing services.

There are many applications for computerized information storage and retrieval systems to help health care practitioners and consumers cope with the rapid expansion in health science literature and information that we discussed earlier in this chapter. There are several different computerized health information systems that have been developed to help users keep informed about relevant health care information. For example, "Medline is an on-line computer-based system to retrieve references to articles in biomedical journals Toxline . . . is an information retrieval system for health professionals and scientists working in the areas of environmental pollution, occupational health and safety, poison control, pharmacology/toxicology, medicine, and related disciplines," and Avline is a computer-based retrieval system designed to help people recover stored information about health care related audiovisual materials.[22]

Interactive computer systems are also useful in health care as diagnostic and educational tools. Computer programs have been designed that allow computers to interview health care clients about their general medical histories.[23] Similar programs have been designed allowing computers to take psychiatric histories.[24] Computers can provide diabetic individuals with dietary counseling and education.[25] Hawkins et al. have developed an interactive computer program designed to adapt to the specific information needs of adolescent users in providing ". . . a number of health related topics such as smoking prevention and cessation, human sexuality, stress management, interpersonal relationships, alcohol and other drug abuse, diet and activity, and body image."[26] Since this program protects the anonymity of its users and there is no human contact in giving or getting health information, the program provides a low-risk means for adolescents to acquire the specific health information they are interested in. Computers offer the greatest potential of any media technology we have discussed in this chapter for providing health care professionals and consumers of health care with high quality health information. As more people have access to computers, computer technology will shift from being a primarily inhouse use of interactive technology to being a public health education tool. The introduction of affordable, easy-to-use computer systems promises the eventual development of the computer as a mass media health communication tool.

Media technologies have provided important health communication tools that enable health care practitioners and their clients to reach beyond their personal ability to communicate to achieve their health care goals. The future development and growth of new media applications in health care promise to introduce exciting and innovative health communication tools and procedures. Media are extensions to our ability to communicate, and the complexities of modern health care demand all of our ingenuity in developing powerful health communication media.

Media play an important role in health promotion campaigns. New health care risks, and prevention methods are presented to the public via a broad range of public media. For example, in October 1982, after a number of people in Chicago died as a result of taking an over-the-counter-medicine, "Extra Strength Tylenol," that had been laced with cyanide, the public and privately operated mass media channels of radio, television, newspapers, and magazines quickly informed the public of the health risk and warned about use of the drug. Within days of identifying the drug as the source of health risk the vast majority of the public had been made aware of the situation. The mass media provided the public with important life-preserving information in this emergency health promotion campaign.

Multi-media health promotion programs, combining mass media, interpersonal, and presentational communication, have been found to be the most effective approach to influencing health care behaviors. Maccoby and Farquhar (1975) reported the results of an effective health promotion campaign utilizing the combined media of television, radio, print, and person-to-person presentational communication to inform people of their susceptibility to heart disease and instigate the development of behaviors that would help people avoid heart disease.[27] The researchers described the communication media they used, in combination with intensive personal health instruction sessions with high-risk adults, in an effective health promotion campaign: "Cooperation from local TV and radio stations enabled us to convey messages using some 40 TV spots, numerous radio spots, and mini-dramas. Space was made available in local newspapers for 'doctors columns' and dietary columns. A number of printed items (a basic information booklet, a cookbook, a heart-health calendar, and so on) were mailed directly to residents. Additional messages were conveyed by business cards and bill-boards."[28]

NOTES

1. McLuhan, 1964, Section N.
2. Cohen, 1963, Section N.
3. Sobel and Brown, 1982, Section L.
4. Schmelling and Wotring, 1976, Section L.
5. Vogel and Krabbe, 1977, Section N.
6. Wright, 1975, Section L.

 7. Emery et al., 1968, Section N.
 8. Harlem, 1977, p. 53, Section A.
 9. Kreps, 1982, Section J.
10. Anderson, 1981, p. 157, Section N.
11. McLaughlin, 1975, p. 184, Section L.
12. Hyman and Sheatsley, 1971, Section N.
13. Maccoby et al., 1977, Section N.
14. Burge, 1981, p. 171, Section N.
15. Elmore, 1981, p. 8, Section N.
16. Ibid.
17. Cassata and Clements, 1978, Section D.
18. Kreps, 1982, Section J.
19. Goodman, 1982, Section N.
20. Park and Bashshur, 1975, p. 161, Section L.
21. Harlem, 1977, p. 39, Section A.
22. Ibid., 35–38.
23. Slack et al., 1966, Section L.
24. Maultsby and Slack, 1971, Section L.
25. Slack et al., 1976, Section L.
26. Hawkins et al., 1982, Section L.
27. Maccoby and Farquhar, 1975, Section L.
28. Ibid., p. 118.

READING

PREVIEW OF READING

The article, "The Doctor Shows," by McLauglin examines the portrayal of medicine in commercial, prime-time television programming. He analyzes the stereotypic treatment of medical personnel, their work, and their relationships with co-workers and clients. The implications of his findings may provide insight into the reasons behind the unrealistic expectations health care providers and health care consumers often have for the outcomes of health care practice.

THE DOCTOR SHOWS

James McLaughlin

Television's doctors, nurses, and patients are cast in situations as patterned as the characters themselves. While a broken bone or a broken heart, a case of cancer, or a case of personal trauma based on untimely death do give some characters and episodes their own identities, the pattern by which doctors and nurses meet the problems of their patients is a neat set of devices continually used and easily abstracted from the specifics of the plays. I shall summarize the major findings of a study based on a sample of 15 network shows broadcast in prime time. Out of the 15 programs, 45 characters were cast in speaking parts as doctors, 12 as nurses, 2 as paramedics, and 23 as patients.

Doctors on television are most often young or middle-aged white males; nurses are most often young white females. All medical professionals are admirable in appearance, demeanor, and personality. They are ethical, kind, responsive to the requests of their patients, honest, and courageous.

Patients are more often female than male. They are 95 percent white and never elderly. Female patients are twice as often bedridden as male patients. An image common to (46 percent of) female patients is that of a bedridden

Reprinted by permission from *Journal of Communication* 25 (1975): 182–84.

woman with a strong man—husband, doctor, or romantic partner—at her bedside.

Doctors on television symbolize power, authority, and knowledge and possess the almost uncanny ability to dominate and control the lives of others. Their power extends not only to medical practice but also to the private lives of their patients. Doctors are always near at hand or easily accessible to patients. While they often advise each other, they rarely receive orders from superiors. Often, as we shall see, the plot pivots on the necessity for the doctor to act on his own initiative and disobey an "order."

Nurses are cast as subservient to doctors and never disobey a command. Thus, the ordering and advising structure concentrates power in the (male) doctors. But all medical professionals, both doctors and nurses, exercise some authority over patients.

In 40 percent of the cases of a medical treatment, a doctor either (a) performed a treatment that was not normally performed due to its high risk, (b) attempted an experimental treatment that was not yet proven fully reliable, or (c) having alternatives to treatment—one a sure, safe thing and the other risky but if successful, a complete cure—chose the latter. The remaining 60 percent of cases involved routine medical practice.

Going beyond strictly physical treatment, in 13 percent of the medical cases in which a doctor was involved he risked personal profit or prestige to act on his own initiative; in 47 percent of the cases he pursued the case into the private life of a patient; in 13 percent he disobeyed a set rule, precedent, convention, or legality to perform treatment not normally performed; and in 13 percent he came into conflict with the advice of a superior, his peers, the patient, or the patient's family or spouse.

Considering both medical and personal involvement, in 40 percent of the cases, the success of the medical treatment was ambiguous but personal conflicts or problems central to the plot were resolved by the doctor; in 20 percent of the cases, even if the medical treatment was a failure, a personal conflict was resolved. The TV doctor has the power to control the emotions and personalities as well as the health, life, and death of the people with whom he deals. There was not one relationship between doctor and patient in which the professional was not successful in resolving some problem for the good of all.

From a strictly medical point of view, the outcome of the doctor's treatment was unquestionably successful in 44 percent of the situations where a medical treatment was performed. With male patients, 70 percent of the medical treatments were successful; with female patients, only 23 percent.

Looking at the entire structure of portrayals, it can be said that in 95 percent of the relationships between a doctor and a patient at least one of the following took place due to the action of the doctor: (a) people have been brought closer to each other; (b) people have worked out a conflict created by the medical treatment; or (c) people have accepted forces they have realized they cannot control. The fact that it is always the doctor who is responsible for working things out creates the symbol of a "necessary outsider"—one who can deal objectively with the facts at hand, interpret and shuffle them, and solve all kinds of problems.

The role of the medical doctor on television is therefore that of a powerful, almost omnipotent, healer who performs his duties above and beyond normally expected capacities. He does so in situations that are exciting or controversial and he deals with not only the physical but also the emotional needs of his patients. If he just followed rules, or left private matters to the patients themselves, or did not risk life, limb, love, or money, things would never work out.

5.

THE INTERPERSONAL HEALTH COMMUNICATION CONTEXT

As a student, I had an experience with a patient, Mr. Burns, that I've never forgotten. When Mr. Burns found out he had high blood pressure, he simply wouldn't believe it. "Change my diet? Never!" he vowed, and turned his back on the nursing team gathered around his bed. I was shocked, yet fascinated, by his behavior. How could an intelligent man like Mr Burns defy sound medical advice?

Every day, I spent a few extra minutes getting to know him better. We chatted about the ball team. We talked about his family. We even touched on the effect of his illness insofar as he might have to reduce his work hours. But neither of us so much as whispered the word *diet*.

By the week's end, we were greeting one another like old friends. And when I least expected it, Mr. Burns turned to me like a woebegone child and asked, "Am I really going to have to quit eating fried chicken?"

"You might," I answered softly, patting his arm.

"But I don't want to," he wailed.

In simple terms, I told Mr. Burns about the effect of fried foods on people with high blood pressure. This time, he listened intently.

When I finished speaking, Mr. Burns, with a shake of his head, said, "Stewed chicken will never replace Kentucky Fried. But I guess I could give it a try."

Later, while I was telling my supervisor about our conversation, I realized with pleasure that I'd been practicing the good communication techniques I'd been taught in class. I cared about Mr. Burns. I wanted to help him feel better about himself, and if possible, help him begin to solve some of his problems. And because I'd taken the time to establish a *trusting relationship*, I'd been able to get through to Mr. Burns. Me—a lowly student.

Communicating isn't so difficult, I realized. But it must be more than reciting verbal techniques. When a nurse really cares about her patient, she should try to ensure an honest exchange of feelings.

That lesson had such an impact on me that I've built my nursing career around the importance of practicing good communications.[1]

PRACTITIONER–CLIENT RELATIONSHIPS

No communication takes place in a vacuum. Human beings are always involved with each other in the communication process. The implications of "together" are multifarious. For example, *all communication takes place within a system*. The individual can be seen at the center of the system (as shown in Figure 5.1). If the individual is a client, in the center ring of the system, he or she is surrounded by health care providers in the next ring and thus the practitioner–client relationship is formed. The client and the health care providers interact within the hospital or other health care setting (third ring), the community (fourth ring), and the other parts of the outside environment which include state and national levels. There is no way to picture a model which would include all parts of the system ad infinitum but this analogy indicates the importance of understanding the impact of the various systems on the individual.

Closed systems are ones in which little or no information, interaction, or exchange takes place within or between parts of the system. A closed system can be compared to an autocratic family in which there is one head of the house, family members' activities take place centrally around the family unit, and little information comes to the family from outside. While a totally closed system could not continue to exist because there would be no information available to direct system responses, various degrees of openness or closedness might be advantageous. A closed health care system, for example, has a clear line of command. There is little question of control or of what duties are assigned to various professionals. New and threatening information which would challenge the system is not allowed in the system or explained. An *open system*, on the other hand, has no rigid structure and is open to information from other systems and subsystems. Thus, it is

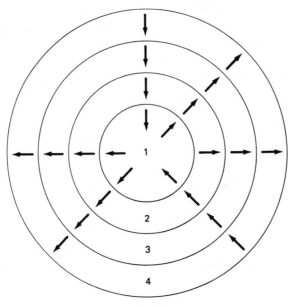

1. The Individual
2. Health Care Practitioners
3. Health Care Setting
4. Outside Environment

Figure 5.1   The Client's Health Communication System.

constantly changing. While that change can often be beneficial it is threatening to the status quo and can cause upheaval. In order for a health system to stay "healthy" it must utilize advantages from both the open and closed approaches.

As systems are complex, so are the contexts of the interaction that occurs among members of the system, particularly in the practitioner–client relationship. For example, a client, whom we shall call McGrady, can be seen at the center of a system that incorporates many relationships. Her relationship with Nurse Bruins is an interpersonal or dyadic one. Client McGrady also has relationships with other members of the health care team who she sees sometimes as a group as well as individually. Additionally, she has relationships with the organization. For example, she deals with her Medicaid representative and her state legislator in order to get better health care. Her relationships are ever-changing due to the environment and the number of people participating in the interaction.

Whether the client is in an open or closed system will also reflect on her care and how she receives information on that care. Again, in a closed system she will clearly understand the hierarchy of her care although there will be limited information exchange. In an open system much more interaction will take place. This background on interpersonal relationships in systems is provided not only to emphasize the complexity of communication but to provide a background for understanding the unique and complicated practitioner–client relationship and underscore the fact that it cannot be isolated from the rest of the health care system or from society as a whole.

The client–practitioner relationship has been a major topic in recent health care literature. Writers discuss such factors as the unequal power relationship between practitioner and client,[2] as well as the mythology of health settings which makes communication more confusing and complex.[3] Double-bind messages are often given to clients in health care. For example, the dentist giving a shot to a child might say, "This doesn't hurt." But, in fact, it does hurt. What the dentist says is true contradicts the child's physical sensations, and the child is put in a situation of deciding which to believe. The dentist's message is antithetical to good communication because of this.

These double messages put people into *double-bind* situations where they receive mutually contradictory messages which confuse the communication situation. Other double-binds include the use of jargon. While needed by the physician to provide accurate instructions and diagnoses for other health colleagues, it confuses and sometimes frightens the client. Jargon, which is discussed in detail in Chapter 2, is one way to have a closed interpersonal communication system where information is not exchanged.

Double-binds continue when we label health care clients. For example, many times the client called "difficult" is the person who has educated him or herself about an illness, who knows enough to ask intelligent questions and who will, on occasion, refuse to undergo certain treatments or tests. This scenario is often compounded when treatment is not working and the health practitioner blames the lack of success on the client's "difficultness."[4]

In contrast health practitioners who work on congruent and productive relationships report that with good communication, problems can be more readily diagnosed, clients can be more easily satisfied, and the work setting can be enhanced for the health professional. The case used at the beginning of the chapter illustrates how communication can enhance a health care relationship and help to facilitate the cooperation so vitally needed between health care providers and consumers in health care.

Establishing an Effective Implicit Contract

Strong interpersonal relationships are based upon the fulfillment of needs by relational partners. Each partner in a dyadic relationship expects the other to act in specified ways. The key to establishing effective relationships is to make expectations clear.

In marital relationships, for example, there are many mutual expectations about the appropriate interpersonal behaviors of the husband and the wife. The husband might expect the wife to wash the dishes, and the wife might expect the husband to vacuum the carpet. Often, however, these expectations remain unspoken. Each relational partner might think that the other should know what is expected without being told. When marriage partners are unaware or unsure of each other's expectations, there is a high probability they will not act in accord with each other's wishes. To complicate this situation further, the expectations relational partners have for one another change constantly, making the potential for the fulfillment of these expectations even less likely.

Inevitably, when people fail to meet the expectations others set for their behavior they disappoint those persons and weaken those relationships. The interpretations most often assigned to behaviors that fail to meet relational expectations are negative. It is often assumed that the person who is not fulfilling the expectations is doing so because he or she is either *mad or bad*. Mad or bad interpretations infer the noncompliant individual is mad (crazy or stupid) or bad (purposefully uncooperative). Mad or bad interpretations weaken the credibility of the communicator and foster suspicion and mistrust within the relationship. The more communicators fail to meet the expectations of those with whom they are in a relationship, the more the relationship is weakened. Communicators are frustrated by the negative responses they receive, and often are unaware they are violating others' expectations. The failure to meet others' expectations can instigate appropriate, often angry and retaliatory, responses. These behaviors, in turn, instigate additional inappropriate behaviors, all of which fail to meet relational expectations, causing a vicious cycle of escalating relational deterioration. For example, a client kept waiting for hours can refuse to pay a bill for months or drop the professional without explanation.

To a certain extent effective relationships are very much like contractual agreements. They aren't exactly explicit legal contracts such as the contracts used in business arrangements (although in the 1960s there was a movement to utilize "marriage contracts" to make marital expectations explicit). Relationships are usually less formal than legal contracts, generally taking the form of unspoken *implicit contracts*. Such a contract *implies* that communicators should act in certain ways toward one another. For example, in a friendship relationship between two nurses working together in the emergency room of a hospital, the implicit contract established might call for informal and playful interaction between the two individuals. The two nurses might tease one another or use lighthearted bantering as a means of relieving some of the tension and stress of their work in the emergency room. This is an implicit contract because it is not formally required by the organization or formally agreed upon by the nurses. The relationship evolves informally out of past interactions between the nurses. The nurses' unspoken agreement to continue fulfilling each other's expectations for lighthearted interaction is an implicit contract.

Effective interpersonal relationships both in and out of health care settings have clearly understood implicit contracts between relational partners. Not only are the communicators aware of the expectations they have of one another, but they work at continually updating their perceptions of each other's expectations. These communicators try to update their awareness of the implicit contract by giving and seeking interpersonal feedback, enabling them to continue to act appropriately with one another as their relationship grows.

Therapeutic Relationships

Interpersonal relationships have many different functions. They can provide communicators with excitement, support, friendship, love, financial gain, intellectual stimulation, as well as serving to increase or decrease their overall state of health. The more therapeutic interpersonal communication is, the more the communication helps individuals involved increase their levels of health.

Therapeutic communication has been defined in many different ways. Fuller and Quesada expressed the clinical perspective on therapy when they described therapeutic communication as ". . . the characteristics of information exchange between therapist and patient that facilitates a mutually gratifying relationship between participants so as to accomplish the primary goal of reduced morbidity for the patient."[5] Their approach to therapeutic communication suggests that it is accomplished only by formally designated "therapists" to help "patients" to prolong their lives. This is a fairly restrictive perspective on therapeutic communication that fails to recognize the wider application of therapy in everyday life.

Pettegrew has broadened the Fuller and Quesada approach to therapeutic communication by identifying a larger range of therapeutic outcomes, although he maintains a somewhat clinical perspective when he defines therapeutic communication as, ". . . the verbal and paraverbal communication transactions between a helper and a helpee which results in feelings of psychological (thoughts), emotional (feelings), and or physical (actions) relief by the helpee."[6] Barnlund further liberates the perspective of therapeutic communication, expanding the range of settings, participants, and applications of therapeutic communication when he explains that interpersonal relationships ". . . are regarded as therapeutic when they provoke personal insight or reorientation, and when they enable persons to participate in more satisfying ways in future social encounters."[7]

Barnlund's approach to therapeutic communication does not limit its application to trained health practitioners, nor does it limit it to health care practice and the preservation of human life. His approach implies that any individual has the potential for communicating therapeutically by helping another person to understand him or herself more fully, thereby aiding that individual in deciding how to direct behaviors to best achieve needs and goals. Furthermore, according to this perspective on therapeutic communication, interpersonal feedback is therapeutic if it informs people about others' perceptions of them, offering them a clearer image about the reactions people have to their communication. Ultimately, therapeutic communication enables individuals to communicate more effectively to achieve their personal goals.

Certainly all interpersonal communication is not therapeutic. Interpersonal communication can often have nontherapeutic effects by confusing and frustrating communicators rather than helping them achieve personal insight and reorientation. Popular evidence about the growing frustrations and dissatisfactions experienced by people involved in the health care system (discussed in depth earlier in Chapter 1) seem to indicate that much interpersonal communication in health care is nontherapeutic. Nontherapeutic communication is counterproductive to the goals of health care because it fosters dissatisfaction among communicators and undermines the spirit of cooperation that is essential to effective health care relationships.

Watzlawick, Beavin, and Jackson have identified several situations where interpersonal relationships can become "pathological" due to nontherapeutic communication.[8] Pathologies are defined as ". . . disturbances that can develop in human communication," and therapeutic communication functions to ameliorate pathologies.[9] Similarly, Ruesch has differentiated between therapeutic communication and disturbed communication, suggesting that human communication can range on a continuum from highly therapeutic to highly disturbed (nontherapeutic).[10] Therapeutic communication can be used in many different health care situations to help individuals grow and adapt, increasing their sense of satisfaction with themselves and with their interpersonal relationships.

Rossiter and Pearce have described honesty and validation as two key characteristics of therapeutic communication; they contend ". . . that honesty accompanied by validation results in psychological growth for persons and that the lack of honesty and validation is likely to retard psychological growth and possibly bring about psychological deterioration."[11] Truax and Carkhuff have identified three key characteristics demonstrated by therapeutic communicators that are similar to those offered by Rossiter and Pearce. Their characteristics include: 1) accurate empathy and understanding; 2) nonpossessive warmth and respect; 3) genuineness and authenticity.[12] Rogers has described therapeutic communication characteristics similarly, identifying such attributes as genuineness and congruence, unconditional positive regard, and empathic understanding.[13] A combination and synthesis of the characteristics of therapeutic communicators advocated by these theorists (Rossiter and Pearce, Truax and Carkhuff, and Rogers) indicates the importance of the following communicator characteristics in communicating therapeutically: *empathy, trust, honesty, validation,* and *caring*.

Empathy refers to the ability to develop a full understanding of another person's condition and feelings and relate that understanding to the person. Health communicators can demonstrate empathy for another person by accurately communicating the other's feelings in interpersonal interaction. Often, empathy can be shown nonverbally as well as verbally, by nodding one's head when the person says something about him or herself and is wondering whether it has been understood, or by maintaining eye contact with the individual with whom one is speaking and mirroring the person's facial expressions in a genuine manner. In health care interviews, mirror questions and reflective probes (discussed in depth later in this chapter) can help communicate empathy by letting the interviewee know the practitioner is following and understanding what is being said.

Trust is a belief that a person will respect another's needs and desires and will behave towards them in a responsible and predictable manner. Trusting behaviors are those that ". . . deliberately increase a person's vulnerability to another person."[14] It is risky to exhibit trusting behaviors to another because that person may not respond in a responsible way. In establishing a trusting relationship it may be necessary for one person to take a chance by disclosing information about themselves to another that might make them more vulnerable to that person. If the other person responds responsibly, and perhaps discloses some risky information of their own in response, the chances that trust will develop are good. If, however, an individual reacts irresponsibly or inappropriately to another's self disclosure trust will not develop. Due to the risk involved in establishing trusting relationships, trust is most often established little by little over long periods of time. In health care, due to the intensity of many interpersonal situations, trust can sometimes be established or destroyed rather quickly depending on the appropriateness of the communicative response.

Honesty refers to the ability to communicate truthfully, frankly, and sincerely. There is never total honesty in any situation, because there is never total truth. People perceive the world according to their own perceptions of reality, and often people perceive the world very differently from one another. Honest communication, however, does not imply objective truth, but subjective truth. It is not purposely deceptive, but is intended to be a truthful representation of information as the individual knows it. "A person communicates honestly to the extent that his messages accurately express his awareness of his experience and invite the listener to share in that experience."[15] Honest self disclosure in health care relationships implicitly invites reciprocal honesty by relational partners.

Validation occurs when a communicator feels as though other communicators accept and respect what he or she has to say. Validating communication affirms the worth of the person and his or her experiences. (Validation is similar to personal communication discussed in depth in Chapter 2.) To validate other people doesn't mean having to agree totally with everything they are saying, but respecting their right to express their opinions and taking what they have to say seriously. Validating communication tends to humanize interaction. It tells the persons you are communicating with that you are willing to be influenced by what they say and their communication is important to you. Health communicators can validate one another in interpersonal communication by listening carefully to what is being said and responding to the other's messages congruently.

Caring refers to the level of emotional involvement communicators express for one another. It is what Rogers calls "unconditional positive regard," the demonstration of interest and concern for the other person's well being.[16] Caring communication must be sincere and appropriate to be useful in health care. Communicators can express caring for one another nonverbally by paying attention to what the other person is saying (maintaining eye contact and nodding when appropriate), exhibiting emotionally congruent facial expressions, and by using their vocal and tactile behaviors to show supportiveness. Health communicators can demonstrate caring for one another by expressing genuine concern over the other's problems and communicating a willingness to help the other person work through their hardships.

Each of the five characteristics of therapeutic communication (empathy, trust, honesty, validation, and caring) are important skills for effective health communication. In many situations the five overlap and merge with one another. For example, empathy and caring can be expressed with the same nonverbal messages of eye contact and head nods; validation, honesty, and trust can likewise be expressed through mutual self disclosure. Empathy, trust, honesty, validation, and caring are also reciprocally occuring human communication behaviors. That is, the expression of empathic, trusting, honest, validating, or caring communications generally induces a reciprocal expression by those communicated with. Due to this reciprocity, the use of therapeutic communication in health care can encourage others to communicate similarly, evoking a spiraling or building effect in therapeutic communication.

In addition to the five characteristics of therapeutic communication, the authors of this book would like to emphasize the importance of humor and listening in health care interaction. The use of humor to reduce stress in health professionals is particularly documented in television comedies such as "St. Elsewhere" and "Mash". Humor in high-stress situations is often cathartic among health professionals, for it relieves the strain. A new hospital in one of our communities is gambling that even the emergency rooms need humor because they put floor to ceiling murals of scenes from "Mash" all over the emergency waiting room walls. Norman Cousins has also emphasized that humor can be useful toward neutralizing stress and changing the meaning of situations so they are less stressful. While cruel or inappropriate jokes are certainly out of place in the therapeutic interaction, gentle humor can be useful in any human exchange.[17]

Listening is also a most important part of therapeutic communication and it is reflected particularly in the caring process. Harlem (1977) emphasizes the importance and difficulty of listening to clients. He says:

> When I was in practice, I found the most exhausting and exacting part of communication was listening to patients, not only to the apparent verbal meaning of what they wanted me to know, or believe and why. It involved trying to enter the patient's world each time, empathizing with him, and reading his body language, those unconscious and often telltale, gestures, mannerisms and expressions . . .[18]

In order to become a better listener, you have to work to improve your listening ability in the areas of sensations, interpretation and comprehension.[19] Sensations are often a barrier to our listening. Construction in the hospital corridor or a crying baby in the nursery can distract both the speaker and the listener. Attempting to converse when these distractions are minimal is important to the listening process. Sometimes this means moving to another area. Interpretation is also important. Prejudging, faking attention and criticizing the person rather than the message are factors that impede the listening process. Additionally, our comprehension must be adequate. Comprehension is improved by concentrating on the speech and by being genuinely interested. We listen best when we do not have any physical constraints or stress and when we are respectful of the listening process.

As reported in Ross (1980) the qualities of an ideal listener have been stated by Pflaumer:

An ideal listener is one who:

- keeps an open curious mind
- listens for new ideas
- relates what is heard to what is known
- is self-perceptive and listens to others from that self
- pays attention to what is said
- does not blindly follow the crowd
- maintains perspective
- looks for idea, organization and arguments
- listens for the essence of things
- stays mentally alert, outlining, objecting, approving
- is introspective but critically analytical
- attempts to understand values, attitudes and relationships
- focuses on the speaker's ideas
- listens with feeling and intuition.[20]

Active listeners additionally incorporate other techniques to be effective. They take notes where appropriate and also paraphrase the material that they heard in order to check out the accuracy of the message with the speaker. In other words, they reflect back what was said to them.

THE HEALTH CARE INTERVIEW

The dialogue between the practitioner and the client, at least initially, usually takes the form of an interview. Interviews can be seen as formal consultations or mutual viewings of data. Usually, in the health care setting interviews are the most formal and encompassing means of consultation between practioners and clients. The perception of the interview by the various participants has a great deal to do with its success. Whereas the traditional interview has long been thought of as the "doctor-client interview," there is now an awareness in health care that all members of the health care team participate in the interview process at some time during client care. The following discussion should be helpful to all health care personnel, as well as to consumers of health care who would like to improve the consultations they have with health care practitioners. The suggestions given for effective interviewing should be incorporated into the elements of therapeutic communication in order to be effective.

Interview Planning

The first part of the interview process is to establish the goal of the interview for both the interviewer (usually the health care practitioner) and the interviewee (usually the client). Generally, the interview takes place because the client is seeking help and the practitioner needs information in order to provide that help. Traditionally, health care practitioners have used a directive approach as their primary interview style. The directive interview is a tightly controlled process used to obtain specific information and to provide the proper course of action that the interviewee should take. The implication of the directive interview is that the client is incapable of identifying the problem or of aiding in the selection of the best solution. There are many problems with the traditional directive interview. Often the client might not agree with the compliance regime or might feel isolated from the suggested solution to the medical problem. Clients have also reported that the practitioner did not hear all of what he or she was trying to express.[21]

In the client-centered interview, based on the theories of Carl Rogers, the practitioner's role is that of a helper who tries to assist the client in achieving his or her own insights and solutions to problems.[22] The client-centered interview is sometimes refered to as a nondirective approach, and is the antithesis of the traditionally used directive approach. In the client-centered interview, the interviewer reflects to the interviewee information he or she has provided—giving the interviewee the opportunity to explore the topic of discussion him or herself. The notion behind this approach is that no one knows more about any person than that individual knows about himself, and by giving an individual encouragement to explore their ideas and feelings about self they can and will solve their own problems. In health care this may become difficult for clients because they often do not know how to express or describe health care symptoms, or may not always have the expertise to diagnose or solve complex health care problems.

The solution to this problem is, of course, to take the best of the directive and the client-centered interviews in order to build a model to fit the client's needs.

Other than identifying the kind of interview (directive or nondirective) that will take place, practitioners and clients should identify such goals as the timing of the interview and the kinds of questions that will be asked and answered. Additionally, interviewers will want to be aware of interview style as well as of interview techniques. Probably the most important goal of the interviewer is to remember that involving the client in his or her own care from the outset of the initial interview will insure a more effective treatment.

Time

As we discussed in the nonverbal communication section of Chapter 2, chronemics or time is an important nonverbal aspect of communication. Time is a factor that will probably affect the interview more than any other factor. Our culture is largely a monochronic one in which time and being on time is valued over relationship factors. The health practitioner as well as the client will make some of their initial judgements of each other based on how they treat the time dimension. The use or misuse of time can become an obstacle—either party if kept waiting for too long, will lose trust or respect for the other.[23]

Pluchman (1978) discussed the issue of time in the health setting.[24] She notes that a time contract between practitioner and client is often one-sided on behalf of the provider. At the time of the scheduling of the interview and again when the interview begins, a realistic contract regarding time should be established to provide a framework for the interview. If time constraints and/or emergency parameters indicate that the interview is going to be a short one, parties to the medical interview have a right to know so that they can structure their questions and answers accordingly. Less repetition as well as structuring of the beginning and the ending of the interview will take place if time is frankly discussed. If other interviews are going to take place in the future regarding health problems this should be made clear. The health practitioner who understands him or herself well will also schedule initial interviews at an appropriate time of day when there are no predictable emergencies. Interviews conducted when there are too many distractions or when the participants are tired will not be successful and the appropriate information will not be obtained. Proper planning and use of time can conserve usable energy.

Practitioners argue that there simply aren't enough hours in the day or that emergencies often interfere with the ideal time constraints of a client's appointment. Clients, on the other hand, often feel that there is not enough time to discuss problems in detail with the practitioner or that the practitioner is too intent on making money or fulfilling quotas to take the necessary time to listen to complaints. Additionally, members of either group might be monochronic. That is, they are clock-watching persons intent on being on time, while the more polychronic are more relationship-oriented persons who finish and complete a prior interaction (despite possibly being late) before they begin a new one.[25]

Space

Space is also an important variable in the interview situation. We are constantly arranging ourselves in relation to others in some spatial context.[26] Space as an internal nonverbal message source can seriously affect communication. Where we sit, how much we distance ourselves from clients, as well as the arrangement of the office or other health care setting are of great importance. Spatial distances, as studied by anthropologist Edward T. Hall, gives us some idea of how much area people in our Western culture need to operate efficiently.[27] Because health practitioners see a vast array of people from many cultures, it is important that they be aware of the client's spatial needs. This can be done by observing the client to see if distances are comfortable or not. Additionally, the interviewer can ask the client where he or she would like to sit or place his belongings. In interviews in which the practitioner wants self-disclosure to take place, it is often more acceptable to sit beside the desk rather than behind it so that space and objects such as desks do not become barriers.

A spatial related disturbance is illustrated by Pluchman; the example would be having the verbal statement, "I'm not afraid of contracting your disease," be accompanied by the health practitioner standing a substantial distance from the client.[28] The message would be perceived by the client as confusing and incongruent.

Space should also be considered in terms of territorial behavior. Clients, like most people, often exhibit territorial behavior regarding their clothes and their bodies. During physical exams where clients are asked to disrobe the perceptive interviewer should be aware of privacy needs and should set up the interview situation so there will be no interruptions.[29]

The Kinds of Exchange

After the time and space guidelines are established, other parameters of the interview should also be discussed. Clients should be given a short overview regarding what is going to happen to them. This should include the kinds of questions that will be asked as well as the kinds of procedures that might be used if the interview is combined with an examination. The practitioner needs to obtain some idea of the language constraints of the client. Is the client aware of medical terms such as penis or vagina if those terms are relevant to the interview? Does the use of those terms embarrass the client? While these kinds of questions should, of course, not be asked at the beginning of the interview, the interviewer should have the level of information exchange in mind. Clients should never be patronized. They should be addressed in language they clearly understand.

As the practitioner–client relationship develops, and possibly in the first interview, truth-telling can become an issue. For example, if the client states that he thinks he has lung cancer and wants to know the probabilities of survival, a decision regarding truth-telling must be made. While not the principal element in the initial interview, it will become increasingly important as the health care relationship continues. Much of the literature on informed consent and truth-telling advocates honest and open discussion for most health care problems but individual health care providers must determine their own stance. Additionally, it is most important to determine the client's point of view. This can best be determined by an open discussion of the issue during one of the interviews. Practitioners sometimes make the assumption that clients do or do not want to know the truth with little data from the client. Chapter 8 will discuss truth-telling and ethics in health care in more detail.

Winning the client's confidence is important in the interview process. This can be done by showing interest, respecting attitudes and ideas, and by stressing the client's physical or mental strengths. It is important not to pry but to let the client choose the rate and amount of self-disclosure.

It is important that interviewers do not probe deeply into subjects in which they have had no training. For example, if the client wants to discuss a serious sexual problem and the health provider has little or no training in this area, the client should not be encouraged to share potentially embarrassing and private data that is not pertinent to the professional's area of expertise and which will have to be repeated to the next professional. It is appropriate in this situation to tell the client that sexuality (or anything else for that matter) is not your area but that you will be happy to put them in touch with the appropriate person.

Watching and listening for nonverbal communication clues is also important. For example, excessive perspiration or wringing of the hands can be viewed as potential signs of nervousness, at which point the interview can be slowed down or redirected until the interviewee is more comfortable. Interviewers are often nervous about the interview, failing to utilize the chronemic (time) aspects of interviewing effectively. Health care interviewers generally overestimate the length of silent pauses by their clients, just as silent pauses in conversation cause many people discomfort on a first date. Pauses in interpersonal conversation are natural and shouldn't be avoided. In fact, in health care interviews clients often may need to pause to be able to interpret their ideas, feelings, and symptoms, enabling them to communicate this information to the health care provider.

Interview Questions

It is important not to have a cookbook formula for the interview. Each client and each professional needs an individual approach. However, the interviewer should be familiar with different approaches and types of questions. An *open-ended question* is one which allows the client to answer without much direction. For example, the questions "How do you feel?" or "What is the matter with you today?" do not direct the answer. Instead they invite the client to give his or her perceptions, views, opinions, thoughts, and feelings. Often an open question can widen and deepen the contact to good rapport.[30] Open questions do have some disadvantages. For example, answers might give superfluous information or take more time than is allocated. *Closed questions* limit options and sometimes specify answers in the questions themselves. They are restrictive by nature. For example, a *moderately closed question* might be, "How long has it been since your last physical?" An example of a *highly closed question* would be to ask the client to pick one of four given answers.

Bi-polar questions are a common type of closed question also used and misused in the interview process. In this type of question the respondent is limited to one of two choices. "Do you drink or not?" is a bi-polar question as is "Do you approve or disapprove of birth control?" The assumptions undergirding bi-polar questions are that there are only two possible answers and that they are totally in opposition to each other.[31]

The advantage of closed types of questions is that the interviewer can control the questions and answers more effectively and that he or she can ask more questions in more areas in less time.[32] It is easier to record and tally answers on closed questions. Disadvantages of the closed questions are that the wrong kind of information can be obtained and that too little data is obtained. The answers to closed questions often fail to reveal feelings or attitudes which might be pertinent to the client's health problem. Additionally, closed questions might force certain positions too early in the interview. These disadvantages and others make the use of the closed question a delicate tool in the hands of the practitioner.

Other kinds of questions which can be asked are *primary and secondary questions*. Primary questions introduce topics or new areas. They can stand alone or out of context. "Where were you when the pain first started?" is an example. Secondary questions attempt to elicit more information and they may be open or closed. Stewart and Cash refer to them as probing or follow-up questions which are used to get more complete or accurate data.[33] They suggest that if the respondent has not completed an answer or is hesitant that the interviewer remain silent while using nonverbal eye contact or head nodding. If the pause does not encourage the respondent to continue such probes as "Go on" can be used.[34]

Mirror or summary questions reflect or summarize a series of questions and answers to make sure an accurate understanding has taken place. "Okay, let's see if I have this accurately. Your headaches always follow exposure to chocolate products?" is an example of a summary or mirror question.

The *reflective probing question* can also be used to help correct real or suspected inaccuracies. For example, the interviewer might say "Didn't you say you had four bouts with the flu?" These kinds of probes must be used carefully so that the respondent's integrity does not seem to be questioned.[35] By knowing a variety of questions and approaches, as well as being aware of proper timing of questions. the interview can be personalized to meet the needs of the client and the practitioner.

A nonjudgmental approach is highly suggested in the interview. By withholding judgment, the interviewer encourages frank and free expression as well as emotional release. Sometimes it is necessary to show disapproval of behavior ("Ten packs a day??") but never of the client. Describing the data and the consequences rather than judging them are helpful techniques. The practitioner can nonjudgmentally say, "The available research data indicates that excessive smoking—and ten packs a day is in that category—is injurious to health," rather than "You are wrecking your life by such irresponsible smoking behavior."

As the interview progresses and trust is established, more directive or secondary questions can be asked. Once again, the nonverbal clues should be used in providing feedback to the health professional. Direct questions can also be asked. It is certainly appropriate to ask the client if they are satisfied with the progress of the interview and an occasional summarizing of what has taken place is also helpful. Often it may be helpful to have the client do the summarizing to make sure that perceptions are mutually accurate.

During the interview, health practitioners should monitor their own behavior. Are they listening instead of talking too much? What nonverbal signals are they sending to the client? Are they aware of prejudices they might have against the client such as size, color of skin, or manner? Are they using language clients understand without being patronizing?

Terminating the Interview

As the interview comes to a close, it is important for the client to know what other steps are required to solve the health problem and what resources are available for the solution. If other interviews or appointments are required they should be clearly stated and agreed to by both parties and clients should clearly understand why they are coming back. They should also be told the cost of all future interviews or procedures. It is important not to coerce the client into returning while making sure they have the necessary information to make that decision. As Enelow and Swisher state, "interviews build on each other."[36] By giving the client information the practitioner encourages client cooperation with their health care regime. (Refer to our discussion of cooperation in health care in Chapter 1.)

One last note. Before terminating the interview, all necessary paperwork should be rechecked to make sure that it is clear and accurate. Material which will be read by other members of the health care team should not violate the client's privacy. Additionally, it should be explained that others might see the records, if that is indeed the case.

Conventional medical records contain the client's history in six parts, usually in chronological sequence. Because this kind of record focuses on a single illness or complaint these records have been replaced in many health care settings by the problem-oriented record more frequently called the P.O.R. The goal of this method of record keeping is to develop a well-defined list of all the problems the client is experiencing with an effective data base. The P.O.R. (or P.O.M.R.) should be done several times in practice settings before being utilized on clients.

Additionally, care must be taken in any record keeping not to prematurely diagnose or label the client without a complete data base.

Foley and Sharf have identified five interviewing techniques that are frequently overlooked in health care interviews; they are: 1) putting the health care consumer at ease; 2) eliciting full and clear information; 3) maintaining control; 4) maintaining rapport; 5) bringing the interview to closure (see Figure 5.2).[37] The effective interviewer is aware of how to structure the interview, the goals to be achieved in the interview, the importance of adapting to the needs and feelings of the interviewee, and the giving and receiving of feedback with the interviewee.

Figure 5.2   The Five Categories of the Most Frequently Overlooked Interview Techniques Self Assessment Checklist

---

A. Beginning of the Interview:
Putting the patient at ease
1. Initiates a visit that puts the patient at ease.
2. Shows respect for patient by attending to needs of privacy and comfort.

B. Middle of the Interview:
Eliciting information
1. Uses open-ended questions to facilitate patient responses when appropriate.
2. Allows patient opportunity to explain story in own words without unnecessary interruptions.
3. Intervenes with appropriate responses when patient is unable to supply relevant information.
4. Rephrases or repeats question if needed to enhance understanding.
5. Clarifies areas of confusion or inconsistencies.
6. Inquires as to how well patient understands present illness.
7. Uses language appropriate to patient's age and background.
8. Aware of verbal habits (continuous okays, uh-huhs, noddings) that may be misunderstood by patient.
Maintaining control
9. Aware of pace of interview.
10. Uses periodic summaries.
11. Makes clear transitions from one step of the interview to another.
12. Interrupts unnecessary patient rambling to maintain focus.
13. Uses pauses to encourage patient response.
Maintaining Rapport
14. Maintains eye contact.
15. Uses nonverbal aspects (office seating arrangement, use of charts, body posture, facial expressions, touch) appropriately.

Fig. 5.2 (*cont'd*)

---

16. Allows opportunities for patient to express feelings about current illness and other problems.
17. Allows for sharing of feelings when appropriate.
18. Accepts patient's values in a nonjudgmental manner.
19. Sensitive to language or behavior that might arouse patient anxiety.
20. Explains the need for requesting certain data in order to reduce patient anxiety.
21. Deals with patient's expressed questions and concerns.
22. Deals with patient's nonverbally communicated concerns.

C. End of the Interview:
   Bringing Closure
   1. Informs patient about next steps when appropriate.
   2. Allows patient opportunity to ask additional questions or add to the interview.
   3. Provides closing statements which facilitate a comfortable ending.

Reprinted with permission from Richard Foley and Barbara F. Sharf, "The Five Interviewing Techniques Most Frequently Overlooked by Primary Care Physicians." *Behavioral Medicine* II (1981): 30–31.

The practitioner–client interview is the most important of health care interactions. The interview should be planned and different questions and techniques made individual for each interview. The practitioner should at all times be aware of the client's feelings, statements, and nonverbal behavior. Additionally, it is important for the interviewer to be aware of his or her own verbal and nonverbal behavior.

While the interview is the most common of all professional-client interactions, there are many other situations in which communication takes place and interviewing is not the main objective. The overall communication behavior of the professional often called "the bedside manner" is a product of the acquisition of good communication skills. As DiMatteo and Freidman state, it is a developed art and the ability of the professional to *learn* to communicate to the patient that he or she is understood.[38] A person who communicates effectively will monitor his or her own cues as well as the patient's, and understand social and psychological conditions such as culture and family experiences. The communication explanations in this and the other chapters of this book were written with these needs in mind.

NOTES

1. Mercer, (no date), Section A.
2. Mendelsohn, 1981, Section A.
3. Barnlund, 1976, Section A.
4. Bandler and Grinder, 1975, p. 13, Section A.
5. Fuller and Quesada, 1973, Section A.
6. Pettegrew, 1977, Section E.
7. Barnlund, 1968, Section A.
8. Watzlawick, Beavin, and Jackson, 1967, Section A.
9. Ibid.
10. Ruesch, 1957, Section E.
11. Rossiter and Pearce, 1975, Section A.
12. Truax and Carkhuff, 1967, Section E.
13. Rogers, 1957, Section E.
14. Rossiter and Pearce, 1975, Section A.
15. Ibid.
16. Rogers, 1957, Section E.
17. Cousins, N., 1979, Section A.
18. Harlem, O., 1977, p. 5, Section A.
19. Ross, R., 1980, Section N.
20. Ibid, pp. 119–120.
21. Enelow and Swisher, 1972, Section D.
22. Rogers, 1961, Section E.
23. Benjamin, 1981, Section D.
24. Pluchman, 1978, Section A.
25. Hall, 1977, Section C.
26. Pluchman, 1978, p. 61, Section A.
27. Hall, 1959, Section C; Hall, 1966, Section C.; Hall, 1977, Section C.
28. Pluchman, 1978, p. 61, Section A.
29. Ibid.
30. Benjamin, 1981, Section D.
31. Stewart and Cash, 1978, p. 66, Section D.
32. Ibid., p. 66.
33. Ibid., p. 69.
34. Ibid.
35. Ibid., p. 71.
36. Enelow and Swisher, 1972, p. 16, Section D.
37. Foley and Sharf, 1981, Section D.
38. DiMatteo and Friedman, 1982, p. 32.

READINGS

PREVIEW OF READINGS

In "I Am Your Patient and I Am Afraid," the client's perspective about the health care system is presented. The fears and anxieties experienced by hospitalized health care consumers are presented in a dramatic first person manner. Some of the situations identified appear unlikely and humorous at first reading, but they are very serious and could happen to you as a health care client. The author identifies several serious health communication problems that confront many consumers. A careful reading of this article will help you understand some of the feelings health care clients experience, aiding you in developing empathy for health care consumers.

In the article "Communication and Pain," the authors examine the way health practitioners communicate about pain with their clients. The article deals with the fact that pain is particularly difficult to explain, both from the client's and the practitioner's view. They suggest that there is a lack of interpersonal skills among health professionals in communicating about pain, and suggest methods for improvement.

I AM YOUR PATIENT— AND I AM AFRAID . . .

You don't know me and I don't really know you, but we've met before. Tens of thousands of times, in fact. I've seen you behind receptionists' counters, cleaning endless corridors, taking samples of my blood, delivering my baby, reading my EKG, filling my prescription, checking me during my physical exam, putting me to sleep for an operation, teaching me to use a wheelchair.

Reprinted by permission from *Coverage*, Kaiser Permanente Hospitals (December 16, 1977).

Yes, we've met under many circumstances, in many moods, for fleeting moments or for an eternity. Ours is a venerable bond, hallowed by an age-old tradition of trust between the sick and the healers. But sometimes I wonder if you comprehend how fragile that bond can be, how susceptible it is to fear. The procedures, tools, even the look, smell and feel of modern medicine that are familiar to you can be terrifying to me.

Every time I come into this alien world, be it clinic or hospital, I feel my heart start to beat a little faster, my mouth goes dry and my jaws tighten. Funny thing, I may not even notice the tension at first. And if you ask, I'd probably deny it. It is all so strange to me, this labyrinth where I seek answers to problems I don't even know I have. Well, maybe I suspect something is not normal, but often I'm afraid to admit it.

You may have to pull that information out of me. In part I may be testing you to see if you merit my trust, but most likely I'm wondering if you really care about me. Sure, I know I am not your only patient, but I want to be certain that if you are tired, super busy, or bored, it is not when I'm one before you. Besides, things I understand when I am well, like long lines for the lab, suddenly become inexplicable irritants when I am sick.

If I must enter your hospital, my fear can only increase. As an out-patient my sojourns into the foreign landscape of the clinic were temporary. In the hospital I feel I am confined to indefinite helplessness. There I am stripped of my family, my friends, money, habits, even my clothes—virtually all the familiar things that help to identify me as an individual. In some cases, even my primary care physician is reduced to a visitor, and I must trust strangers with my health, perhaps my life.

Most of the time I do rely on your professionalism and skills, but the psychological price I pay in anxiety and alienation can make me difficult to handle. If I complain about the cold coffee or bland meals it's possibly because I miss the warmth of breaking bread with loved ones, or chatting with coworkers on the coffee break. A sympathetic ear or a word of understanding can bolster my spirits better than any pain-killer; your frown or hurried indifference will deepen my isolation.

You may know every nook and cranny in this unit, on this floor, throughout this massive hospital, but I don't. Even when I'm ambulatory I feel akin to the rat in the maze; confined to my bed I worry that should anyone come to visit they'll never find me. All those stainless steel machines, coils of tubing, syringes, bottles, pills—they may comfort you with the strength of technology, but they're a constant reminder of how sick I am.

I don't know your land of starched white uniforms, waxed floors, and sterile walls, nor do I want to inhabit it. I do want information to interpret what is happening to me; I also need to feel that I am more important than your routine duties. Please don't think of me as a fascinating gallbladder or a stubborn tumor. Beneath this plastic ID band pulses a human heart.

That heart is connected to a brain and it requires attention, too. Explain things to me. I don't know your medical terminology, your abbreviations and initials, so let us communicate in plain, simple language. At the same time realize that I am having trouble giving voice to my fears, and I may not be able to take everything at once. Piecemeal may be best, and allowing family and friends to convey some of the hard news can help. Openness is essential to holding my trust.

Repetition also helps me master my fears. Many patients comprehend written explanations better because they can be studied at leisure. However, it is not enough to list, for example, all of the possible dangers of an operation. I want the questions raised by the possibilities also answered. So please forgive my continual "whys" but understand that they are necessary to my acceptance of events.

Honesty and humaneness combined with empathy for my problems—these are the qualities I look for in you. Help me take the necessary risks by caring about each individual who passes through your hands.

You don't have to love me; I realize you are a sensitive person who has feelings to protect. But don't deny your humanity either. Don't try to hide your feelings under a hard exterior. Treat me and care for me as you would want for yourself. It is a just and ethical principle as true today as when the ancient healers first handed it down.

Sensitivity to people's psychological needs has always been essential to healing the sick. Under today's pressures and urban stresses the patient requires reassurance of compassionate care from everyone in the medical environment. The plea here is the plea of everyone: Care for me as an individual in a setting that scares me, makes me feel lost and alone, and is as foreign to me as it is familiar to you. We hope that this dramatization will reinforce the dedication of our clinic and hospital staffs, no matter what your jobs, to the patients' well being.

COMMUNICATION AND PAIN

Lillian Dangott
B. C. Thornton
Paul Page

The sensation of pain is difficult to communicate, even though it is an almost universally shared experience. Research indicates that individual pain levels vary so drastically that there is confusion in establishing common reference points (15, p. 9; 20, p. 20). As shown by communicators' general concern and research on health related matters (see 6), it has been recognized that the health professional needs to discover ways to communicate about pain in such a way

Reprinted with permission from the authors from *Journal of Communication* 28 (1978): 1.

that supportive interaction, commonality, and rapport are established while the health care is being administered.

Clinical observations of patients suggest that the experience of pain is highly related to the individual's personal anxiety level, anticipation, and personal pain thresholds (2, 15, 19, 20, 24). Equally important are environmental distractions, security, and trust, which play a major part in the degree of pain experienced by the patient. Additionally, social interactions, both verbal and nonverbal, can weave together the patient's physiological and psychological experiences to either subdue or exaggerate pain sensations (17, p. 283).

Research on the interaction between the health professional and patient on the subject of pain is in preliminary stages. Baer, Davitz and Lieb (1) administered a hypothetical paired-item scale to 74 social workers, nurses, and doctors to study how the health professional reacted to verbal and nonverbal pain indicators. The results of the study indicated that of the three groups, the social workers were more attentive to pain indications because, the authors suggest, the latter group has closer contact with the patient and is supposedly trained to be aware of both verbal and nonverbal communication signals. Other signals confirm that there are nonspecific clues regarding pain which are given to the attending health professional (3, p. 119).

In a more general research project on nonverbal cues in a dental office, Plainfield (16) found that the decor and arrangement of the office, as well as the nonverbal messages the patient receives from the manner, the facial expressions, and the gestures of the dentist, influenced behavior.

Coulthard and Ashby concluded from their study that "the most frequent types of exchange are doctor-initiated information-seeking exchanges rather than patient-initiated information-giving exchanges . . . the development of the discourse is tightly controlled by the doctor . . ." (7, p. 142). At the same time, the role of expressive and communicative aspects of the patient relationship are underestimated in importance by the medical profession (8).

The difficulties in the communication between health professional and patient were accentuated in a detailed report by Nash (14, p. 81). This hospital-based study of emotional communication between client and professional indicated that ill patients often do not hear what is said to them by the health professional, which suggests that the presence of pain itself hinders communications.

The professional has an additional communication problem with patients: that of not sharing the same language. Vowles (26) describes the common prefessional school situation where the student spends his/her academic career learning to speak technical jargon which consequently decreases the ability to communicate about illness with patients in language they can understand. Jan (12) states that in the medical-dental setting there is a misunderstanding of the way words are used, and suggests avoiding words that suggest pain or which increase anxiety. Spaan (23) re-emphasizes that a word used in a medical office may not mean the same thing to the professional as it does to the patient.

Other studies which indicate that communication is affected by the use of technical jargon include Collins (5); Skipper, Mauksch and Tagliacozzo (22); Korsch, Gozzi and Frances (13); Boyle (4) and Golden and Johnson (10).

Boyles' research found that even simple terms such as heartburn, palpitations and jaundice were understood differently by doctors and patients. An additional finding was that doctors did not share the same meanings of these terms *within* their profession. Golden and Johnson (10) reported on observations of 25 physician-patient interactions. They found that only one physician of the 25 made any attempt to determine if the patient had understood explanations or prescriptions correctly. This study emphasizes the contention of Fuller and Quesada (9) that most health professionals do not understand the process of feedback or reciprocal communication. Rossiter (18) explores several key issues which must be considered in defining "therapeutic communication," one of which is that communication itself can have healing effects. The literature suggests the serious communication problems existing between the health providers and patients and the need for development of a more effective paradigm of interaction.

A group of 20 dentists and a control group of 10 other professionals (physicians, nurses, and medical technologists) were interviewed. In order to analyze the information from the interviews, we chose the "confirming and disconfirming classification scheme" suggested by Sieburg (21, p. 129) because it provided for both nonverbal and verbal reported behaviors and an interactional perspective of the communication process. According to Sieburg a confirming situation describes "a whole constellation of behaviors that have a postive or therapeutic effect upon the receiver." For interactions to be positive, a feeling of recognition, acknowledgement, and endorsement must be conveyed (21, p. 131). Although this does not necessarily mean praise or agreement, and includes struggling through pain and disagreement, a confirming communication recognizes other persons as unique, with an acceptance of individuality, and expresses concern and a willingness to become involved with the other person.

A disconfirming communication, by contrast, expresses indifference, misunderstanding, and a denial of the other's experience. It reflects "unawareness of others, misperception of them, rejection of their attempt to communicate, denial of their self-experience or disaffiliation with them" (21, p. 138).

In a pilot study using this categorization scheme, we developed a third category, the category of "mixed messages," which indicates messages that were in part both confirming or disconfirming.

Thirty persons from the health professions were interviewed, 20 of whom were dentists. The dental profession was emphasized since this specialty is often associated with discomfort or pain. The ten other professional included lab technicians, physicians, and nurses.

Each person was interviewed by individuals trained in interviewing techniques, the average interview lasting at least 30 minutes. The interviews were tape-recorded with permission. In each of the interviews, persons were asked what they "said and did to a patient when they were going to have to inflict pain." They were then asked if they "communicated differently with a child than they did if the patient was an adult." They were allowed to respond to these questions in an open-ended manner. Interviews were transcribed and categorized according to confirming, disconfirming, or mixed messages.

For example, if the style of the professional was to use disconfirming messages for the adult, this kind of message was also used for the child. The messages were similar throughout the sample for both adults and children for 29 out of the 30 professionals interviewed.

A second finding was that only three of the professionals referred to the use of nonverbal behaviors in communicating about pain. Eighty percent of the professionals in our sample had a prevalent attitude of *denial* of patient pain. For example, one dentist said, "My patients don't have pain." Another dentist stated, "Only once every five years or so do I have a patient who has pain."

Even those professionals who recognized the patient's pain often used communication styles which were disconfirming in other aspects. For example, they said they often limited themselves strictly to transmitting information to the patient with no expectation or desire for feedback. One said: "You just tell them that it is going to hurt and they accept it. You are factual about it." Another said: "Try to be straight-forward and tell them that it is going to hurt a little bit. They understand usually." Both examples show the health professional's primary concern with giving information only. Emotions, questions, empathy, or reactions are not encouraged.

The health professionals who used the disconfirming approach carefully avoided the word "pain." "Bee sting" or "pinch" were the most commonly used euphemisms. Discomfirming communication was the mode of communication most often categorized. The authoritarian nature of that kind of communication is seen in the following examples:

> "*I assume that I am not going to inflict pain and I treat the patient that way.*" (dentist)
> "*I don't think you really have to inflict pain* . . . *physicians really hurt patients more than dentists.*" (dentist)
> "*The patient's mental attitude is the biggest problem. I don't think there is that much pain involved with it, but* they think they are going to have pain so some of them actually feel pain when they don't have any." (dentist) (our emphasis)

These disconfirming communications do not allow the other person the opportunity for a response. Rather, the patient is told how he/she should feel.

Social values and attitudes can reinforce the difficulty that professionals have in this area of communicating about pain. Ivan Illich, in his recent controversial book *The Medical Nemesis* (11), speculates that our culture ignores the reality of pain and has made pain into a technical matter. It, therefore, can become almost a sign of failure to the health professional.

Denial of the existence of pain and disconfirming messages obviously do not solve the patient's pain problem, for pain is a reality that is inescapable in many health situations. And a cook-book approach to interactions between the health professional and patient would simply imply mechanical and impersonal communication. However, we would like to suggest that therapeutic messages derived from a positive model would be something like: "This shot is uncomfortable (or painful) for some people; let me know how it is for you," or, "It is difficult for me to know how this is going to feel to you; I want you to let me know."

In situations where the patient is unable to talk, the professional can communicate using nonverbal interactions. "Yes-no questions" can be utilized to understand the patient's situation. The patient can then reply to the questions by blinking the eyes, nodding the head, etc. A straightforward message is not suggestive to the patient as long as it inquires into the patient's experience and does not indicate specifics. In these example, not only is information transmitted, but the patients are encouraged to express themselves, thereby establishing a two-way interaction which allows them to communicate their experience in their own terms. These behaviors we have suggested can be utilized in developing a more confirming paradigm for communication in health care.

REFERENCES

1. Baer, Eva, Lois J. Davitz, and Renee Lieb. "Inference of Physical Pain and Psychological Stress." *Nursing Research* 19, 1970, pp. 388–392.
2. Baldwin, DeWitt and M. Weisenberg. "The Role of Psychological Factors in Reducing Patient Reaction to Pain." Unpublished paper, University of Nevada, Reno, April 1977.
3. Blitz, Bernard. "The Role of Sensory Restriction in Problems with Chronic Pain." *Journal of Chronic Diseases* 19, 1966, pp. 119–125.
4. Boyle, C. M. "Differences Between Patients' and Doctors' Interpretation of Some Common Medical Terms." *British Medical Journal* ii, 1970, pp. 286–289.
5. Collins, E. "Do We Really Advise The Patient"? *Journal of The Florida Medical Association* 42, 1955, pp. 111–115.
6. Costello, Daniel E. "Health Communication Theory and Research: An Overview." In Brent D. Ruben (Ed.) *Communication Yearbook I.* New Jersey: Transaction Books, 1977, pp. 557–567.
7. Coulthard, Malcom and Margaret Ashby. "Talking with the Doctor, I." *Journal of Communication* 25, Summer 1975, pp. 140–147.
8. Daly, Mary and B. Hulka. "Talking with the Doctor, 2." *Journal of Communication* 25, Summer 1975, pp. 148–152.
9. Fuller, David S. and Gustavo M. Quesada. "Communication In Medical Therapeutics." *Journal of Communication* 23, 1973, pp. 361–370.
10. Golden, J. S. and G. D. Johnson. "Problems of Distortion in Doctor-Patient Communications." *Psychiatry In Medicine I,* 1970, pp. 127–149.
11. Illich, Ivan. *The Medical Nemesis.* New York: Pantheon Books, 1976.
12. Jan, Howard R. "General Semantic Orientation in Dentist-Patient Relations." *Journal of the American Dental Association* 68, 1964, pp. 424–429.
13. Korsch, B. M, E. K. Gozzi and V. Frances. "Gaps In Doctor-Patient Interaction and Satisfaction." *Pediatrics* 42, 1969, pp. 855–871.
14. Nash, Helen. "Perception of Vocal Expression of Emotion by Hospital Staff and Patients." *Genetic Psychology Monographs* 89, 1974, pp. 25–87.
15. Pace, J. Blair. "Psychophysiology of Pain: Diagnostic and Therapeutic Implication." *Journal of Family Practice I,* 1974, pp. 9–13.
16. Plainfield, S. "Communication Distortion: The Language of Patient Practitioners of Dentistry." *Journal of Prosthetic Dentistry* 22, 1969, pp. 11–19.

17. Riegel, Michelle Galler. "Pain Control Through Hypnosis." *Science News* 110, 1976, pp. 283–285.
18. Rossiter, Charles M. "Defining Therapeutic Communication." *Journal of Communication* 25, Summer 1975, pp. 127–130.
19. Serjeant, Richard. *The Spectrum of Pain.* London: Rupert, Hart-Davis, 1969.
20. Shealy, C. Norman. *The Pain Game.* Millbrae, California: Celestial Arts, 1976.
21. Sieburg, Evelyn. "Confirming and Disconfirming Organizational Communication." In James Owen, Paul Page, and Gordon Zimmerman (Eds.) *Communication in Organizations.* San Francisco: West Publishing, 1976, pp. 129–149.
22. Skipper, J. K., H. O. Mauksch, and D. Tagliacozzo. "Some Barriers Between Patients and Hospital Functionaries." *Nursing Forum* 2, 1963, pp. 14–23.
23. Spaan, Robert C. "A Tooth Is a Tooth . . . Aristotle; A Tooth Is Not a Tooth . . . Korzybski." *Journal of the Oklahoma Dental Association* 68, 1964, pp. 424–429.
24. Sternbach, R. A. *Pain: A Psychophysiological Analysis.* New York: Academic Press, 1968.
25. Stewart, John. *Bridges Not Walls,* Menlo Park, California: Addison-Wesley, 1973.
26. Vowles, Keith O. "Development of a Communication Course for Undergraduate Dental Students." Unpublished master's thesis, San Francisco State College, 1970.

6.

THE GROUP HEALTH COMMUNICATION CONTEXT

Dr. G. S. Edwards is a well-known oncologist who is determined to make the detection and treatment of cancer bearable and even humane. She has developed an effective team approach, utilizing the particular skills of a receptionist with counseling training and three nurses trained in oncological nursing. This approach is designed to do much more than treat the purely physiological aspects of the tumor and to include the patient and his or her family's well-being.

The doctor's office serves as the hub of a wheel. The receptionist and chemotherapy room are within steps and Dr. Edwards is almost instantly available for consultation if necessary. The nurses and the receptionist-counselor are trained by the doctor in communication, cancer, and chemotherapy. These members of the team often answer initial client questions or serve as intermediaries if the doctor is out of the office. Clients calling the office are always able to talk to a member of the oncology team. Quite often, Dr. Edwards will interrupt whatever she is doing to take these phone calls. At least a majority of the same staff sees the client on each visit.

The examining room is in the doctor's cheerful office and family members stay in the room with a curtain separating them from the doctor and the client during the examination unless the client directs otherwise. Notetaking is common. Family members are encouraged to accompany the client. Often, hours are spent educating the family regarding the various treatment alternatives. The theory utilized is that well-educated clients and family members can be capable participants in the decision-making and treatment phases. Families are taught to become active in the treatment process. If shots are required, for example, they learn to give these shots in Dr. Edwards' arm, which psychologically removes much of the threat of this procedure. During the twenty-four hours after the first treatment, the doctor often makes a house call to check on both client and family. Later, during treatment, the receptionist-counselor might also visit the client in home or hospital settings.

The members of the oncology team are chosen carefully. The receptionist-counselor has conducted support groups and worked in other health care settings. The nurses were carefully picked for their concern about clients, their relaxed manner, and their ability to communicate. The team members report that they like each other and feel trust in their professional relationships. Meetings are held on a daily basis and the doctor listens carefully as well as participates. She is quite aware that the client provides different kinds of information to each team member and it is during the meetings that all the information is integrated and put to use for the client's benefit.

Family members also report feeling part of the extended family effort. They credit the initial time spent educating them regarding the illness as reassuring during the whole treatment. Additionally, being involved gives them something to do at a time when most of them are feeling useless and frustrated. They also note that neither they nor the client have to call the doctor often during the treatment process because of the adequate preparation (even though the doctor has provided them with her home telephone number).

The report of the client and the family, however, is most important. Dr. Edwards' clients do not follow the usual national pattern where large numbers drop out of chemotherapy during the treatments. Rarely do her clients refuse to complete the treatments. In addition, they report reduced side effects. The clients credit open communication and the team process with giving them needed support and more bearable treatments.

Dr. Edwards is candid about the advantage of the team system. Time spent initially with the client and the family prevents excessive phone calls to the physician, and having a fully functioning team shares pressure, and allows her to supervise and be more aware of the overall client regime and profile. It also frees her to keep up to date professionally and to work with her colleagues. She particularly stresses that the time taken with clients by team members induces client cooperation during the treatment regime, which in turn reduces morbidity and raises the response rate to the treatment because of better patient toleration. Clearly, this physician's office operates as an effective health-related small group.*

GROUP COMMUNICATION IN HEALTH CARE

The small group has been a fascinating element of social organization since people learned that working together for a goal could be beneficial.

In health settings there are many different kinds of groups. One of the most important of these is the health team where professionals work together for the client's benefit, often with the client and family as members of the team.

Other innovative groups are the many self-help groups. Alchoholics Anonymous and La Leche are examples of how people are organizing groups around their needs. These groups are often started by persons anxious to find others who share the same problems they do. Problem-identification and solution are important parts of self-help groups. Additionally, the groups' strength lies in giving the members a chance to share case histories and personal problems. Self-help groups do not always involve the health professional even though the group's reason for being is health related. Often, however, groups are also being formulated and utilized in health care settings. In these groups health providers work with families or clients regarding special problems. Colostomy groups and rehabilitation groups are examples. In these groups patients are provided with important support mechanisms.

The material presented in this chapter on such variables as leadership and roles should be applicable to all facets of group communication in the team, self-help, and educational group settings. The information provided in this chapter is designed to help all health related small groups function better and more efficiently.

Usually some kind of thought is given as to whether a problem can best be solved by an individual or a group before a group is formed. Figure 6.1 gives some assistance in making a decision of this kind.

Note that the problems that are best suited to group solution are more complex, demand more expertise, and generally require a higher degree of responsibility than do the problem situations that are better suited to an individual problem solver.

---

*This health care team is based at the Santa Barbara Clinic in Santa Barbara, California. Actual names are used.

Figure 6.1   Criteria for Choosing a Group or Individual Problem-Solving Technique

Group Solutions are Best	*Individual Solutions Are Best*
1. If there are many steps to the solution.	1. If there are just a few steps to the solution.
2. If there are many aspects to the problem.	2. If there are just a few aspects to the problem.
3. If the problem is impersonal.	3. If the problem is personal.
4. If the problem is of moderate difficulty.	4. If the problem is simple.
5. If several people are needed to provide the information to solve the problem.	5. If information to solve the problem can be provided by one person.
6. If the problem requires divisions of labor.	6. If the problem does not require divisions of labor.
7. If the problem requires several solutions.	7. If the problem requires just one solution.
8. If a great deal of time is required for solution of the problem.	8. If a small amount of time is required for solution of the problem.
9. If individuals have to assume a great deal of responsibility for the solution.	9. If individuals do not need to assume a great deal of responsibility.
10. If attitudes regarding the problem are going to be many and complex.	10. If attitudes toward the problem are going to be simple.
11. If it is likely group members will engage in task oriented behaviors.	11. If individuals will not be task oriented.

Social and Task Dimensions

While groups are usually established for a particular purpose such as providing health care to a client or serving as a management team for a health organization, every group has two built-in tasks: completing the group assignment and maintaining the group's process and "social being". These tasks are often called the *social* and *task* dimensions. The social dimension is often overlooked in planning and research indicates that this lack of planning is always a mistake. Humans are social beings and they have many relationship needs such as the expression of emotion. The *socio-emotional* climate which takes these needs into consideration is very important if the group is to function effectively. To determine the social, emotional and/or psychological needs of individual members of the group, time has to be allocated within the group to explore these needs. The communication process is the vehicle by which members can do this. As group or team members understand the needs of others, behaviors interlock and members constrain their behavior while fitting into the group patterns. As the group develops, certain members will play roles that help or hinder the socio-emotional dimensions of the group. The socio-emotional factors are often overlooked by health professionals, though they are the most important part of the group, on the grounds that they are too busy to participate.

In the task dimension, groups are able to move efficiently only if they have *not* been negligent of the socio-emotional aspects. Research indicates that groups that work well together can perform more difficult tasks than those that do not. Additionally, groups that offer satisfaction to their members either through having a job done well or through simple task achievement are more successful. The three factors associated with group interaction that have some bearing on personal satisfaction and group effectiveness are:

1. Opportunities for participation
2. Effectiveness or quality of participation
3. Perceived consequences of participation.

A communication climate which is *supportive* rather than *defensive* produces groups that fulfill the task and socio-emotional dimensions of the group more productively. Supportive climates are characterized by

Figure 6.2   Supportive and Defensive Communication Climates

Supportive Climates	Defensive Climates
1. Description	1. Evaluation
2. Problem Orientation	2. Control
3. Spontaneity	3. Strategy
4. Empathy	4. Neutrality
5. Equality	5. Superiority
6. Provisionalism	6. Certainty

From Gibb, Jack R., "Defensive Communication." *Journal of Communication* 11, 1961, p. 147.

being nonjudgmental, cooperatively independent, empathetic, and willing to experiment and be spontaneous. They reinforce participative planning and actions. Defensive climates are the opposite. They are judgmental, manipulative, emotionally neutral and dogmatic.[2] (See Figure 6.2.) Unfortunately, most health related settings are defensive ones; however, the oncological office of Dr. Edwards, discussed at the beginning of the chapter, exemplifies a supportive climate. The people who work in that office have a daily morning or evening meeting to discuss work allocation and client needs. When clients come to the office they are questioned by all members of the health team and the important information is later informally or formally shared. All of these are supportive rather than defensive activities.

Roles

Roles in groups emerge around the social and task dimensions. A *role* is a position in an interlocking network of positions in a group. Generally a role is defined in terms of the person occupying the role rather than by preordained actions. For example, nurses have roles to play in hospitals but each nurse in the hospital enacts that role in a different way.

Roles are often categorized as *task, maintenance,* or *self-centered.* Role emergence takes place over time and often group members play several roles. Roles can also change over the group's life span. Task roles involve such actions as initiating, giving information, seeking opinions, and being the person who elaborates and clarifies. Examples of task roles can be seen in Figure 6.3.

Maintenance roles involve the socio-emotional climate. Here group members support, harmonize, and give expression to relationship feelings. Persons playing these roles sometimes act as "gatekeepers" who keep channels of communication open as tension relievers or compromisers. Examples of maintenance roles can also be seen in Figure 6.3.

Another group of members will play self-centered roles such as dominator or confessor. Self-centered roles often disrupt the effective functioning of the group and detract from group effectiveness. Self-centered roles should be discouraged in groups, while task and maintenance roles should be encouraged. (See Figure 6.3 for examples of self-centered roles.)

While many roles are necessary for a fully functioning team, it is important to recognize that each member does not need to play all roles. In fact, in some of the most effective health care groups, roles are clearly delineated even when they overlap. In the oncology office referred to in this chapter, the physician has the medical knowledge and is the

Figure 6.3   Group Roles

Group task roles help the group accomplish its jobs; group maintenance roles help the group solve its socio-emotional problems.

Group Task Role Examples

1. *Initiator-Contributor*: Contributes ideas and suggestions; proposes solutions, decisions, new ideas, or restates old ideas in novel ways.
2. *Information Seeker*: Asks for clarification in terms of the accuracy of comments, asks for information or facts relevant to accomplishing group tasks, suggests information if needed for decisions.
3. *Information Giver*: Offers facts or generalizations which may relate to personal experiences and are pertinent to the group task.
4. *Opinion Seeker*: Asks for clarification of group members' opinions, and asks how group members feel.
5. *Opinion Giver*: States beliefs and opinions about suggestions made, indicates what the group's attitude should be.
6. *Elaborator-Clarifier*: Elaborates ideas and other contributions, offers rationales for suggestions, tries to deduce how an idea or suggestion would work if adopted by the group.
7. *Coordinator*: Clarifies relationships among information, opinions, and ideas, or suggests an integration of ideas.
8. *Diagnostician*: Indicates what the task oriented problems are.
9. *Orienter-Summarizer*: Summarizes interaction, points out departures from agreed upon goals, brings group back to the central issues, raises questions about the direction in which the group is headed.
10. *Energizer*: Prods the group to action.
11. *Procedure Developer*: Handles routine tasks such as seating arrangements, obtaining equipment, and handing out pertinent papers, etc.
12. *Secretary*: Keeps notes on the group's progress.
13. *Evaluator-Critic*: Analyzes the group's accomplishments, checks to see if consensus has been reached.

Maintenance Role Examples

1. *Supporter-Encourager*: Praises, agrees with, and accepts the contributions of others; offers warmth, solidarity and recognition.
2. *Harmonizer*: Reconciles and mediates differences, reduces tensions by giving group members a chance to explore their disagreements.
3. *Tension Reliever*: Jokes, or in some other way reduces formality of interaction, relaxes the group members.
4. *Compromiser*: Offers to compromise when his or her own ideas are in conflict, admits own errors so as to maintain group cohesion.
5. *Gatekeeper*: Keeps communication channels open, facilitates interaction between some group members and blocks interaction between others.

Fig. 6.3 (*cont'd*)

6. *Feeling Expresser*: Makes explicit the feelings, moods and other relation-ships in the group; shares own feelings with others.
7. *Standard Setter*: Expresses standards in evaluating the group process and standards for the group to achieve.
8. *Follower*: Goes along with the movement of the group passively, accept-ing the ideas of others, sometimes serving as an audience for group interaction.

Self-Centered Role Examples

1. *Blocker*: Interferes with progress by rejecting ideas or taking the negative stand on any and all issues; refuses to cooperate.
2. *Aggressor*: Struggles for status by defining the status of others; boasts; criticizes.
3. *Deserter*: Withdraws in some way; remains indifferent, aloof, sometimes formal; daydreams; wanders from the subject; engages in irrelevant side conversations.
4. *Dominator*: Interrupts and embarks on long monologues; authoritative; tries to monopolize the group's time.
5. *Recognition Seeker*: Attempts to gain attention in an exaggerated manner; usually boasts about past accomplishments; relates irrelevant personal experiences, usually in an attempt to gain sympathy.
6. *Confessor*: Engages in irrelevant personal catharsis; uses the group to work out own mistakes and feelings.
7. *Playboy*: Displays a lack of involvement in the group through inappro-priate humor, horseplay, or cynicism.
8. *Special-Interest Pleader*: Acts as the representative for another group; engages in irrelevant behavior.

Source: K. Benne and P. Sheats, "Functional Roles of Group Members." *Journal of Social Issues* 4 (1948): 41–49, with permission from the Society for the Psychological Study of Social Issues.

group leader. The receptionist-counselor is in charge of business details and the client's statistics, and the nurses give efficient and caring treatment. However, all team members overlap in providing social and emotional support to the clients, the families, and each other.

Leadership

Nowhere in America is hierarchy and status more evident than in health care. In most small groups in the health care area the physician is auto-matically the leader through ascribed status. That is, he or she is made leader by simple virtue of occupation. This is not the case in most groups, however, where leadership emerges over time. In fact, groups such as health care teams with designated physician leaders often develop informal leadership which bypasses the physician.[3]

In this case the leadership role is usually given by the group to the person who has provided the group with the most assistance in meeting its goals. While there are many kinds of leaders it is important to recognize how each leader uses his or her power. For example, does the leader have the ability to coerce others or to provide the leadership that allows latitude among members in decision-making? Gouran sees a leader as a person using his or her power to move or influence a group toward perceived goals through verbal and nonverbal communication[4]

Power in small groups has been studied and it has been determined that there are many kinds. It is important that leaders be able to recognize their own power as well as the power of group members. Some leaders, in fact, achieve a *halo effect* in which all their personal attributes are desired by others to the point where values formerly denigrated become valued.[5] An example of this would be the venerated surgeon in the hospital setting.

There are generally three major leadership styles; autocratic, democratic, and laissez-faire. These three leadership styles vary in the degree of control they exert over group process and decision-making. Each of the three leadership styles have marked advantages and disadvantages for different group situations.

Autocratic leaders are very dominant and wield strong authority over group members. Autocratic leaders tell group members what to do and how to do it. Sometimes autocratic leaders even watch the group members work to make sure they follow orders correctly. Autocratic leadership is probably the most common form of leadership in most health care settings, due to the high pressure climate and the control the doctors and administrators hold over others.

The major benefits of autocratic leadership are clear lines of authority, strong control, quick decisions, quick response time of group, and the ability of an expert leader to direct novice group members in complex or emergency tasks. However, the detriments of autocratic leadership may often outweigh its advantages. Some of these disadvantages include the hindering of creativity by group members, failure to utilize the knowledge and expertise of group members, dehumanization of group members, and resultant lack of motivation by group members to abide by decisions. Autocratic leadership should only be used in emergency health care situations or where group members lack adequate knowledge of health care methods.

Democratic leadership attempts to share authority appropriately with all group members. The democratic leader elicits information from all group members and asks for their participation in decision-making. Often the democratic leader seeks consensus among group members for decision-making, or if consensus is unreachable, he or she seeks a majority vote.

Some of the advantages of democratic leadership include active participation by all members, sharing of member expertise, generating a great deal of information, and motivating involvement and support of membership. Disadvantages of the democratic style include the generation of extensive conflict by airing different perspectives, the length of time required to hear all member opinions, the frustration of slow, labored decision-making, and the potential for majority cliques outvoting and manipulating smaller cliques. Democratic leadership is best used in complex problem-solving situations where a great deal of information and expertise is needed to make nonemergency decisions. For example, long range planning for an urban medical center should utilize democratic group processes with group members representing several relevant groups within the hospital and its environment. Democratic leadership is also prevalent in most self-help groups.

Laissez-faire leaders delegate authority to group members. Of all of the leadership styles, laissez-faire is the most misunderstood and maligned. Often it is thought of as a "weak" form of leadership. In practice, however, laissez-faire leadership often requires the greatest strength of a leader. The leader must be confident enough in his or her group members to allow them to make decisions on their own. The leader provides the group members with information and is available for problem solving but generally gives authority to the group for taking care of business.

Advantages of laissez-faire leadership inlcude encouraging the growth and development of group members and the fostering of creative decision making. Disadvantages of laissez-faire leadership occur when the leader doesn't adequately prepare group members to work on their own or when group members are unable to handle the demands of the job and either take advantage of the situation or flounder in the performance of the job. Laissez-faire leadership is best suited to well-trained, sophisticated, professional groups of people who can handle the demands of their jobs. An example of laissez-faire leadership might be in an occupational therapy department of a community health organization, where the department head assigns each therapist a case load and allows them to decide the best means of treatment but remains available to help with problem-solving.

No one leadership style is ever correct for all health care situations. The most competent leaders are able to adapt their leadership style to the particular group of people they are working with and the specific situations they are confronting. Situational leadership enables the leader to utilize the strengths of each style.

Lastly, one of the most important functions of the leader is to encourage group members to have responsibility for the group's success. This can be done in part by clarifying group responsibility and member roles to the satisfaction of group members during different phases of the group's existence.

As mentioned earlier, there can be separate task and socio-emotional leaders in groups though effective leaders are often efficient in both dimensions. Leadership emerges over time along with roles, conflict, and other aspects of group life. Leadership skills can be learned, particularly through a study of communication processes.

CONFLICT IN GROUPS

The perspective group members have regarding conflict greatly affects group life. If conflict is seen as being constructive the group will attempt to understand and manage it; if it is seen as destructive, it must be quickly resolved and controlled. The first approach allows for management, the second calls for dissolution.

Conflict in groups (or for that matter interpersonal conflict) is caused by many external and internal factors. Controversies over attempts to influence group members as well as attempts to influence a group's direction are often responsible for conflict. In the process of creative conflict resolution communication needs to be encouraged. What is initially important, is to decide who and what is in conflict.[6] Conflict is observable and can be studied. For example, one can look at the interaction patterns of groups.

In defining a type of conflict it is important to note if it is *affective* (emotional) or *substantive* (intellectual opposition).[7] It is, however, only in climates of mutual regard that conflict can be seen as issue-oriented, which is the most useful kind of conflict. Strategies used by people facing conflict are many. They have been reviewed by Frost and Wilmot (1978) and much of the following material is abstracted from their book.[8]

There are four primary conflict strategies people employ. *Avoidance* excludes active struggle. Those practicing this strategy sometimes refuse to talk, or they leave the conflict setting. The avoidance of conflict in initial stages is common in health organizations where the benefits of conflict are not recognized. Changing the subject is a common avoidance tactic. *Escalation* can include such tactics as labeling, increasing the intensity of the struggle, and yelling or violence. It can also include a purposeful expansion of the issue beyond its legitimate limits. Coalition formation can also cause escalation. *Reduction* is a conflict strategy designed to lessen the conflict. Again, if one's perspective is that conflict can be healthy and creative for a group this is not always an effective technique since issues and needs need to surface before the problem can be understood and resolved. A nurse who tells his or her colleagues that a breakdown in communication is not important is using a reduction technique. *Maintenance*, the last conflict strategy we will discuss, keeps the conflict at a tension level which is manageable to each of the combatants. Maintenance tactics are designed to equalize the power of the participants or to gain symmetry. An example of a maintenance technique is the "quid pro quo" in which each party gets something for something.[9] Hospitals and other health care settings need to train their employees to recognize and use useful conflict strategies.

All of the conflict strategies discussed can be utilized by dyads as well as by small groups. Group conflict, however, becomes more complicated when different members are using different conflict strategies and the strategies are accompanied by emotions such as anger. Anger is usually the vehicle by which conflict is expressed in groups and while it can sap energy from groups it can also galvanize conflict resolution. In order to be used in a positive way, anger needs to be recognized as a legitimate emotion which will not destroy the group or its members if it is used ethically. Anger is particularly difficult to deal with in hierarchical settings such as health care where power resides at the top. Subordinates fear expressing anger because of unequal power, yet suppressing anger may be more detrimental to the group than expressing it. As hospitals and private offices deal with the problem of nurse retention it is important that they realize the anger nurses have toward their place in the health care hierachy. Dealing with this anger would be cost efficient for these organizations.

Conflict can be both productive and destructive for groups. The destructive aspects of conflict are usually emphasized more than the positive aspects. Often people fail to recognize the opportunities afforded by group conflict. In fact, in the case of "group think," where group members go along with what they think is the will of the group, conflict is crucial if the group is to make a good decision. Conflict over a problem solution will allow group members to see different aspects of the solution and will offer the group different individual evaluations.

There are six primary benefits of group conflict that people normally do not consider. They are:

1. Conflict acts as a smoke-detector for the group, often helping group members to identify larger underlying problems that should be addressed by the group.
2. Conflict acts as a safety-valve for the group, releasing tension and anger for the group and its membership.
3. Conflict encourages interaction and involvement of group members in discussing issues of concern to the group.
4. Conflict promotes creative behavior by group members, encouraging group members' search for solutions to problems.
5. Conflict promotes the sharing of relevant information among group members, by encouraging the voicing of disparate ideas.
6. Conflict tests the strength of group members' ideas and their potential problem solutions under fire, by arguing the relative merits of proposed ideas and solutions.

One of the most effective techniques for looking at anger, power, and thus conflict in small groups is *process observation*. As discussed in Chapter 2, there are two levels of each communicative act: content and relationship. The content level focuses on how members of the group present the basic information in the message. The relationship level refers to the feelings expressed, particularly through nonverbal channels. Process observation provides the group with a means of evaluating group communication by having an observer assess the group at both content and relationship levels. The observer can be a member of the group who acts as an observer for a particular session, or an outside observer who has no ties to the group. This observer reports back to the group at the end of the session on what he or she saw happening within the group. Process observers need some training in observation techniques; at the minimal level their need is to understand what the group wants from the observation.

Sometimes checklists or interaction analysis schemes are used for the observation. Most important, the processor must be nonevaluative and be able to describe what he or she saw. This material, presented to the group in a fair manner by an unbiased observer can often be the starting point for effective discussion of the conflict. It should be noted here that the role of the process observer should be clearly negotiated and understood by all the group members before process observation begins. The process observer and third-party negotiator roles can be separate or one and the same. If the observer is trained in negotiating skills, the two roles can sometimes be effectively combined. However, persons unskilled in arbitration should not undertake to solve a group's problem. Additionally, while members of the group can often undertake the observer's role, they cannot effectively act as negotiators of a conflict of which they may be part.

The negotiator has many strategies available for helping the group with conflict. First, he or she can assist the group in clarifying their goals as well as in the implementation on those goals. The negotiator can provide a safe atmosphere in the group for effective feedback. He or she can also assist group members in prioritizing and dealing with the problems as well as in equalizing power within the group at least for conflict resolution purposes. Techniques such as role reversal can sometimes be effective.

In attempting to resolve the conflict or to come to some form of conflict resolution, group members or the negotiator must think of strategies. Should everyone that is part of the conflict "win" in some way or should there be a *win–lose* outcome? It is even possible to structure a conflict situation in which everyone loses. These solutions are based in part on the solutions analyzed in game theory.[10]

Understanding the structure of the conflict assists in determining the solutions necessary. It also makes clear that parties to the conflict must have an equal say in determining the choices and the payoffs if the solution is going to be effective and permanent. It is important to develop a climate of openness, honest acceptance, and cohesiveness for conflict resolution. Getting to the roots of conflict in a group can be important. As Mabry and Barnes state, "Ultimately, members should feel good about their personal contribution to a group."[11] This feeling can take place in an atmosphere of debate or strong feelings as long as individual differences are respected.

Ethical conflict behaviors are also important to discuss in this closing section on conflict. In conflict situations, arguing the specific issue at hand rather than hidden agendas is an important fair-fighting technique. Additionally, in a supportive group atmosphere, violence, character attacks and "dirty-fighting" techniques should be avoided. On the positive side, it is important to construct reasonable arguments rather than emotional, unsubstantiated positions. Lastly, a "gamesman" win-at-all-costs mentality can be avoided by being open to the ideas of others for a *mutual-win* solution. Conflict is rarely a *zero-sum game* where one person must win at the expense of others.

Dealing with conflict in health care or other settings is time-consuming, but can be beneficial to the group if conducted ethically. Participants need to be educated in how to handle conflict well. We suggest that the time taken to educate individuals in effective conflict communication skills is overall very cost and energy efficient.

GROUP DECISION MAKING

As groups become more prominent in health care, decision making and problem solving become important. There are many models for understanding the process of making group decisions. It is important to remember that decision making is not always problem solving. For example, a decision by a group to disband their work fifteen minutes early on a Friday afternoon does not always have to do with a problem! Decisions have to do with the outcome of group interaction. A decision is the choice made by group members from alternative proposals available. A group reaches a decision as its members come to consensus. *Consensus has many meanings.* It can imply unanimous agreement, the will of the majority, or implicit agreement. *For practical purposes, it means a commitment to the decision reached.* It should be emphasized that commitment to a decision is a different step than the making of a decision.[12]

Groups, as well as individuals, go through processes or phases to reach their decisions. In Fisher's decision emergence scheme, ideas pass through the *orientation phase* where members socialize and relieve primary tension. In the *conflict phase* there is dispute and ideas are tested while coalitions develop. In the *emergence phase* there is much ambiguity in the group as members try to arrive at the "best" decision. This third and crucial stage marks the beginning of the eventual outcome of the group. In the *reinforcement phase* unity of opinion usually pervades over the decision as courses for group action are prescribed.[13]

Decision making is the first part of any problem-solving process. Problem solving usually involves several group decisions. *Problem solving is the name for communication techniques used for the purpose of decision making as well as for the carrying out of the decision.* We will discuss some decision-making techniques useful to all decision making in health care.

Communication problem-solving techniques are important for health care groups and for health care professionals. Some problems are best suited to group solution, while others are best suited to individual solution. We will examine problem solving from both an individual and a group perspective. These problem-solving techniques should be not confused with health oriented techniques such as the P.O.M.R. (Patient Oriented Medical Record). It is our intent here to discuss the particular formats that can enhance decision making in health care settings.

The problem solver must first decide what constitutes a problem. For example, the hospital administrator must decide whether tardiness of employees in the spring is due to a temporary change in the weather or whether it is indicative of an overall pattern more serious for the institution. A problem exists for an individual when he or she becomes aware of the obstacle or obstacles to obtaining an objective or goal. Problems can involve familiar or unfamiliar material as well as subjective or objective material. Problem solving is both an ability and a process. One of the most successful problem-solving methods has the following steps which are adapted from John Dewey's reflective thinking by Tubbs (1978):

I. Problem Phase

    A. Identification of problem area, including such questions as:

        1. What is the situation in which the problem is occurring?
        2. What, in general, is the difficulty?
        3. How did this difficulty arise?
        4. What is the importance of the difficulty?
        5. What limitations, if any, are there on the areas of our concern?
        6. What is the meaning of any terms that need clarifying?

    B. Analysis of the difficulty:

        1. What, specifically, are the facts of the situation?
        2. What, specifically, are the difficulties?

    C. Analysis of causes:

        1. What is causing the difficulties?
        2. What is causing the causes?

II. Criteria Phase

    A. What are the principal requirements of the solution?

    B. What limitations must be placed on the solution?

    C. What is the relative importance of the criteria?

III. Solution Phase

    A. What are the possible solutions?

        1. What is the exact nature of each solution?
        2. How would it remedy the difficulty? By eliminating the cause? By offsetting the effect? By a combination of both?

    B. How good is each solution?

        1. How well would it remedy the difficulty?

2. How well would it satisfy the criteria? Are there any that it would not satisfy?
3. Would there by any unfavorable consequences? Any extra benefits?

C. What solution appears to be best?

1. How would you rank the solution?
2. Would some combination of solutions be best?

IV. Implementation Phase

What steps would be taken to put the solution into effect?[14]

The single question form of problem solving is another alternative which has been researched by Larson and his colleagues. Looking at high-success and low-success groups, Larson derives this formula which Tubbs (1978) presents:

- What is the single question, the answer to which is all the group needs to know to accomplish its purpose?
- What subquestions must be answered before we can answer the single question we have formulated?
- Do we have sufficient information to answer confidently the subquestions?
- What are the most reasonable answers to the subquestions?[15]

Assuming that our answers to the subquestions are correct, what is the best solution to the problem?

The single question form emphasizes successful problem solving which focuses on obtaining solutions rather than getting bogged down with the trivial detail for the discussion.

Whatever decision-making strategy is used, brainstorming can be an important part of the decision-making process. This technique is used to generate ideas and to avoid polarized yes–no answers to problem-solving. Brainstorming encourages unique and creative solutions to problems. Ideas for brainstorming sessions are as follows:

Brainstorming

When brainstorming, it is important to get the group to abide by the following rules:

1. *Anything goes.* Get your ideas out and on paper. Sometimes wild ideas are the best ones or can be combined with other ideas for innovative solutions.

2. Don't be *evaluative* as the ideas are being presented. Just listen!

3. Think of as many ideas as you can. Allow the session to go on as long as possible. Brainstorming doesn't work when members have to rush to another meeting!

4. Record all ideas so that everyone can see them. Newsprint or blackboards are helpful.

5. Take a break between brainstorming and evaluation. When evaluation does take place be positive, fair, and go slowly toward your solution.

Because brainstorming starts out as nonevaluative it can prevent many of the difficulties that occur in groups when judgment of individuals or ideas is formulated in the early stages.

In summary, understanding group phases as well as such factors as leadership, conflict maintenance, role emergence, decision-making, and problem-solving are important to everyone who has ever been a part of a small group. Much of our work and play in today's world takes place in cooperative effort with others. An understanding of what makes people work well together is vital in order to be an effective group member. Continued research on the complexity of group phenomena is also important to help us identify and understand the interrelated group communication processes.

SPECIAL PROBLEMS OF HEALTH PROFESSIONALS IN TEAM SETTINGS

As can be seen from the previous discussion of small groups, interacting with others is complex. This complexity often becomes even more complicated in health care settings where high emotions, status differences, and time pressures interact. One of the major problems is that members of the health care teams often ignore the need for understanding when dealing with the important socio-emotional needs of team members such as power, roles, and feelings.

Additionally, there are two aspects of team decision making which are of particular importance. They are the structure of the team and the team barriers to communication. The structure refers to whether the team is hierarchical or egalitarian. (See the discussion of leadership in this chapter for an analogy.) Barriers to communication include many factors. For example, team members often have different perceptions of health which greatly affect team communication, particularly regarding service and inquiry. Even in the same field, some health training institutions emphasize service while others highlight research and verification. The two orientations provide much conflict.

In addition to different orientations, health providers working in groups often have different perceptions, methods, and treatment modalities. Blocks and distortions in communication have been reported.[16] Researchers found that persons from various professions even differed in their perception and evaluation of clients and their health conditions.

Another important point that affects communication in teams and groups is the information flow regarding the knowledge of another's field. Nagi (1971) postulates that because of the hierarchical status of health care team members, information is influenced by the relative status of the fields. He contends that the articulation of roles on teams comes about primarily as a result of accommodation of the lower status professions to those team or group members of higher status, a form of "legitimate power" referred to earlier in this chapter. His conclusion is that this limits the possibilities of reexamining the roles and realigning the boundaries of the different fields and professions for effective health care.[17] These factors mentioned are just a few of the many that cause problems for people working together in health groups or teams.

The focus in health team literature in the last ten years has been on decision-making and conflict management. Sources on health teams stress the importance of team members spending time with each other in order to better understand each other's planning. This, of course, provides another double-bind for health care providers who feel that their time should be spent in actual care giving rather than in solving team problems.

More recent literature stresses the problems of turf management and overlapping roles. As the team concept matures, innovative teams are learning to do rounds together, integrate chart notes and have weekly meetings.[18] Other information on health teams stresses the importance of teaching the team concepts in educational as well as practice settings.[19]

After three years of research on health teams, Thornton and her colleagues found that most of the team energy is spent trying to manage relationships within the teams. Team members are so concerned about structuring their interactions that not enough time is spent on the task or the social-emotional aspects of team development. A balance is certainly needed on teams between structure, content and process. Additionally, this research demonstrated that team training is vitally important for effective functioning.[20]

Whatever the problems of health teams, they have become important to client care. Health and medical literature abounds with references to teams. In additionally, all health professions are beginning to demand input into client care and the team is a vehicle for this input.

McGregor identifies eleven characteristics of effective teams:

1. The atmosphere tends to be informal, comfortable and relaxed.
2. There is a lot of discussion in which virtually everyone participates.
3. The task or the objective of the group is well understood and accepted by the members.
4. The members listen to each other.
5. There is disagreement.
6. Most decisions are reached by a kind of consensus.
7. Criticism is frequent, frank, and relatively comfortable.
8. People are free in expressing their ideas as well as their feelings.
9. When action is taken, clear assignments are made and accepted.
10. The chairman of the group (or team) does not dominate it, nor on the contrary, does the group defer unduly to him or her.
11. The group is self-conscious of its own operations.[21]

Source: From Douglas McGregor, *The Human Side of Enterprise.* Copyright © 1960 by McGraw-Hill. Reprinted by permission of McGraw-Hill.

NOTES

1. Mabry and Barnes, 1980, Section N.
2. Gibb, 1961, Section A.
3. Thornton, 1977, Section F.
4. Gouran, 1974, Section N.
5. Mabry and Barnes, 1980, pp. 155–157 Section N.
6. Fisher, 1974, p. 104, Section N.
7. Ibid., p. 105
8. Frost and Wilmot, 1978, Section N.
9. Ibid.
10. Ibid.
11. Mabry and Barnes, 1980, p. 193, Section N.
12. Fisher, 1974, p. 104, Section N.
13. Fisher, 1974, Section N.
14. Tubbs, 1978, pp. 229–30, Section N.
15. Ibid, pp. 232–233.
16. Frank, 1961, Section F.
17. Nagi, 1975, Section F.
18. Ibid.
19. Thornton et al. in Baldwin, Rowley and Williams, 1980, Section F.
20. Ibid.
21. McGregor, 1980, Section N.

READING

PREVIEW OF READING

The article, "The Hidden Barriers to Team Building," examines the process of developing team work among group members. Some of the problems hindering the development of teams are identified, and strategies for overcoming these problems are identified. The authors suggest the best groundwork for team building involves the establishment of shared knowledge, shared territory, equal status, and availability to interpersonal communication between all group members.

THE HIDDEN BARRIERS TO TEAM BUILDING

Patricia Palleschi
Patricia Heim

The room could have been any conference room. There were stark walls, no carpets and from the window a delightful view of an industrial park. The leader had arranged the chairs in an arc around the slide projector. As participants filed in, each left an empty spot as a buffer against the strangers already seated. Several had on business suits, some had on jeans and sneakers. One or two had on leisure suits. The purpose of the meeting was to engage in long-range planning, but even as the meeting began, problems arose. Mr. Hart, who had pulled his seat back from the group, began to add his own critical commentary to the leader's opening dialogue. Several of his colleagues took exception to his commentary. Two hours later, what had begun as an exercise in building a team through participation in goal setting had ended up as a free-for-all!

There are hidden barriers to team building in this scene. Unless we address these hidden barriers before we try to pull a group together, our efforts will be

Reprinted by permission from American Society for Training and Development, *Training and Development Journal* 34 (1980): 14–18.

sabotaged from the outset. These barriers may be thought of as a lack of groundwork; the groundwork beneath a cohesive group. This groudwork consists of: (1) shared knowledge, (2) shared territory, (3) same stature, and (4) same communication availability. Without each of these, a team won't make it because a group must have this shared information.

Think about all the groups which you think are characterized by "team spirit." Chances are that the individual members of those teams are very much like one another. Sure, you can pinpoint differences in some areas, but the similarities are more astounding. For instance, think about your management group. Most likely you share the way you treat your spouse, the way you spend your money and your time, as well as sharing a general philosophy about work life. The ultimate team, a sports team, has individual members who share such minutiae as the color of the socks they wear, the food they eat for breakfast, and even how they will act at parties.

The "sameness" of group members does not occur haphazardly. Operating within a group whose members exhibit commitment to group goals are a set of unwritten rules called "norms." Schein defined a norm as an assumption or expectation concerning what kind of behavior is right or wrong, good or bad, appropriate or inappropriate, allowed or not allowed.[1] Being the same as other group members, following the norms of the group, is one way an individual communicates commitment to a group's goals.

There are many obvious norms such as the unwritten dress code in the business world, the sexual codes, the code concerning the proper place to eat lunch. There are also many subtle norms which are equally powerful in groups. We recently observed a staff meeting in which one group member began to verbally attack the others. Gradually, as a heated discussion ensued, all the arms and legs of the other group members were crossed away from the offending member. Through this display of body orientation, the group communicated, albeit unconsciously, that this group member was violating the norm that group members never attack other group members.

Just as a group member is punished for violating norms, a group member may also be rewarded for a contribution to group cohesion via adherence to norms. Such rewards can be verbal or nonverbal. A smile, a pat, a playful shove can all be rewards.

Awareness of norms in four key areas can help you build effective teams. For team spirit to emerge, individual group members must feel that they all have the same level and type of knowledge, the same territory, the same status, and the same ability to communicate with one another. Lack of any one of these erects a hidden team building barrier.

Shared Knowledge

Taking a few liberties with an old aphorism, "What you see is what you know," is a good way of describing a rather complex process. What we "see" or perceive does have a sneaky way of becoming what we "know" *and* what we believe to be true. In an employee relations office, the staff member who comes in with a gripe against a malicious boss is often perceived as the "victim." If the next week the "malicious" boss tells the employee relations director about a lazy staff member, a new "truth" emerges.

But, before we dismiss the process too simply, what we perceive is often predicated on the labels or names we have readily available for the thing within our perceptual field. If the last bicycle you rode was your old Schwinn, you may look in the bicycle shop and see nothing but a bunch of bikes. The enthusiast, who has ridden a Colnago and has the names of 40 foreign brands at his or her fingertips, may look in the bicycle shop and see several touring bikes, several childrens' bikes, one or two good racing bikes and a bicycle shop owner who doesn't know what he's doing because a beloved Italian brand is nowhere in sight. The more words we have to describe our world, the more sophisticated we become and the more we will "see.".

It is important, therefore, for a group to have the same vocabulary and level of sophistication. The person who is given knowledge about management will become a manager. The institution of management cannot exist without that particular vocabulary which has been designated "managerial." What is usually called "orientation" is actually schooling in how to *label* the organizational environment.

Knowledge—or lack thereof—builds an "out-group" as well as an "in-group."

Making it difficult to gain knowledge, by holding secret meetings or sending confidential memos makes those with that knowledge value their group membership even more. Such secret knowledge builds greater group cohesion in much the same ways that secret pledges and codes of adolescent groups work. You may have observed people returning from a seminar joking with one another about "being in a parent state" or exhibiting "control needs." This sounds like so much jibberish to the outsider—and it is supposed to. This group has acquired common intellectual property which reinforces that these individuals belong together as a group.

Jargon may include derogatory labels for competitive groups within or outside the organization. The "other" advertising agency may be called "the Huns." The "other" sales force may be "the thugs." The language creates an "Us vs. Them" world, where no such separation may actually exist.

Jargon may be formally accepted by groups in a written "manifesto" or "statement of philosophy." An organization may state its philosophy in the employee handbook or via a column in a newsletter. Such formally accepted jargon also may indicate something of the shared world view of the group. If the newsletter is replete with "game" metaphors, there is a likelihood that the organization will be seen as participating in a high-stakes game. If the manifesto exhibits military metaphors, one may make some assumptions about the way the group is run or their common past experiences. Once the individual begins to use those metaphors, he or she is buying into that perception of the world. And on a more subtle level is saying "I buy into this group."

Shared Territory

In the same way that we don't feel as comfortable in the home of another as we do in our own homes, we don't feel as comfortable in other people's offices. We tend to be on "better behavior," to not challenge, disagree or argue because we are not in our own territory. Jack Anderson pointed out Chief Justice Burger's use of territoriality to gain an edge: "He has now annexed to his personal offices, the courts conference room, the inner sanctum where the justices meet in secret to thrash out their decisions. He has even installed a desk so there can be no mistaking that the court convenes in Burger's lair."[2]

The implications for building a team are myriad. Groups need to carefully consider where their meetings are held. A free exchange of information may be inhibited by the sense of being in another's territory. On the flip-side, one member may be exerting an inappropriate amount of power because the meetings are always held in his or her territory.

Indeed, rather than assigning individual territory, areas may be designated formally or informally as "belonging" to that group. For instance, an executive dining room tells outsiders that those inside are members of an established elite group. To the executive, the dining room serves as a constant hidden reminder of membership in that elite group. The people in the dining room meet frequently on an informal basis. This dining room says, "We are a group," and a special group at that.

Informal territories may also involve a table in the cafeteria, a seldom-used conference room or the chairs by the water cooler which may gradually become a place where a group gathers. A strong sense of "ours" develops concerning these locations. As a group differentiates more between "ours" and "not ours," cohesion within the group grows.

A team-building effort may falter because a group has not found a neutral area in which it can meet and call its own. Also, consciously seeking out a territory for a "homeless group" may contribute significantly to a team-building effort.

Same Stature

Whether John sits around a table with the group or behind his desk effects the group social structure. One director in a large manufacturing company held his staff meetings in his office. The director sat behind his desk with his four direct-reports sitting in chairs facing him. As a result, the director easily dominated the meetings and communication among his staff was kept at a minimum both in the meeting and out. Also, by distancing himself physically from the group, the director was able to maintain a psychological distance. His people rarely came to him for help. This failure at team building could have been drastically changed if only the director had moved to the other side of his office where there was a round table.

The historical value of a round table goes back to the era of King Arthur. A cultural norm also seems to accompany the position at the head of a rectangular table. If someone is the elected group leader, the most likely position to assume is at the head of the table. Strodtbeck & Hock created experimental jury deliberations and found that the person sitting at the head of the table was chosen significantly more often as the leader, especially if perceived as a person from a high economic class.[3] In addition to the quality of leadership, dominance and status also tend to be associated with the end position.[4] Because of the perceived importance afforded the position at the head of a table, a group needs to consider who tends to sit in that position and what effect it has on the group structure. That seat may afford one member the de facto leadership of the group or it may allow that person to dominate and sway group decisions—solely because of the seating arrangement.

In addition to the arrangement and shape of furniture in an office, the comfort of furnishings may affect group interactions. A spartan office with hard wooden chairs may make for short and to-the-point meetings. Both the atmosphere and the physical discomfort preclude the kind of nontask communication which allows group members to get to know and like each other. Physical comfort and aesthetically pleasing surroundings may cause people to spend more time together expanding the necessary social dimension of process that fosters cohesion.

Much has been written about the communication of status through office furnishings. Many companies delineate quite clearly the acquisitions one is entitled to on each of the management levels: size of office, carpeting, windows, desk (size and materials), chair (arms and height of back), etc. While there is a tendency to laugh at these antics, employees are fiercely aware of the furnishings of others and when they are being slighted in this fashion. In the company in which one of us works, a manager complained because another manager had wood paneling and he didn't. (One is only eligible for wood paneling at the director level.) Maintenance promptly came out and painted the wood paneling, to maintain "equality."

Groups are also very cognizant of the status that is communicated by their physical surroundings. As cited earlier, the plush executive dining room tells those both outside and inside the group that these people are different and unique; an elite. Uncomfortable, unpleasant surroundings may also tell all that this group really isn't too important, powerful or desirable. In the same way that the executive dining room fosters cohesion, the unpleasant surroundings make group cohesion more difficult to attain and maintain. A dumpy lounge may be a large but hidden barrier to group cohesiveness. Who wants to commit themselves to such a low status group?

Group networks also affect team interaction, cohesiveness and productivity. For instance, if a member of a five-person team has an office on a different floor than the other team members, that lone member may not really feel like a team member. Or, if all the group's internal communication is required to go through one member for that person's secretary to type before distribution to other group members, an inordinate amount of power and control is placed on one group member. The remaining team is at his or her mercy for communication.

Other factors that can affect communication networks are, as suggested earlier, proximity and gathering places. We tend to talk more frequently with those who are physically near us. Also, places that create physical proximity, such as the water cooler, foster communication. The problem with these tendencies is that one may frequently be near and therefore talk with some members of the team and not others. This lopsidedness tends to make some of the members feel excluded, thereby destroying group cohesiveness.

The importance of team building is rapidly growing as our companies grow larger and the employees demand more personal satisfaction on the job. Belonging to a team not only facilitates getting the work done faster and better, but it also allows one to feel "connected" in what may be an impersonal atmosphere.

Many team-building techniques may be employed, but first the groundwork must be assessed. Is there a common base of knowledge from which to draw? What about some common territory? Are there significant status differences? And does everyone have the same access to communication? Not until you've answered all these questions can you really start building your team.

REFERENCES

1. E. Schein, *Process Consultation* (Reading, Mass., Addison-Wesley Co., 1969).
2. N. M. Henley, *Body Politics* (Englewood Cliffs, N.J.: Prentice-Hall, 1977).
3. F. L. Strodtbeck and L. H. Hook, "The Social Dimensions of a Twelve Man Jury Table," *Sociometry* 24 (1961): 397–415.
4. A. P. Hare and R. F. Bales, "Seating Position and Small Group Interaction," *Sociometry* 26 (1963):480–486; B. S. Lott and R. Sommer, "Seating Arrangements and Status," *Journal of Personality and Social Psychology* 7 (1967): 90–95; N. F. Russo, "Connotation of Seating Arrangement," *Cornell Journal of Social Relations* 2 (1967): 37–44.

7.

COMMUNICATION IN HEALTH CARE ORGANIZATIONS

There was trouble at Glenview County Hospital. The morale of hospital employees was at an all time low. Several key staff members had tendered their resignations, and there was a rumor circulating among the hospital staff that widespread administrative changes and restructuring were in the offing. Low morale was affecting the quality of health care, due to poor staff attitudes and internal squabbles. Bob Wilson, the chief administrator of the hospital was worried. He didn't know what was going on at the hospital nor what he should do about it.

Bob Wilson had been hired three months ago by his predecessor, Frank Hyatt, who retired after 14 years with the hospital. Before coming to Glenview, Bob had been the assistant administrator at a nearby hospital for a little less than two years. Prior to that he had received a master's degree in health administration from the state university. Neither his past employment nor his education had prepared him for the low morale situation at Glenview.

Bob decided to bring in his two assistant administrators to discuss the morale situation and find out what was at the root of the problem. They both corroborated the fact that there was a problem and in fact told Bob that they both had heard from several "reliable sources" about the upcoming administrative layoffs. The more Bob denied the layoffs, the more suspicious the assistant administrators became. They wanted to know why he couldn't confide in them, and tell them what was "really" going on. Eventually they began to assume that they were both potential victims of the administrative restructuring they were certain was being planned.

Bob was even more concerned about the morale situation after talking to his assistants. It seemed that no matter what he did, the people working for him were becoming more and more paranoid. He gave Frank Hyatt a call and asked if Frank had any idea what was going on at the hospital. Frank said he had never encountered a serious morale problem in all his years as an administrator at Glenview. In fact, he had always felt that morale at the hospital was excellent, like a big happy family. This didn't make Bob feel any better about the situation.

Bob decided to call in one of his former professors from the university, who was an expert in organizational behavior, as an external consultant to solve the morale problem. The consultant began his work by interviewing different members of the hospital staff. Again and again he heard the same story; they believed the new hospital administrator was planning a major administrative reorganization, including massive layoffs. When asked where they had heard of this reorganization several different names were mentioned. One name, however, was identified as a source of information by almost everyone the consultant spoke to: Horace Jackson, a hospital janitor.

Horace was 64 years old and had been with the hospital for more than thirty years. He was well liked within the organization, and, in fact, spent a good deal of his time each day wheeling a large plastic trash container around the hospital and visiting with members of each hospital department. When the consultant interviewed Horace, he claimed he hadn't heard of any layoffs. The consultant recognized the contradictions between the report he received from Horace and those he had received from other members of the hospital staff, and realized that Horace was probably the initial source of the rumor about layoffs.

When the consultant informed Bob Wilson of what he had found, Bob reacted angrily and wanted to fire Horace. The consultant warned against hasty action and told Bob that firing Horace would only serve to confirm the false rumor about layoffs. If Horace, who had been with the hospital for thirty years, was expendable, then the hospital staff would really be convinced the rumor was true. Instead, the consultant suggested that Bob recognize that Horace was an informal leader in the organization and could be nurtured as an organizational ally rather than an enemy.

Bob called Frank Hyatt again and asked what he knew about Horace Jackson. Frank replied that Horace was one of his most trusted employees—in fact, that he had taken special care of Horace. He had invited him into his office every once in a while and asked him how things were going. Horace provided Frank with information about what was happening behind the scenes at the hospital. Frank said he usually sought advice from Horace about problems at the hospital and administrative decisions, and was generally given good advice. Every Christmas Frank made sure to give Horace a bottle of scotch as a present.

Bob began to realize how important an individual Horace was in the hospital. He recalled how curt he had been when Horace had dropped by his office during his first week and asked if he needed any help. Bob was busy with some details and had offhandedly dismissed Horace's offer of help. Bob realized that Horace had probably been insulted and had retaliated by starting the rumor about hospital layoffs.

Bob followed the consultant's advice and began to nurture his relationship with Horace. He invited Horace to have lunch with him at the hospital cafeteria and asked for the janitor's advice about improving hospital morale. He shared some of his ideas about improving the quality of health care at the hospital with Horace. Over the next month Bob encouraged Horace to drop by his office to discuss any problems or ideas he had. Over this same time period the rumor about layoffs began to subside and morale began to improve. Horace was now sending new information through the organization about what an excellent administrator Bob Wilson was!

In this case history much of the hospital's informal communication was working against the goals of the organization. To solve the morale problems in the organization the hospital administrator had to redirect organizational communication. In this chapter we will explore the different ways communication affects organizational activities. We will see how important communication is in effective health care delivery.

Human beings organize their activities with one another to accomplish complex tasks. As the modern world has grown more and more complex the need for organized human activities has grown, as evidenced by the great abundance of organizations that affect our lives. Some of the most important organizations in our lives are health care organizations.

The health care organization is the primary setting for health care practice. Hospitals, medical centers, health maintenance organizations, clinics, nursing homes, and convalescent centers have developed as centers for health care delivery in the modern world. Human communication in these health care organizations enables health professionals, health care support staff, and patients to coordinate their activities to accomplish health care goals.

Communication in organizations enables organization members to share important information about the goals, structures, problems, and strategies of the organization. Yet ineffective communication can block the fulfillment of organizational goals and further complicate the health care delivery system by distorting information, blocking the exchange of important messages, and alienating health care workers from one another. In this chapter we will examine the development of effective communication in health care organizations.

ORGANIZATIONAL COMMUNICATION AND THE SYSTEMS PERSPECTIVE

As we mentioned earlier in Chapter 2, an organization is a social system composed of interdependent groups of people sharing the performance of commonly recognized goals. *Organizational communication refers to human communication between organization members (as well as between organization members and related others) during the performance of organizational tasks and the accomplishment of organizational goals.* Organizational communication allows organizations to exist by providing people with the ability to coordinate their behaviors and to organize their tasks.

Organizational communication can best be viewed from a system perspective. *Systems theory* represents the organization as a complex set of interdependent parts which interact with one another to adapt to a constantly changing environment and achieve its goals. As we indicated in Chapter 5, communication occurs at various levels within the system. There is communication between the different parts of the system; there is communication within each system part, as well as there being communication between the system and its *environment*. In this chapter we will be using some systems terminology in an effort to explain this view of looking at organizations.

The organization is a system. Every system inputs resources from its environment and exports products to its environment. The *output* of a system is never the same as the system *input*. The mediating process of interaction among system parts and between the system and its environment allows the organization to create an output that is more than just the materials and information that the organization started out with as input. The combined and coordinated activities of all the system parts creates a *synergy* or an added energy to the output of the system allowing the system to transform raw materials into advantageous finished products.

System processes are *nonsummative*. Nonsummativity implies that the synergistic aspects of system processes are not merely additive but the individual processing of each system part combines to accomplish far more than they could individually. *The whole is equal to more than the sum of its parts.* Or, by working together members of the health care system can do far more to achieve health care goals than they might have by working independently, emphasizing once again (as we did earlier in Chapter 6) the importance of teamwork in health care delivery.

Futhermore, the systems theory principle of *equifinality* infers that the final state of a system's output is not determined by the initial conditions or inputs confronting the system but the same final conditions can be reached by the system from different initial conditions in many different ways.[1] The interaction among system parts allows the system to be creative in the processing of different inputs in different ways to achieve appropriate outputs for achieving the goals of the system. This indicates that health care organizations have the ability to provide health care services for different people with different health care problems by adapting the activities of its personnel and utilizing its health care resources flexibly. Communication is the means by which the health care organization can adapt its personnel and processes to specific health care situations and problems.

As we have indicated, the system (or organization) transforms raw materials (inputs) from its environment into finished products (outputs) that help the system achieve its goals. This is known as the *transformation model* (see Figure 7.1). Every organization must input information and raw materials from its environment whether these inputs are customers, clients, technologies, materials, foods, or personnel, and export products to its environment including such outputs as retail goods, entertainment, processed information, or treated clients. The system

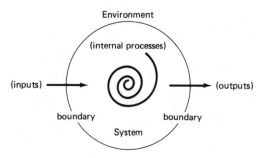

Figure 7.1   The System Transformation Model.

imports and exports materials through its *boundaries*. As we will describe in more depth later in this chapter when we consider Weick's model of organizing, the boundaries of the system play an important role in selecting, evaluating, and utilizing the inputs and outputs of the system.

As we briefly discussed in Chapters 2 and 3, there are several hierarchical levels to systems analysis. Any organism or mechanism that processes raw materials into finished products through the combined efforts (processing) of its component parts is a *system*. These internal component parts of the system that do the active processing of inputs into outputs are known as *subsystems*. Each of the subsystems work interdependently with other subsystems in the accomplishment of system goals. In a health care organization (system) the component parts (subsystems) might be the various departments or units of the organization such as nursing, medicine, administration, maintenance, pharmacy, and social work. Each of these health care subsystems are dependent on one another in the delivery of health care services. Every system is itself a part of a larger system known as the *suprasystem*. Even though we have only identified three successively larger levels of systems analysis, subsystem – system – suprasystem, this does not mean there are ever only three levels to any organization. Any of the system levels can be viewed as either subsystem, system, or suprasystem building *macroscopically* to larger and larger levels of organization, or dissecting *microscopically* to smaller and smaller units of organization. This is one of the major attributes of systems thinking—it allows the organizational analyst the opportunity to examine both the "big picture" view of organizations and the component parts view of the organization (see Figure 7.2 for system levels).

The system's *environment* plays a large role in system functioning by both providing the system with materials and information for processing and by creating markets and outlets for system outputs. Furthermore, the environment surrounds the system and affects the goals and operation of the system. Every system strives for survival, even though environmental demands challenge its survival. This indicates the constant struggle in systems between *entropy* and *negative entropy*. Entropy is the tendency that all systems have to disorganize and wear down over time, while negative entropy is the system's ability to develop organization and grow. Negative entropy allows the organization to survive, while entropy causes the organization to deteriorate.

As we discussed in Chapter 6, every system ranges from being relatively *open* to being relatively *closed* to information from its environment. No living system is ever totally open or closed to its environment. It is impossible for an organization to totally ignore all messages from its environment, or to perceive all messages from its environment. Sys-

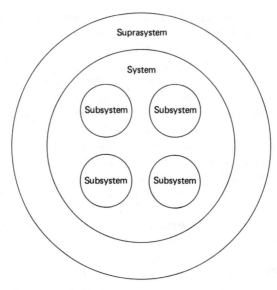

Figure 7.2   Hierarchical System Levels.

tems are also relatively open or closed to their environment in terms of the amount of information they export. As we discussed in Chapter 6, it is not always best to be too open or too closed in giving or receiving information, but to adapt the system's level of openness or closedness to its environment in response to the given situation at hand. For example, in times of great social turmoil and change it is wise for the organization to closely monitor social changes and the affects of these changes on its operations. In this situation relative openness is an effective communication strategy for the organization to adopt. While in times of complex internal operations within the organization it is best for the system to expend its energy concentrating on coordinating its own processes rather than monitoring and communicating exclusively with its environment. In this situation relative closedness is an effective communication strategy for the organization to adopt.

It is, however, important for the health care organization to be aware of what is going on in its environment to help plan for future demands. Being aware of the kinds of health care problems indigenous to the people in the immediate vicinity of a public health center will help the organization gather appropriate personnel and resources for serving these people. As the population of this community changes the hospital should make changes in its operations and resources to meet new needs. Often it is too late to merely react to environmental changes and demands in health care. By the time the health care organization has gathered new resources and devised new plans for meeting changing health problems many people may have been unable to obtain needed health services and suffered unnecessarily. The modern health care organization must learn to be *proactive*, to gather information from its environment about imminent health care problems and plan organizational strategies for meeting these problems. An example of this is the development of specialized triage methods for processing and treating flood victims in an area where flooding is a strong possibility in the future. It might be too late to develop and implement these specialized methods when a flood occurs but having the methods available makes the health organization better able to cope with potential health care demands brought on by its environment.

WEICK'S MODEL OF ORGANIZING

Karl Weick presents an innovative behavior-oriented model of organizing, stressing human interaction as the central phenomenon of organization. He contends that organizations do not exist but are in the process of existing by continually organizing human activities.[2] Human communication is the crucial process performed by organization members enabling ongoing organization to occur.

An important part of Weick's model is the organizational environment. Environment, according to Weick, is not the physical surroundings (buildings, offices, equipment, people, etc.) that organization members encounter but instead is the information to which organization members react. *Organizational environment is an information environment, based on the messages organization members perceive and the meanings they create in response to these messages.*

Organizations rely on a variety of sources of information in organizing, such as interviews, sales calls, letters, documents, telephone conversations, or group discussions. In a medical organization, health care personnel rely heavily on medical records and practitioner–client interviews as sources of information in performing their organizational tasks. There are many other sources of information in health care organizations, in fact, the wide range of messages interpreted by organization members in the performance of their health care tasks is the information environment the health care organization resides in.

Weick argued that since human beings actively create the world around them through perception, organization members do not merely react to an objectively accepted physical environment but *enact* their environment through information and the creation of meaning. The organization's environment is derived from the exchange of messages and creation of meaning by organization members. Organizing occurs within the context of human interaction.

A crucial part of Weick's model of organizing is information *equivocality*. Equivocality is the level of understandability of messages organization members respond to. Some aspects of equivocality include the level of ambiguity, complexity, and obscurity of messages. The level of equivocality of a message relates to the level of certainty with which an organization member can decode that message.

Organizations are necessary because they help people deal with complex phenomena. Weick asserts it is the task of organizations to process equivocal information. Organization members perform communication processes designed to cope with information equivocality. It is this ability to cope with equivocal information that Weick refers to as the process of organizing. "The activities of organizing are directed toward the establishment of a workable level of certainty. An organization attempts to transform equivocal information into a degree of unequivocality with which it can work and to which it is accustomed."[3]

Organizations must react to message inputs with the same amount of equivocality that is present in the messages themselves. This is known as the principle of *requisite variety*. To deal with a highly complex situation an organization should perform a highly complex communication process in response to adequately handle the input. Conversely, to deal with very understandable information an organization should react with very clear, simple behaviors.

Weick identifies two related communication processes used by organizations to cope with the level of equivocality of information

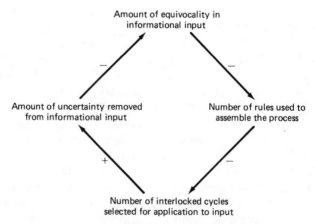

Figure 7.3 Sequence of a Subprocess. (From Karl E. Weick, *The Social Psychology of Organizing*, Copyright © 1969 by Addison-Wesley. Reprinted by permission of Addison-Wesley.)

inputs. These two processes are *rules* and *cycles* (see Figure 7.3). Rules prescribe the activities organization members perform in response to information inputs. Cycles are a series of interlocked communication behaviors between organization representatives that allow the organization to process information.

Rules are developed by organizations to direct organizational behaviors in response to common inputs. Form letters, rate sheets, and written directions are some examples of how rules are often used in organizations to direct action. Simple (unequivocal) message inputs can usually be responded to by the organization with pre-set rules. For example, when a client goes to a health care clinic complaining of a head cold (a common ailment) the health care practitioner can react to the client with several rules such as, "Get plenty of bed rest, drink a lot of fluids, keep warm," and so on. If a client goes to the same clinic complaining of loss of gravitational pull and weightlessness (a very uncommon ailment) the practitioner probably does not have any rules for reacting simply to the situation. Since this is a highly equivocal input, the practitioner must react to the client in an equivocal manner.

Cycles are communication tools the organization uses to process equivocality out of inputs. Weick describes a cycle as a double-interact, a three part exchange of messages, act—response—adjustment. Each cycle processes some equivocality out of the input, making the input more understandable to the organization and enabling the organization to apply rules for responding to the input. Taking the previous example, in reacting to the weightless client clinic representatives will probably perform many communication cycles, such as questioning the client at great length, conferring with one another, asking the opinions of other professionals, consulting books, and so forth. Each of these cycles will help the health practitioner de-mystify the client's health problem until a course of treatment (rules) can be applied to the problem.

In summary of our discussion of equivocality, rules, and cycles, if the information input into the organization is highly equivocal the organization must rely on performing cycles to cope with the input; if the information input into the organization is unequivocal the organization can apply rules to the input for guiding organizational response to the input.

There are three major phases the organization goes through in the process of organizing: *enactment*, *selection* and *retention*. Rules and cycles are used in each of these phases, where the level of equivocality of the input is ascertained, appropriate rules are selected (if available to the organization), or communication cycles are performed (if the input is too complex to be handled by rules).

The enactment phase of organizing is where the organization attends to the information environment that surrounds it. The organization recreates (or enacts) its environment in the sense that organization members assign meaning to information events as they try to understand them. During this enactment phase the organization is made aware of changes in its information environment, the level of equivocality of information inputs is determined, and appropriate rules and cycles are called upon to process the information inputs.

In the selection phase of the model of organizing decisions are made determining how the rules and cycles used by the organization have affected the equivocality of the information inputs and which cycles should be repeated by the organization to further process the inputs. According to the decisions made in the selection phase, rules and cycles are selected and repeated to continue reducing the level of equivocality of the messages input into the organization, enabling the organization to better understand and react to the inputs.

In the retention phase of organizing, information is gathered and stored about the ways the organization has responded to different inputs. The various communication cycles developed and used by the organization to process equivocal information are evaluated for their usefulness to the organization and if deemed to be successful, strategies for coping with equivocal situations are made into rules for how the organization can respond to similar inputs in the future. A *repertoire of communication rules* is developed during the retention phase to be used as a form of *organizational intelligence* to guide organizational actions.

The enactment, selection, and retention phases of organizing work together in the process of organization, and *feedback loops* between the phases are used to coordinate their activities. Feedback loops are message systems connecting the phases, allowing communication between the phases. Weick identifies two feedback loops in his model of organizing, one connecting retention to enactment and the other connecting retention to selection. In this way the retention phase, which contains the organization's intelligence, can be used to guide the enactment and selection activities.

There are two different types of messages sent via the feedback loops, *positive feedback* and *negative feedback*. Positive feedback messages request the performance of more new behaviors, and negative feedback messages request the discontinuance of any new behaviors. In essence, positive feedback messages are used to elicit information from the retention phase for use in selection and retention, as well as to seek information from enactment and selection for storage in retention. Negative feedback messages are used to stop the flow of information from retention to enactment and selection, halting the performance of new behaviors. Negative feedback is also used to halt the flow of information about

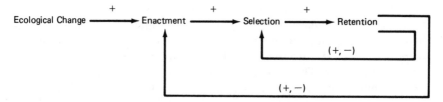

Figure 7.4   Organizing Phases and Feedback Loops. (From Karl E. Weick, *The Social Psychology of Organizing*, Copyright © 1969 by Addison-Wesley. Reprinted by permission of Addison-Wesley.)

enactment and selection activities to the retention phase. (See Figure 7.4 for a diagram of organizing feedback loops.)

In the enactment phase of organizing, message inputs are perceived and evaluated for their level of equivocality by the organization. Feedback loops between enactment and retention allow the organization to both utilize the information from retention to guide the evaluation of messages and to store the information about the messages enacted for future reference. While in the selection phase where communication rules and cycles are chosen and created in response to information inputs, feedback loops from retention to selection are used to guide the organization in deciding how to process message inputs by drawing upon organizational intelligence and the repertoire of communication rules stored in the retention phase. The retention phase constantly draws information from enactment and selection through feedback loops to update its information about message inputs and organizational response strategies.

In a hospital a health care practitioner will search his or her past experiences in deciding how to diagnose a health care problem a client is having. Hopefully, the practitioner can find some precedent in his or her past experiences (repertoire of rules) for the problem at hand and use this stored information to treat the client's ailment. The past experiences that are accepted as being relevant to the health care problem are accepted through a positive feedback loop. Of course, there will be past health care experiences the practitioner has had that do not relate directly to this problem. The practitioner will reject these past experiences in diagnosing the problem, because the information they offer is of little value in ascertaining the current client's problem. The health care practitioner rejects these past experiences through use of negative feedback loops. Health care diagnosis depends on the effective coordination of enactment and retention phases of organizing.

During the course of health care treatment the practitioner must monitor the responses of the client to determine the efficiency of the health care regimen. If the client manifests unpopular side effects in response to health care treatment the practitioner must search for alternative treatments. These alternative treatments will be identified in the practitioner's repertoire of rules or as part of the repertoire of rules that are part of the hospital's organizational intelligence. If there are no rules to cover the side effects the client is manifesting, the practitioner along with the rest of the health care team will have to develop new behavior cycles to treat the patient. Advantageous cycles (those that adequately treat the client's problem) will become part of the practitioner's and the hospital's repertoire of rules to be used in future health care situations. Effective health care treatment depends on the coordination of selection and retention phases of organizing.

Although the health care diagnosis and treatment examples just discussed primarily involve one practitioner, in health care practice many people are usually involved in the organizing process. Doctors, nurses, therapists, aides, clients, client's families, health care administrators, and others constantly interact with one another to provide health care. Often, organizational intelligence is distributed throughout the health care organization, and in order to make a knowledgeable decision about diagnosis or treatment the health care practitioner must rely on obtaining information from other organization members. Moreover, in highly equivocal health care situations the practitioner must interact with others to process the information down to an understandable level through the performance of communication behavior cycles.

In the case history at the beginning of this chapter the hospital administrator was faced with a highly equivocal problem of low staff morale. He had never encountered this problem before and therefore had no rules available for dealing with this situation. To resolve the equivocality of the morale problem the administrator initiated several communication cycles, including conferencing with his assistant hospital administrators, calling the retired administrator and asking his advice, hiring a consultant who interviewed members of the hospital staff—all helping to clarify the low morale situation and indicate means for resolving the problem. The administrator then initiated several communication cycles with Horace, the janitor, further reducing the equivocality of the situation and solving the morale problem. The use of communication cycles with Horace proved so successful in coping with the problem that the administrator probably made them part of the organizational intelligence and used them as an organizing rule. If the past administrator, Frank Hyatt, had only retained the rule of communicating with Horace by sharing that information with the new administrator much of the ensuing problem might have been avoided.

The organizing model stresses the importance of organizational response to the information in its environment. Earlier in this chapter the organization's boundary was identified as the point where the organization exchanges information with its environment. It is at the organization's boundary where enactment processes occur. The proactive health care organization must keep on top of changes in its information environment by paying particular attention to its boundary spanning mechanisms and personnel. In health care organizations the boundary spanning personnel are often the receptionists, admission clerks, emergency room employees, and outpatient clinic staff. These organization members must be trained to evaluate information from the environment and be given the organization resources to respond to information inputs intelligently and effectively. (See Figure 7.5 for the organizing model.)

In summary, recommendations for health care organizational supervisors include the following:

1. Allow adequate communication contact between organization members particularly when they are processing equivocal (uncertain) information.

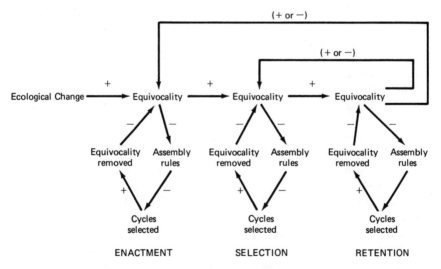

Figure 7.5   Weick's Model of Organizing. (From Karl E. Weick, *The Social Psychology of Organizing*, Copyright © 1969 by Addison-Wesley. Reprinted by permission of Addison-Wesley.)

2. Foster interaction between employees by encouraging workers to ask questions, particularly on difficult tasks.
3. Use groups of workers to deal with tasks too complex for individuals to comprehend easily.
4. Concentrate on the relationships and interlocked communication between organizational members because the process of control within organizations is accomplished through relationships between individuals rather than by individuals.
5. Develop training programs stressing teamwork and have daily and weekly meetings when necessary.
6. Problem-solving groups can be formed to provide the necessary interlocked communication behaviors necessary for organizational adaptation.[4]

MESSAGE FLOW IN HEALTH CARE ORGANIZATIONS

Message flow in organizations has traditionally been described in terms of *formal organizational structure*. The formal structure of an organization follows the *organizational chart*, which maps the prescribed hierarchy of power relationships that exist within an organization. Depending on the job titles and job descriptions people have within their organization, certain formal relationships are prescribed between them and other organization members in the performance of their job responsibilities. For example, the people to whom you must report, the people who must report to you, those you supervise, those you work directly with, all have formal communication relationships that will show up on an accurate organizational chart. (See Figure 7.6 for an example of an organizational chart.)

The three major forms of formal message flow are *downward communication, upward communication,* and *horizontal communication.* All three of these forms of message flow follow the relationships between organization members prescribed by the organizational chart and all three forms of message flow perform important functions for the organization.

Downward communication flows from upper management down to lower levels in the organizational hierarchy. Downward communication is the most basic type of formal message system. Several of the key organizational functions of downward communication include sending orders, giving job related information, reviewing job performance, and indoctrinating members toward organizational goals. Downward communication is an important management tool for directing the

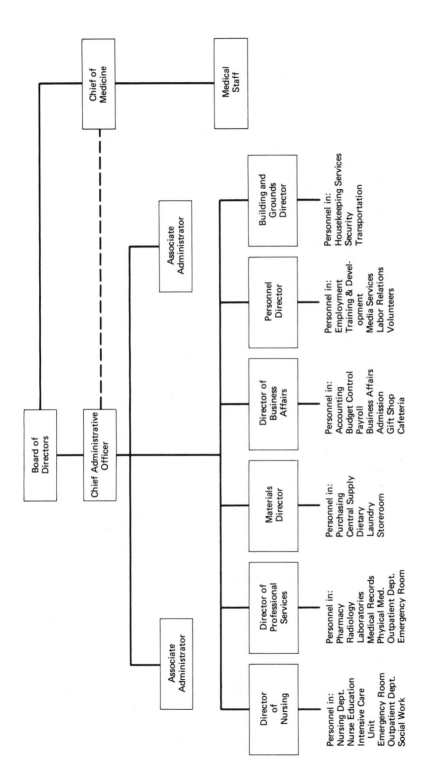

Figure 7.6   Organizational Chart for a Mythical Health Care Organization.

performance of workers in their organizational tasks. There is usually a great abundance of downward communication in health care organizations. As we will discuss in more depth, however, the prevalence of downward communication messages does not infer organizations' effective use of downward communication.

Upward communication flows from lower level employees within the organization up to management personnel. Upward communication is the primary source of feedback management has for determining the effectiveness of their downward communication. Additionally, upward communication messages function by providing management with information about the day-to-day operation of the organization to use in making decisions, encouraging employee participation in the organization (thereby enhancing organizational cohesiveness and relieving employee tensions). Channels for upward communication are often underdeveloped in health care organizations causing a variety of organizational communication problems for the delivery of health care. We will discuss the problems of insufficient upward communication later on in this chapter. The case study at the beginning of this chapter provides one example.

Horizontal communication flows between members of the organization who are at the same hierarchical level; it is basically peer communication between organization members. Horizontal communication functions by allowing task coordination, providing a means for sharing relevant information, as well as providing a channel for problem solving and conflict maintenance. Although horizontal communication is an important formal channel of organizational communication it is often overlooked and underused in organizational practice.

Even though downward, upward, and horizontal channels of organizational communication provide important communication functions, in organizational practice formal message flow is often poorly utilized. Downward communication, although heavily utilized, is often overplayed by management. In Chapter 2 we differentiated between content and relationship aspects of messages and in downward communication the content information of explaining procedures and goals can be overshadowed by the relationship information of establishing power and control. Overdependence on continually giving orders and instructions to workers can alienate workers from management, causing employee resentment toward management and the organization. Additionally, downward communication is often unclear and contradictory, causing confusion and anxiety for organization members. Later in this chapter we will discuss the problems of contradictory downward communication messages in health care organizations, which causes role conflict for many health care workers.

There are several factors in organizations that cause upward communication channels to be underdeveloped. First of all, since people higher up in the organizational hierarchy wield power over those people holding lower positions within the organization, it is very risky for workers to tell their bosses about problems that exist in the organization or gripes they have with management's downward communication. If a worker's upward communication evokes the wrath of his or her boss, the worker's job might be jeopardized. Because of the risks of upward disclosure of unpopular information workers often communicate only favorable messages to their bosses, a syndrome known as the *mum effect*. Moreover, management is often unreceptive to honest employee feedback and reacts angrily and defensively to upward communication. The story about the ancient Greek monarach who would slay the messengers who brought him unfavorable news about military campaigns is similar to the more current story about a nurse who informed hospital management about questionable health care procedures leading to a baby's death and was fired for her troubles. Certainly situations such as this one strongly discourage other hospital workers from coming to management with unfavorable information.

The greatest problem with horizontal communication in most organizations is management's failure to recognize it as being useful. In many organizations peer communication is discouraged and sometimes it is punished. Horizontal communication is often thought of as merely being small talk and fraternizing between workers. At management levels organization members often become so busy working within their own area of the organization they have little time for communicating with other personnel at their same hierarchical level. Yet, as we discussed earlier, horizontal communication provides organization members with useful information allowing them to solve problems and coordinate activities.

To effectively utilize downward, upward, and horizontal message flow in organizations, management must become aware of the importance of formal message flow in their organization. Downward messages must be clear, informative, and sensitive to adequately prepare organization members to perform organizational tasks without alienating them. Management must demonstrate genuine receptiveness to open and honest upward communication to provide them with feedback necessary to help them direct organizational performance. Workers should be encouraged to share their ideas with management. After all, those health care workers directly involved with the performance of organizational tasks know first-hand what works and what doesn't work in health care practice. Management can tap into the knowledge health care workers have by eliciting feedback. Horizontal communication between organization members should be encouraged by management especially in complex situations where task coordination and problem solving skills are most necessary.

Some communication strategies for improving formal message flow in organizations include the use of group meetings to facilitate interaction among organization members, regular performance review and problem solving interviews between management and workers, formal training procedures and orientation programs for workers, suggestion boxes and worker idea reward systems, as well as briefing sessions during shift changes. Organizational media such as newsletters, memos, taped messages, training films, and bulletin boards can be used to augment formal message flow in organizations. The key, however, to effective formal message flow in organizations, whether it be downward, upward, or horizontal, is the development of meaningful interpersonal relationships between organization members. Only through the development of effective human relationships can organization members learn how to trust one another and communicate meaningfully with each other.

In addition to formal message flow systems that have been prescribed by the formal hierarchy of the organization, an informal message flow system emerges naturally through human interaction within the organization. *Informal message flow* refers to the communication that develops between organization members that is not necessarily prescribed by the formal goals and hierarchy of the organization but develops out of interpersonal attraction, shared social interests, and non-task oriented interaction among organization members. As we mentioned, informal message flow does not necessarily follow the organizational hierarchy but instead develops its own social structure. Often this informal channel of communication in organizations is referred to as the *grapevine* and is usually composed of social groups, cliques, club members, family relations, and other informal relationships that develop between organization members.

One of the primary reasons for the development of informal communication systems within organizations is the need organization members have for information about the organization. Organizations are often large, complex, and multifaceted systems and in order for members of organizations to behave effectively within their organizations they need information about what is going on behind the scenes and what is being planned by other members. The grapevine provides organization members with information about who is doing what and what changes are occurring within the organization, affording information about organizational functioning that can help them direct their activities.

In organizations information is powerful and whoever possesses information about the organization and is willing to barter that information can exercise power within that organization. Often individuals who seek organizational power, especially those who are not afforded power through the formal organizational hierarchy, attempt to gain power by gathering information through their activities within the grapevine. Those organization members who possess a great deal of information and utilize their information to direct the grapevine are known as *informal leaders*.

Informal leaders wield a great deal of power within organizations, yet, strangely enough, they are seldom recognized by the formal power structure of the organization as being either legitimate or powerful. Due to this management oversight, the formal and informal systems within the organization are often in competition with one another. For years organizational theorists have been planning to stamp out the grapevine, not realizing the grapevine is a naturally developing part of organizations based on human beings' quest for organizational information. Paradoxically, the more strongly the management attempts to rid itself of the grapevine, the more it grows and flourishes. This was exemplified by the case study at the beginning of the chapter. The more uncertain and turbulent the communication climate of the organization becomes, the more organization members feel the need for information about the organization.

A more effective strategy for utilizing the informal message flow in organizations is to coordinate formal and informal communication systems. Organization members usually become informal leaders because of their extreme desire for power and recognition within the organization, often known as *Machiavellian* tendencies. Management can feed the Machiavellian tendencies of their organization's informal leaders by keeping these leaders informed about important happenings in the organization and developing a trusting relationship with them. By feeding these informal leaders with honest and important information about the organization the management can enlist these leaders and their informal channels of communication to spread information through the organization, supplementing formal downward message flow channels. Furthermore, management can elicit useful upward communication from the informal leaders, who know a great deal about organizational operations. Perhaps even more importantly, management can eliminate the spread of dangerously untrue rumors and replace them with organizationally approved information on the grapevine.

In the case history at the beginning of this chapter Horace Jackson was identified as an informal leader in the hospital. Although his formal position was that of a janitor, his informal position was extremely influential due to the information he had gathered and relationships he had developed working at the hospital for more than thirty years. When the new hospital administrator ignored Horace, he was really ignoring the informal communication system within the hospital. Since the new administrator wasn't cultivating the grapevine and feeding it with accurate information, Horace took it upon himself to feed the grapevine with false information, information about massive layoffs at the hospital. Eventually the new administrator was made aware of the importance of the informal communication system in the hospital, and began to integrate formal and informal organizational communication systems by providing Horace with relevant and accurate organizational information.

ROLE CONFLICT AND MULTIPLE AUTHORITY IN HEALTH CARE

Hospitals have developed as the primary health care organization in the modern world. As such they embody the wide variety of health care personnel, technologies, and services that are part of the modern health care system. In the delivery of health care services the activities of many individuals are coordinated, necessitating the development of extensive administrative and control systems in hospital organizations. In fact, many hospitals tend to become top-heavy. That is, hospital organizations often develop disproportionately extensive hierarchies of control. The overdevelopment of hierarchical levels in health care organizations contributes to the development of several administrative problems for health care workers.

As House (1970) points out, the overdevelopment of hospital hierarchies violates two basic principles of management, *chain of command* and *unity of command*.[5] The principle of chain of command asserts that organizations should have a clear hierarchy of control where each level of the organization holds the responsibility for directing the activities of people at lower levels, with authority flowing directly from the top of the organization to the bottom. The principle of unity of command relates closely to chain of command, asserting that within organizational hierarchies subordinates should receive a command from only one supervisor to minimize confusion in directing organizational activities.

In hospital organizations there are usually at least two major sources of control—hospital administration and medical administration. Additionally, the professional standards of each of the health practitioners, whether they be pharmacists, physicians, nurses, dentists, therapists, or social workers, in effect, directs the performance of health care professionals. These different sources of hierarchical control complicate the direction of organizational activities. The hospital chain of command is often bypassed because of the many sources of control. For example, a physician who is not a full-time member of the hospital staff but is there treating one of his or her clients may order a nurse to treat that client in a manner that is contradictory to the general rules of hospital administration or medical administration. The nuse is put into a double-bind and must decide whether to disregard the doctor's instructions and perhaps jeopardize the well-being of the client, or follow the doctor's orders and violate the regulations of the hospital administration. The nurse may wonder who is in control in that situation. Must he or she answer to the doctor, to the hospital administration, or to her own professional judgment? The chain of command is not clear and can cause ambiguity, frustration, and health care activities that do not meet the standards of all parties concerned.

In the same health care situation unity of command may also be violated. The nurse is given mutually contradictory orders by the medical staff, the administrative staff, and perhaps the nursing hierarchy as well. This puts the nurse in a classic double-bind situation. No matter what the nurse decides to do, at least one of his or her bosses' instructions will be disobeyed.

The situation of multiple authority in health care organizations puts many health care workers in an untenable situation where they are uncertain about their health care duties and their health care roles. This uncertainty about the clear definition of the health practitioner's role is known as *role ambiguity*. Role ambiguity results from unclear and ambiguous information about how the professional is to do his or her job. *Role congruence* is the degree to which the health practitioner's job performance matches the role expectations of both administrator and practitioner. Certainly in situations of multiple authority the health care organization suffers from insufficient role congruence. Lack of role congruence, in turn, puts the health practitioner in a situation of *role conflict*, where the practitioner is caught between two or more mutually exclusive expectations for job performance. Of course, all organizational members have a certain amount of role conflict in the performance of their jobs, due to differing expectations. But in health care organizations role conflict abounds, causing employee frustration, confusion and, in many cases, poor job performance.

The problem of multiple authority and role conflict in health care organizations is a clear situation of too many chefs and too few cooks. There are too many people giving orders about the administration of health care to a small number of health care workers. This situation is caused by the growing complexity of the health care delivery system.

As health care knowledge develops, new specialized areas of health care practice are added to the repertoire of hospital services, increasing the number of specialized personnel and administrators to coordinate their activities in the health care organization. The ever increasing specialization of health care practice has resulted in the growing departmentalization and decentralization of health care delivery organizations. Health care organizations generally have many middle management personnel wielding a rather narrow *span of control*, or the number of health care personnel they directly supervise. Narrow span of control is a characteristic of *decentralization*, while *centralized organizations* usually have fewer bosses having the responsibility of directing the activities of many subordinates. Generally, a centralized organization has a narrow chain of command, while a decentralized organization has many different divisions, each with management personnel who have formal organizational responsibility. Centralized organizations have relatively few power and decision points, while decentralized organizations have many points where formal power is wielded and decisions are made.

Decentralization is often advantageous for complex organizations because it relieves the extreme organizational responsibilities of top management, spreading decision-making responsibility among middle managers who are directly involved in the operation of the organization. Certainly decentralization is beneficial in health care organizations such as hospitals because it puts the responsibility for specialized health care decision making on the health care professionals who are most knowledgeable and more involved with the specific health care situation.

On the other side, however, decentralization has the disadvantage of giving middle managers decision-making responsibilities when they often do not see the larger organizational picture and the implications of their decisions on other organizational divisions or personnel. In health care organizations the decision makers are often so involved with their own immediate health care delivery problems they may not recognize the repercussions of their decisions on the rest of the hospital. Moreover, as we have already pointed out, since health care areas overlap in the delivery of health care services, there is great opportunity for contradictory decisions and directives from different sources of authority in decentralized health care organizations. Once again, multiple authority in health care can lead to role conflict, which in turn can lead to frustration, confusion, and inefficient health care services.

Decentralization, multiple authority, and role conflict have become an inevitable part of organizational life in health care practice. To minimize the problems of role conflict in organizations several authors have suggested the use of management personnel to serve as integrators and liaisons in complex organizations.[6] These integrators will help connect the different divisions of the organization, allowing specialists to understand the larger picture implications of their specialized decisions. Ombudspeople, or people appointed to hear, investigate and ameliorate complaints of organization members, can often help health care personnel work out role conflicts between them and their supervisors. Communication between health care personnel across hospital divisions and hierarchical levels can break down role conflict and help foster cooperation between members of the health care organizations.

COPING WITH ORGANIZATIONAL BUREAUCRACY

The ever increasing complexity and specialization of health care delivery has caused health care organizations to become very bureaucratic. *Bureaucracy* refers to the level of formalization of rules and processes within an organization. Although in modern word usage bureaucracy has gotten a bad name, classical organizational theorists have for many years advocated bureaucratic models for administering organizations.[7] The bureaucratic organization exhibits the following characteristics: *rules* and regulations, *division of labor, hierarchy* of formal organizational power, *interchangeability of personnel in relatively self-perpetuating organizational roles, impersonality* in interpersonal relationships, and *rationality* and predictability in the accomplishment of organizational goals. Modern health care organizations are designed to embody these characteristics of bureaucracy.

The bureaucratic model has gotten a bad public image in recent years due to extreme formality of bureaucratic organizations. The word bureaucracy has become almost synonymous with organizational inefficiency, red tape and insensitivity. Bradley and Baird report that "complaints against bureaucracy have been numerous: it has been accused of stifling individual creativity, encouraging conformity and modifying the personality."[8] Certainly hospitals have had many of these same criticisms leveled at them. Health care organizations are notorious for their red tape. Stories of dying patients who were denied treatment in public hospitals until they filled out forms or identified their method of payment or insurance abound. Stories like these attest not only to the red tape and insensitivity of bureaucracies but also to the ways that the overdevelopment of bureaucratic structures can become self-defeating to the accomplishment of organizational goals.

Bureaucracy, however, offers many advantages to large complex organizations such as hospitals. Precision, speed, clarity, continuity, discretion, unity, and strict subordination of personnel are reported as benefits of bureaucratic structure.[9] Bureaucratic structure adds predictability to organizational behavior by prescribing rules and procedures for dealing with tasks. As we discussed in our section on Weick's model of organizing, rules help organizations cope with low equivocality inputs, indicating that bureaucracy is useful for handling normal, predictable organizational tasks. Yet, rules are not useful in responding to highly equivocal inputs, suggesting the bureaucratic model is inappropriate for use in response to complex organizational problems. Bureaucracy does not lend itself to creativity, yet many hospitals must react creatively to the unpredictable health care problems presented to them by consumers. In retrospect, bureaucracy can offer many strong advantages to organizational practice, yet can also be very constraining for the organization.

The strengths and limitations of bureaucracy for organizational functioning underscore the ongoing tension in organizations between *differentiation* and *integration*. Differentiation refers to the needs organizations have for specialized personnel and processes. Health care organizations utilize specialized health professionals, technologies, and procedures in the delivery of health care services, thereby exhibiting differentiation. Integration refers to the needs organizations have for coordinating the many different activities and processes of organizing in achieving their goals. Hospitals strive to coordinate the activities of doctors, nurses, pharmacists, therapists, support staff, and clients in the delivery of health care services, thereby exhibiting integration. Differentiation and integration are often mutually competing processes in organizations. The more differentiated (specialized and departmentalized) a health care organization is, the more difficult it becomes for the organization to demonstrate integration (coordination and cooperation) and conversely, the more integrated an organization is, the more difficult it is for the organization to differentiate. In a similar manner bureaucracy helps an organization respond in regulated, ordered, predictable ways but often makes it difficult for organizations to develop innovative patterns and processes.

Organizations must develop a workable balance between differentiation and integration to remain viable and they also must maintain a healthy balance between bureaucracy (structure) and adaptability (flexibility and creativity). The organizational balance between differentiation and integration and between bureaucracy and adaptability is achieved through the ongoing maintenance, evaluation, and development of organizational processes by management. The formal organization leaders should continually seek feedback from organization members, as well as customers (in health care the management should seek feedback from clients) to evaluate the function and relational effectiveness of organizational processes and structures, utilizing the information gathered to update and develop the organization so it may operate more effectively in the future.

On an individual level, organization members can best cope with the rigidity and impersonality of highly formalized health care bureaucracies by becoming familiar with the rules and regulations and hierarchical power relationships that make up the bureaucratic structure of the system. By learning the "ropes" of the system the individual can utilize organizational structure to their best advantage. Knowing who has the authority and power to get things done in an organization, as well as finding out the procedures and mechanisms for initiating changes and facilitating organizational action can help the organization member achieve personal, professional, and task-related goals within the organization. As we mentioned earlier in this chapter, information is extremely powerful in organizations and knowing who to speak with and what channels to utilize in an organization can be very powerful information for an individual to possess. Additionally, the development of good working relationships with fellow organizational members at all levels of the hierarchy can help an individual achieve his or her goals. It is especially useful to establish communication relationships with formal and informal organization leaders who can provide other members with important information about the operation, present condition, and future actions of the organization. By learning the rules and structures of the organization and establishing effective interpersonal relationships with organization members, individuals can help direct activities within bureaucratic organizations, rather than being manipulated by the bureaucracy.

NOTES

1. Von Bertalanffy, 1969, Section N.
2. Weick, 1969, Section N.
3. Ibid, p. 40.
4. Kreps, 1980, pp. 397–98, Section N.
5. House, 1970, Section N.
6. Casella, 1977, Section A; see also: Fisher, 1981, Section N.
7. Fayol, 1949, Section N; Taylor, 1911, Section N; Weber, 1948, Section N.
8. Bradley and Baird, 1980, p. 10, Section N.
9. Tortoriello et al., 1978, Section N; see also: Taylor, 1911, Section N.

READING

PREVIEW OF READING

In "Conflict in Hospitals," Schulz and Johnson review research on organizational conflict and identify the underlying forces fostering conflict. Conflicts involving hospital administration, medical staff, nursing groups, and hospital clients are examined. The authors suggest several organizational approaches to dealing with conflict, including goal setting, creative problem solving, constructive confrontation, participative management, and team training.

CONFLICT IN HOSPITALS

Rockwell Schulz
Alton C. Johnson

Evidence of conflict in hospitals is readily apparent. Nurse and nonprofessional hospital employee strikes receive wide publicity. Periodically, administrator-medical staff conflicts break into public view. Furthermore, hospital-client conflicts seem to be increasing as consumers of hospital service level charges of inefficiency and inattention to consumer expectations. Internally, the administrator is continually faced with eruptions of personal or departmental conflicts.

The first step in resolving conflict is to identify the underlying forces fostering it. This paper reviews empirical research reported in management, sociological and hospital literature for insight into some of these underlying forces. The scope of this review includes a brief consideration of hospital-client, interpersonal and individual conflicts. Conflicts related to administrators, medical staff and nursing groups are discussed in somewhat greater depth. Finally, some mitigators of conflict are suggested.

Modern management literature describes benefits that are derived from a reasonable amount of organizational and individual conflict.[1] Indeed, confron-

Reprinted with permission from the quarterly journal of the American College of Hospital Administrators, *Hospital Administration*, 16 (1971): 36–50.

tation is sometimes necessary in order to achieve overdue reforms. Just how serious, then, is conflict in hospitals?

One might expect conflict to affect quality of patient care adversely. This tends to be confirmed by studies of Georgopoulos and Mann, who found higher quality care in hospitals where physicians and nurses had a greater understanding of each other's work, problems and needs.[2] Studies in mental hospitals report patients are affected adversely by staff conflict.[3] While conflict might foster institutional innovation and progress, the welfare of the individual patient is served more effectively with institutional stability and harmony. Moreover, conflict can be debilitating for participants, rigidify the social system in which it occurs, and lead to gross distortions of reality.[4] Thus, this paper assumes that minimizing conflict is an important goal and it suggests sources and mitigators of conflict.

Institutional Conflict

Evidence of client-hospital conflict is increasing; however, few empirical studies have been conducted to examine this problem. Patients have very little voice in hospital matters, nor, until quite recently, have they seemed to desire one; largely we suspect, because they've assumed that professionals know what's best for them. Etzioni notes that only in public monopolies (e.g., the post office) do clients have less influence than in hospitals.[5] Apparently, he does not see current constituencies of hospital governing boards as an effective voice for the client. The recent report by the Urban Coalition tends to support the view that patients, especially the poor, do not have a proper voice in decision making.[6]

A lack of clearly defined community service goals could be an underlying factor in hospital-client hospital conflict. Etzioni suggests that "sometimes an organizational goal becomes the servant of the organization rather than its master . . . Goals can be distorted by frequent measuring of organizational efforts, because as a rule, some aspects of its output are more measurable than others."[7] Certainly, hospitals are susceptible to this inversion of ends and means. The hospital financial statement, for example, is one of the few easily understood measurements available to trustees and administrators and it usually stresses institutional goals as opposed to patient goals.

Conflict or competition between hospitals is evident from the major programs, such as comprehensive health planning, designed to reduce it. However, there appears to be little empirical research on the seriousness, underlying sources, or measurable effects of such conflict. It can be assumed that displacement of community service goals by institutional goals would be an important factor in such conflicts. What is best for an individual hospital is not always best for the society it serves.

Conflict Within Institutions

Certain internal characteristics inherent in the hospital organization foster conflict. For example, interdependence, specialization and heterogeneity of personnel and levels of authority, all appear to be related positively to conflict.[8] In fact, few organizations are composed of as many diverse skills as the hospital, which generally has nearly three employees for each patient and a heterogeneous health team influenced by over 300 different professional societies and associations.

Individual Conflict

An individual's role in the hospital can have a major effect on conflict to which he is subjected. His personal characteristics and past environment will determine the impact and his coping mechanisms to role conflict. Role theory, including role conflict, has received considerable study, although not in a hospital setting. It is easy to imagine role conflict faced by physicians, nurses and administrators. The physician, for example, functions as an agent for an individual patient, his specialty, his profession, his staff, his institution, his community and his own welfare as an individual practitioner. The welfare of these individuals and groups and obligations of the physician to them and to himself are periodically in conflict. The nurse is frequently caught between multiple lines of authority. The administrator usually functions in a boundary role; that is, he is frequently in a position between the nurse and physician, two physicians, patient and employee, etc.

Role ambiguity is related to role conflict. Role ambiguity can be defined as uncertainty about the way one's work is evaluated superiors, uncertainty about scope of responsibility, opportunities for advancement, and expectations of others for job performance. A variety of studies have demonstrated that there is frequently a wide disparity between what a superior expects of his subordinate and what the subordinate thinks the superior expects of him. In an industrial setting Kahn found the individual consequences of role ambiguity generally comparable to individual effects of role conflict. They include, "low job satisfaction, low self-confidence, a high sense of futility, and a high score on the tension index."[9]

A Coping Mechanism: Retreat

Surveys in industrial enterprises found that tension and strain increase directly with occupational status. Individuals in professional and technical occupations experienced the most tension followed by managerial, then clerical and sales.[10] However, Kahn found the medical administrator in the industrial plant who works under conditions of high role conflict scored low on tension.[11] In a case study he found the administrator kept potential conflicts in a delicate balance by retreating into his own section of expertise, i.e., statistical and financial management. The obvious implication is that the administrator can minimize conflict and tension by restricting his role. While this represents one case study in a non-hospital setting, one can logically assume a relationship between the scope of an administrator's role and his effort to effect changes and administrative conflict. Such a coping mechanism may aid the equanimity of the administrator but will not help him fulfill his broader obligations and responsibilities. Kahn's studies also relate personality variables to experiences of strain from conflict.[12] He found tension more pronounced for introverts, for emotionally sensitive people, and individuals who are strongly achievement-oriented. Personality characteristics also affected exposure to role conflict and tension. Individuals who are relatively flexible and those who are achievement-oriented are more subjected to conflict pressures.

Interpersonal Conflict

Interpersonal conflict is defined broadly to include both (a) interpersonal disagreements over substantive issues, such as policies and practices, and (b) interpersonal antagonisms, that is, the more personal and emotional differences which arise between interdependent human beings.[13] Both forms are broadly evident in the hospital setting. Interpersonal antagonisms would seem to be more prevalent in hospital operations because by nature they deal with emotions. However, no studies were found related to relative frequency, severity or source of interpersonal conflict in hospitals.

Administration-Medical Staff Conflict

Whereas in industry top executives usually enjoy both formal and informal power and status, power and status do not appear to be centered in the same individuals in the hospital organization. This characteristic, rather unique to hospital organization, is a basic source of administration-medical staff conflict.

Power has been defined as the maximum ability of a person or group to influence individuals or groups. Influence is understood as the degree of change that may be effected in individuals or groups. Authority has been defined as legitimate power.[14] In reviewing a variety of authors, Filley and House have summarized the basis of power being derived from (1) legitimacy, (2) control of rewards and sanctions, including money, (3) expertise, (4) personal liking, and (5) coercion.[15] Observation tells us that the hospital administrator usually has (1) legitimacy from delegated authority for hospital affairs from the governing board, (2) effective control of funds, beds, and other resources, (3) increasing expertise, particularly as management information systems improve, (4) personal liking, and (5) ability to coerce through demands of such sources as the Joint Commission on the Accreditation of Hospitals. Studies by Perrow and Georgopoulos and Mann tend to confirm the increasing dominance of the administrator.[16] Recent demands by the American Medical Association and medical staffs in many hospitals for medical staff representation on hospital boards tend to confirm their protestations of declining influence.

The Factors Of Status

Other studies are somewhat conflicting; however, they appear to relate more to factors of status. For example, Georgopoulos and Mann, after describing the administrator as most influential, describe his source of influence as delegated authority from trustees, while sources of physicians' influence include their expertise, prestige, status and power among patients and the community.[17] A recent survey reported that "trustees and medical staff do not view the administrator as a leader, but as a generally passive influence caught between the board and doctors."[18]

Goss suggests that physicians tend to view administration as a less prestigious kind of work.[19]

The hospital administrator's drive for professionalism and his desire for more prestigious titles such as president or executive vice-president, tend to suggest that he believes he needs to improve his status. As physicians attempt to maintain or increase their power, and administrators improve their status, presumably, both tend to feel threatened. Under such circumstances conflict increases.

Physicians and nurses, like professionals in other fields, have primary allegiance to professional status rather than to organizational status.[20] Hence, the potential for professional-institutional goal conflict is present.

The hospital organization is sometimes referred to as a duopoly with essentially autonomous administrative and medical staff organizations. Croog suggests that each system is oriented to a different set of values, one emphasizing provision of service, one emphasizing maintenance of operation of organization.[21] The Barr report related hospital inefficiences to this dual management authority.[22] Other studies tend to confirm the presence of a conflict between bureaucratic routine and individualized patient care.[23] Perhaps a more flexible organizational structure with emphasis upon project teams would reduce this type of conflict.

Nursing Conflict

Considerable basic conflict in nursing is evident from many studies. Most of these inquiries indicate that nurses are satisfied with their vocation, but dissatisfied with specific conditions of salary, work load, working hours, etc.[24] However, Argyris suggests more basic problems, such as frustration of the dominant predispositions of nurses.[25] He reports nurses in the hospital he studied were not able to fulfill effectively important predispositions, such as being self-controlled, indispensable, compatible, and expert. Findings of Corwin, Taves and Scott, reported later in this paper, seem to support these conclusions.

Status may be a source of basic conflict among nurses. In years past, nursing was one of the few careers a woman could enter and attain some degree of professional prestige. Today, more vocational opportunities are opening to women as sex discrimination continues to decline. Women can, or at least sometimes believe they can, gain greater recognition in such fields as business, government, medicine and teaching.[26] Whereas nurses had been virtually the only professionals in the hospital outside of the physicians, they are now receiving increasing competition for status from a proliferation of allied health professionals, many of whom have higher standards of education, pay, and autonomy. In his survey of student nurses and personnel in three major hospitals, Taves found that "compared to student nurses who have a relatively high image of nursing on the average, the image that the general duty nurse holds seems to be especially low . . . Head nurses have a somewhat better image of nursing than general duty nurses." He also found that other hospital personnel had an even lower image of nursing.[27]

Struggle for Professionalism

Frustrations are evident in nursing's struggle for professionalism. Corwin and Taves suggest that "the drive to gain professional status and achieve a unique place of importance within the hospital's division of labor, inevitably brings the group into conflict with the lay administration and physicians who are jealous of their prima donna status within the hospital scheme."[28] Scott states that the nurses' drive for professionalism may be based on carving out a special niche for themselves in which they can operate relatively independently from control by other groups and which allows them some claim to superior status.[29]

Organizational factors present conflicts for nurses. Nurses' career advancement has shifted from an individual to an organizational context wherein a nurse must move through the bureaucratic hierarchy to gain recognition. Rewards in this hierarchy, however, do not reflect professional patient care, but administrative duties. Argyris suggests that nurses believe that an administrator is a second-class citizen. He also suggests that the only area where a nurse is free to "blow her top" is in the administrative area and this adds another factor which keeps administration in a low status function.[30] On the other hand, Taves found that nursing personnel who have higher ranking official positions in the organization are more satisfied with their jobs than lower ranking personnel.[31]

The Need to Mitigate and Control Conflict

Others suggest sources of nursing conflict can be a lack of role and job concensus,[32] type of care,[33] and dislike of working with nonprofessionals.[34]

Regardless of the source, it is evident that a considerable degree of conflict exists in hospitals. The problem then, is one of developing ways and means of mitigating or at least controlling conflict. The next section suggests some approaches to the resolution of this problem.

ACTION PROGRAM

Figure 1 presents a decision model related to diagnosing and mitigating conflict. It lists conflict participants and some of the underlying sources of conflicts presented in this paper. A brief description of the mitigators listed in the exhibit follows.

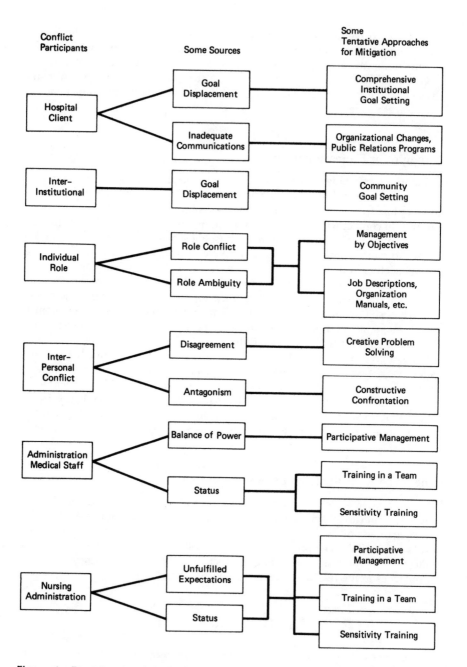

Figure 1   Decision Model for Diagnosing and Mitigating Hospital Conflict.

Comprehensive Institutional Goal Setting

Comprehensive institutional goal setting is a formalized program to define goals and objectives *explicitly*. Too often goals are defined implicitly, such as "high quality care at low cost." Explicit goals state measures affecting quality and costs. Often goals can be stated in terms of specially attainable objectives.

Goal definition should begin with a study of the needs of the society the institution intends to serve in order to obviate displacement of goals. Medical staff members and employees, in addition to administrators and trustees, should participate in setting goals. Sociologists, political scientists and economists, as well as planners and citizens of the publics served, can provide appropriate resource personnel to deliberations. Explicit institutional goals aid community understanding, assist internal and external evaluation of outputs reducing over-emphasis on inputs such as costs and facilities, help to sublimate personal differences by focusing efforts on end results, and help to marshall required resources for attaining goals.

Organizational Changes, Public Relations Programs

Communications can be improved by broadening official lines of communication with citizens served by the institution. Policies for governing board membership might be revised to represent more appropriately the constituencies served. Or, an advisory board might be established to review expressed needs of constituencies and hospital programs to meet needs. A public relations program based on appropriate client attitude surveys can be beneficial.

Community Goal Setting

While many communities are preparing plans for community health services, few have effectively articulated explict goals and objectives that plans should serve. The City of Dallas is a notable exception.[35] There, community goals for health services provide a framework for institutions to coordinate individual goals and plans.

Management by Objectives and Role Definition

Management by objectives is the participation between the subordinate and his superior in setting the subordinate's goal.[36] Through interaction and discussion, a subordinate can determine precisely what is expected of him, thus reducing anxiety resulting from ambiguity, while at the same time improving worker independence in task performance and at the same time increasing accountability.

Role definition through job descriptions and administrative manuals can also help to reduce role conflict and ambiguity. These tools are familiar to most administrators.

Creative Problem-Solving

Creative problem-solving utilizes techniques that sublimate antagonistic conflict and fosters creativity in participative problem-solving. Maier notes the distinction between "choice behavior" which is an examination and a selection from the alternatives, and "problem-solving," which is a searching or idea getting process.[37] By turning choice situations into problem-solving situations, participants are more apt to focus on end results rather than on who is presenting or standing for what. It maximizes creativity and sublimates hostility, self-pity and rigidity. Creative problem-solving promotes end results wherein everyone wins, rather than a choice situation in which there is a winner and loser or a compromise wherein everyone loses.

Constructive Confrontation

Issues of conflict tend to proliferate when there are interpersonal antagonisms between individuals. A manager can take steps to avoid issues that may result in open interpersonal conflict between individuals. However, indirect effects of interpersonal antagonism will frequently persist and in the long run may be more damaging than an open confrontation. Walton suggests using constructive confrontation with third party intervention, particularly by consultants from outside the institution.[38] Components of confrontation include, 1) clarifying the issues with parties, 2) expressing feelings descriptively, 3) expressing facts and fantasies, and 4) resolution and agreement. It would appear, however, that third party intervention should be utilized sparingly.

Participative Management

Participative management is a philosophy of management in which hospital employees and physicians participate in a meaningful way in the administration of the hospital. It is a philosophy espoused by Rensis Likert and by the late Douglas McGregor, who wrote of "theory X and theory Y."[39] Studies by Coleman, Gamson and Corwin support the view that broad participation in authority systems minimizes major incidents of conflict, although minor incidents may be more frequent.[40] Management by objectives and comprehensive institutional goal setting are examples of participative management. The administrator does not abdicate his responsibility, he shares it. By sharing planning, coordination, control and management information, the administrator can actually gain more control over his responsibilities.[41]

Sensitivity Training

Sensitivity training, with emphasis on institutional social system development, can help to overcome "hang-ups" related to conerns over status.[42] Laboratory training based on the more traditional group dynamics training is suggested rather than the recent individual self-awareness training which at times borders on therapy. It is the latter, personal development training, that has been maligned recently.

Training in a Team

Health workers are expected to function as a team, yet they are seldom trained for this role. Hospital administrators spend more time with physicians and nurses than any other group. It would be beneficial if they had meaningful dialogue in the formative educational period. This could be easily arranged through seminars or research projects on such subjects as ethics, legal problems, group dynamics, contemporary problems in health, to name just a few. Opportunities for informal as well as formal associations should be arranged. Interdisciplinary study or informal association can also be arranged through the work environment.

Combined degree programs between medicine and hospital administration and/or nursing and hospital administration should be considered seriously. In addition to improving team associations at the educational level, it would help to improve administrative skills of those who actually administer a large part of health service and health team.

In Summary

Conflict in hospitals is an incredibly complex issue. While it deserves considerably more research, much can be done to apply current knowledge of sources and mitigating activities. In general, increased demand for services and attempts to diagnose and lessen conflicts will result in new policies and procedures. Among these will be research studies to identify the impact of various conflict situations. In addition, one can expect to see changes in goal setting, planning, organizational relationships and training programs.

NOTES

1. Among them are: Amitai Etzioni, *Complex Organizations*, Holt, Rinehart & Winston, 1961, pp. 124–26; Mason Haire, *Modern Organization Theory*, Wiley, 1965; and Robert L. Kahn, *Organizational Stress*, Wiley, 1964.
2. Georgopoulos, Basil S. and Floyd C. Mann, *The Community General Hospital*. Macmillan Co., 1962, p. 400.
3. Stanton, Alfred H., and Morris S. Schwartz, *The Mental Hospital*. Basic Books, 1954, pp. 342–65; and William A. Caudill, *The Psychiatric Hospital as a Small Society*. Howard University Press, 1958, pp. 87–127, as reported by Peter M. Blau and Richard W. Scott, *Formal Organizations*. Chandler, 1962, pp. 53–54.
4. Walton, Richard, *Interpersonal Peacemaking*. Addison Wesley, 1969, p. 5.
5. Etzioni, Amitai, *Modern Organizations*. Englewood Cliffs, N.J.: Prentice-Hall, 1964, p. 95.
6. *Rx for Action*, Report of the Health Task Force of the Urban Coalition. John Gardner, Chairman. Washington, 1969.

7. Etzioni, *op. cit.*, pp 4–11.
8. Thompson, Victor, "Hierarchy, Sepcialization & Organizational Conflict," in *Administrative Science Quarterly*, p. 519, and Corwin, Ronald, "Patterns of Organizational Conflict," *Administrative Science Quarterly*, Dec. 1969, pp. 507–21.
9. Kahn, Robert L., *Organizational Stress*. Wiley, 1964, p. 380.
10. *Ibid.*, p. 144.
11. *Ibid.*, pp. 362–71.
12. *Ibid.*, pp. 225–335.
13. Walton, *op. cit.*, p. 3.
14. Filley, Alan C., and Robert J. House, *Managerial Process and Organization Behavior*. Glenview, Ill.: Scott, Foresman & Co., 1969, p. 55.
15. *Ibid.*, p. 61.
16. Perrow, Charles, "Goals and Power Structure," *The Hospitals and Modern Society*. Eliot Friedson, editor. Free Press, 1963, pp. 112–46, and article in *Handbook of Organizations*; and Georgopoulos, *op. cit.*, p. 567.
17. Georgopoulos, *op. cit.*, p. 567.
18. "Trustee's View of Administrators Told," *Modern Hospital*, October 1968, p. 29.
19. Goss, Mary E. W., "Patterns of Bureaucracy Among Staff Physicians," *The Hospital*, p. 180.
20. Argyris, Chris, *Diagnosing Human Relations in Organizations: A Case Study of a Hospital*. New Haven: Yale University, Labor and Management Center, 1965, p. 62; and W. G. Bennis et al., "Reference Groups and Loyalties in the Outpatient Department," *Administrative Science Quarterly*, March 1958.
21. Croog, S. H., "Interpersonal Relations in Medical Settings," *Handbook of Medical Sociology*, H. E. Freeman, S. Levine, and L. G. Reeder, editors, Prentice-Hall, 1963, p. 256.
22. Secretary's Advisory Committee on Hospital Effectiveness, Department of Health, Education, and Welfare, 1967.
23. *Abstracts of Hospital Management Studies*, Vol. IV (June 1968). University of Michigan, pp. 137–40 and 196.
24. Corwin, R. G., and Marvin J. Taves. "Nursing and Other Health Professions," *Handbook of Medical Sociology*, pp. 187–212, and Argyris, *op. cit.*
25. Argyris, *op. cit.*, p. 189.
26. Corwin, and Taves, *op. cit.*, note that studies in two states indicated teaching out-ranked nursing in prestige (p. 193).
27. Corwin and Taves, *op. cit.*, p. 189.
28. *Ibid.*, p. 206.
29. Scott, W. Richard, "Some Implications of Organization Theory for Research on Health Services," *Milbank Memorial Fund Quarterly*, Vol. XLIV, No. 4, Part 2 (October 1966), p. 52.
30. Argyris, *op. cit.*, pp. 67–69.
31. Taves, *op. cit.*, p. 51.
32. *Ibid.*, p. 74 and p. 205. Georgopoulos, *op. cit.*, p. 398, and Argyris, *op. cit.*, p. 10.
33. Perrow, *op. cit.*, p. 965. Perrow reported a study by Coser which found nurses giving only custodial care were alienated because they were "unable to implement a single goal."
34. Argyris, *op. cit.*, p. 70.
35. *Goals for Dallas*, Dallas, Texas, 1966.
36. Odiorne, George, *Management by Objectives*, Pitman, 1965.
37. Maier, Norman F., "Maximizing Personal Creativity Through Better Problem Solving," *Personal Administration*, Vol. 27 (1964) and Filley, Alan C. and Andre Delbecq, "On the Possibility of a Better World," University of Wisconsin (unpublished).

38. Walton, Richard E., *Third Party Consultation*, Addison-Wesley, 1969.
39. Likert, R., *New Patterns in Management*, McGraw-Hill, 1961; and McGregor, D., *The Human Side of Enterprise*, McGraw-Hill, 1960.
40. Coleman, James S., *Community Conflict*, Glencoe, Ill., Free Press, 1957; William Gamson, "Rancorous Conflict in Community Politics," *American Sociological Review*, Vol. 31, pp. 71–81; and Ronald G. Corwin, "Patterns in Organizational Conflict," *Administrative Science Quarterly*, December 1969, pp. 507–20.
41. Tannenbaum, A. S., "Control in Organizations: Individual Adjustment and Organizational Performance," *Administrative Science Quarterly*, September 1962, p. 236.
42. Buchanan, Paul C., "Laboratory Training and Organization Development," *Administrative Science Quarterly*, September 1969, pp. 466–77; Lewin, Kurt, *Resolving Social Conflicts: Selected Papers on Group Dynamics*, Harper, 1948.

8.

INTERCULTURAL AND ETHICAL COMMUNICATION IN HEALTH CARE

Obi Nahito was studying electrical engineering at a small college in the western United States. He was from the central part of Africa and was the only person from his country studying at this small college.

In the midst of his junior year his father died in Africa. With a small inheritance and a collection of money from various family members, his mother was sent to be with him in the United States, as her only wish after the death of her husband was to be with her youngest son.

Although she could not speak English, she was content to stay in the small apartment where she cooked, cleaned, and was slowly introduced to the world of American technology while her son attended classes.

In the middle of the semester, Obi's junior engineering class was required to take a three-day wilderness field trip. He was hesitant to leave his mother since she could not communicate with anyone, but the field trip was required for course completion and his mother assured him she could manage.

The day after Obi left, however, his mother became terribly ill. After several hours of agonizing pain, she managed to get to the apartment door and open it. A next door neighbor found her shortly afterwards and rushed her to the hospital. She was terrified and she understood nothing. She was mortified when strangers removed her clothes and started probing her body. She was of no assistance in indicating where her pain was located, and the emergency room doctor finally prescribed a tranquillizer. When the nurses tried to give her the medicine in pill form, she became further agitated and would not take the medicine. The doctor then prescribed an injection. When she refused to lie still for this, she was tied down while the shot was given. From that point onward, she huddled in a ball under the covers of her bed and the head nurse observed that this patient was likely to have died from fear if not from her mysterious illness.

Obi's mother's condition worsened and exploratory surgery was scheduled. The physician was hesitant to proceed, however, until he had informed consent from the client or from the son. He tried to explain nonverbally what he was going to do to the patient, hoping he could secure her cooperation. Taking a knife, he gestured over her stomach. She began moaning and screaming. This continued for four hours until the son finally reached the hospital.

As details were given to the son he was horrified. His mother's beliefs were still firmly rooted in an African culture which believed that medicine in pill form was white man's magic and should never cross the lips of a true believer. Additionally, in her view she had been threatened by the knife-holding physician as it was taboo in her country to penetrate the skin with a knife. Two of her important beliefs had been threatened by the well-intending health professional.

Later, with the son's help it was determined that the woman had appendicitis and that an operation was indicated. What are the intercultural and ethical decisions that health providers should consider as they advise a family such as this one?

In this chapter we will discuss intercultural, interprofessional and ethical concerns in health care practice. Cultural sensitivity and ethical behaviors are prerequisites for effective health communication. It is our contention that culture and ethics are linked in many important ways. What is and is not ethical is largely determined by the cultural orientations of communicators. An understanding of culture will help us understand ethical aspects of health care practice.

CULTURE

Culture is particularly important in health care if effective communication is going to take place. If health care personnel have a poor understanding of their own culture, let alone the culture of the client, their intervention can often do more harm than good as they misinterpret behavior (communication).

The word culture is often vaguely and unexplainably used. We talk about the "black culture," the "drug culture" or the "culture" of the community without defining the meaning of any of these terms. Edward T. Hall, a foremost anthropologist, defines culture as communication[1] and Karl Deutsch concurs.[2] Deutsch says that culture is based on the community of communication which consists of socially stereotyped patterns. These stereotypes include habits of language and thought which are carried on through various forms of social learning, particularly through methods of child rearing. One country can be host to many cultures or subcultures within its geographic boundaries. Within the United States for example, women have a somewhat separate culture from men, blacks from Indians and children from the elderly. In the area of health care, physicians have a culture difference from that of other health care providers. Language, friendship, eating habits, communication practices, music, social acts, economic and political activities, and technology dictate culture and its different groupings.[3]

Culture is intriguing, but it is also difficult to study and understand. Why someone eats certain foods, wears certain clothes, and uses certain language would be far easier to investigate if each person belonged to only one culture but frequently cultures overlap. It is possible to be a sixty-year-old female American Indian physical therapist living in England. In such a case, many cultural influences would interplay.

Often in the past, the importance of culture has gone unrecognized, particularly in regard to such areas as health care. However, a recent emphasis on the many facets of culture has stressed the importance of studying intercultural communication. Not only does the study of culture bring fresh insights into the variability of human beings but it aids us in studying and solving communication problems between different groups.

Cultures are difficult to understand and study because we subconsciously absorb cultural constraints. Culture becomes a form of conditioning which is so subtle it cannot be isolated for independent study. It must be remembered that this conditioning shows itself through behavior which is a product of culture. For example an American doctor or a nurse might be offended by a client who tried to stand too close to them, whereas in an Arab culture close proximity would be expected.

The difficulty of studying and researching culture is further compounded by the many subcultures to which we belong. *For our purposes a subculture is defined as a group of people with clearly identifiable values that exist within the geographical boundaries of a dominant culture.* In the United States for example, some of these subcultures would be based on religious or regional definition, as well as the definition of groups which deviate by choice from the national norms or culture. In discussing the subculture of white middle-class males, Kalish and Collier state:

> Among middle-class males of White or European ancestry will be found homosexuals, persons living on rural communes, militant advocates of Black supremacy, men who want to father children without marrying the mothers, men who wish to bake bread rather than buy it, men who refuse to eat meat, men who are in training to serve as guerilla fighters when the Communists take over the country and men who are addicted to heroin. The degree to which a culture will tolerate deviation and accept the conflicting values of its sub-cultures depends on the values of the culture. Vegetarians are more tolerated than homosexuals; workers on communes are more tolerated than advocates of violence.[4]

As the quote indicates, the complexity of studying cultures and subcultures is formidable but not impossible.

Intercultural Communication

Intercultural communication, also called cross-cultural or transcultural communication, occurs whenever the two people interacting are members of different cultures or subcultures. For example, a Spanish speaking nurse and an East-Indian speaking client are an intercultural combination as is a husband and wife or two family members from different age groups. There is a cultural variance between members of any interaction when their perception of social objects and events as well as their use of the language is different because of their acculturation. *Acculturation refers to the process of absorbing cultural traits by transference from others.*

When the acculturation of two people who are trying to communicate has been different, these two people talk with differing perceptions of a situation and often they do not take enough time to understand each other's perceptions. *Intercultural communication can best be understood, in fact, as cultural variance in the perception of social objects and events.* Human perception (discussed in detail in Chapter 2) is often distorted or exaggerated if perceptual frameworks are complicated by intercultural variables such as beliefs, values, attitude systems, world views, and social organization.[5]

Beliefs, Values, and Attitude Systems

Beliefs, values, and attitudes have a strong impact upon health care for both the practitioner and the client. *Beliefs* are basic units of thought establishing a relationship between at least two entities. They are thoughts people hold on the truth or falseness of a given topic. Virtually any idea that begins with the phrase, "I believe that . . ." is a belief. Verbal beliefs are called opinions. *Values* are beliefs that evaluate or judge. Values are judgements of the worth of something. They often involve good or bad or right or wrong statements. *Attitudes* become the cluster of beliefs relevant to some central object of judgment. For example, if I believe that cancer is contagious (a *belief*) I will think that it is bad to visit hospitals (a *value*) and my *attitude* toward visiting or being with anyone who has cancer will be negative. Attitudes are predispositions people have about whether to react positively or negatively to something. Beliefs are organized in a hierarchy that ranges from shared primitive beliefs that seldom change to beliefs that are less rigid. However, beliefs and values that are primitive and rigid in one culture often change in another. What is more, values can change within a culture itself over different time frames. For example, in India in former periods a high cultural value was placed by the majority on having large families. Now because of the need for population control in that country, the values are changing and the emphasis is on smaller families.

Attitudes have the components of cognition, affectiveness, and intensity or expectancy. These three elements interact to create the psychological state needed to react to objects and events in our environment. For example, if we believe that mental or physical pain should never be endured and we have no prejudices against pharmacological drugs, then our attitude system might be favorable to using pharmacological products such as Valium and Demerol without much discrimination. It is important to remember that attitudes are cultural learnings.

World View and Social Organization

Two other organizing principles for intercultural communication are world view and social organization. Both are important because they affect our perception of others. *World view*, for example, *deals with one's attitude toward religion, the nature of humans, and of the universe.* How a culture is organized affects how members of the culture perceive and develop their world. Attitudes on one's world view are subtle and do not reveal themselves easily as they go about influencing belief, values, and attitudes as well as such things as the use of time and space. "Our world view is so deeply imbedded in our psyches that we take it completely for granted and assume that everyone views the world as we do."[6]

Social organization concerns how a culture organizes its members and its institutions. Geography and roles are an important part of social organization. The institutions of society such as schools, churches, the universities, armies, prisons, mass media, and the health system convey the values of a certain world culture. Through unwritten codes of laws as well as written ones values and stereotypes are conveyed by these institutions. For example, the unwritten codes of health care in the United States have always included a provision that physicians "always know best" and should have major control over areas in the realm of medicine. Not realizing how rigid this unwritten code still is, a young midwife in Nevada recently started delivering babies in a rural area. The state medical profession protested, stating that midwifery was the practice of medicine. The midwife, her attorney, and many supporters of the community disagreed with this definition insisting that childbirth, of itself, is not a medical matter. When the courts decide this case, they will have to interpret unwritten as well as written social codes and concepts, for at the present time there is no mention of midwifery in the Nevada statutes as either a medical or nonmedical matter. The courts will have to decide what is in part a cultural matter.

Social organizations especially define the role each of us must play within the culture in such institutions as families, churches, and hospitals. In the past these roles have been rigid and rather inflexible. The advantage of inflexibility is that clear information about the role is conveyed. The disadvantage is that it is difficult to change the role as society changes. Examples in point would be the attempts to change the role of nurses in today's society.

Roles can stay the same across geographical boundaries though extenuating circumstances can change the roles. For example, the fact that 90 percent of Russian physicians are female would make the role of the physician different in the Soviet Union than in the United States. Sexual status as well as the low status of medicine in Russia would make role communication confusing for an American doctor visiting in that country. Health professional organizations such as medical or nursing associations are prime arbitrators of professional socialization for the roles of their members. Not only do they govern who can or cannot belong to their organization, they govern much of the unwritten code regarding the conduct of their members.

Disseminating Intercultural Information

In addition to understanding intercultural communication through beliefs, values, attitude systems, world views, and social organizations, it is important to understand that views regarding these variables are disseminated through *socialization, the process by which members of a culture receive continuous, usually unanimous, reinforcement to behave in culturally approved ways.* Socialization is conveyed through stereotyping, ethnocentrism, proselytyzing, and metacommunication. *Stereotyping is the process that occurs when we as individuals convey our beliefs regarding such issues as equality, individuality, and social status and expect others to agree with us in some way.* "Indians are always drunk," "Blacks are inferior," and "blonds are dumb" are examples of painful and undocumented stereotypes still held by some people.

As can be seen, *stereotypes are symbols intended to identify ethnic groups, races, or subcultures.* Generally, they are standard mental pictures used to oversimplify the characteristics of members of another group.

Stereotyping is done because it makes communication easier. Through stereotyping we feel we know which groups we can feel more comfortable with and which groups are more likely to share our values. We develop stereotypes regarding status and role as well as ethnicity. For example, seeing the physician as "godlike" is a stereotype, sometimes harmful to both physician and client but it serves as a way to make the health care hierarchy clear to all parties.

Health care workers from other cultures are particularly annoyed by the stereotyping that locks members of their culture into simplistic groupings. One clinical worker was annoyed by the local residents' tendency to say "Haitian is like that, Hispanic is like that, you know those Italians are all alike . . ." She felt these stereotypes blinded people to the diversity within such groups.[7]

Ethnocentrism, like stereotyping, is a major barrier to cultural understanding. *It is the tendency to interpret or to judge all other groups, their environments and their communication according to the categories and values of our own culture.* Americans are seen as particularly ethnocentric by many groups. We are both benevolently ethnocentric, that is, we judge others by our standards but still tolerate them, and militantly ethnocentric, in that we frequently force our values on others. Everett Klunjans, a Chancellor of the Honolulu East West Center proposed that Americans should stop playing God and join the human race. He has indicated that he thinks it is time for Americans to develop a more humble style of relating to people.[8] Ethnocentrism can be a serious problem in health care when the health practitioner is relating to someone from a different culture and is not accepting of them. Getting impatient with a Hindu who won't eat meat or an African who wears an amulet are examples of ethnocentric behavior. A political example of militant ethnocentrism was the terrible anger felt by many Americans at all Iranians in the country during the hostage crisis in 1980. Though the Iranians in America were obviously not responsible for the crisis in Iran many thousands of miles away, several Iranians were shot, houses burned, and individuals attacked. While these were isolated incidents, they did happen and they show the misunderstanding that can occur when cultures do not share the same perception. The reverse of course was also true for Americans in Iran. There, the Iranians felt superior to all Americans including the hostages and treated them in an ethnocentric manner.

Proselytyzing is an attempt to force an intercultural perspective on others. It is the process of advocating that members of other cultural groups should adapt your view on religion, politics, government, or whatever else is at stake. Proselytzing takes place in health care when providers, or other clients for that matter, attempt to force their views regarding health or medicine on others. This is often done in an effort to get clients to "comply" rather than cooperate.

Finally, metacommunication is a vehicle for socializing others to one's point of view. As was discussed in Chapter 2, *metacommunication should be remembered as the method of sending messages about the "correctness" of a person's communication.*

In summary, the socialization that takes place through stereotyping, ethnocentsm, proselytzing, and metacommunication is important to understand for intercultural communication in health care and elsewhere.

Nonverbal Communication and Intercultural Variables

Edward T. Hall wrote a book aptly entitled *The Silent Language*.[9] The major thesis of the book is that the nonverbal or silent language that exists in every country of the world and which is the basis for intercultural communication is not understood by most people. Hall sees it as imperative that we learn about the nonverbal aspects of culture in order to survive. Although studied intensively, nonverbal communication is still not clearly understood. (Recall our in-depth discussion of nonverbal communication systems in Chapter 2.)

HOW TO MEDIATE INTERCULTURAL DIFFERENCES

To improve intercultural communication we need to know about the culture of others and they need to know more about ours. We need to take time to study and interact with people so that we can learn and understand the perceptions that differ from our own.

In working with clients or with health personnel who are members of other cultures, there are many steps that can be taken to facilitate better communication. Most important, time must be taken to discover what kinds of special verbal or nonverbal information is necessary to establish effective interaction. What are the space needs of the individual from the other culture? Do they respond to touch? What kind of eye contact is considered appropriate to establish trust? Are there any special rules of protocol that should be followed? In the case study at the beginning of this chapter, a realization of cultural differences would have been helpful.

When the cultural differences are quite disparate, care should be taken with the interviewing process discussed previously in Chapter 4. One of the best ways to gather information about clients is to listen to their stories, which can provide useful clues to areas important to the client. While this may seem to be time-consuming, in the long run it probably saves time and gives the information necessary to provide a higher overall quality of care for the client. Time becomes important in the establishment of trusting relationships. The female proctologist and the male client need to establish trust before an examination. The traditional Chinese female and the hurried American male gynecologist must also do the same. A black health provider tells of the mistrust black people have of many health professionals because of the conception they have that members of their race have been used as guinea pigs in medicine. In all of these examples of different cultural relationships, only time taken to establish trust can prevent potential problems. The professional must be aware that if mistrust is present in the relationship, several patterns can occur which are generally geared to telling the professional what the client perceives he or she wants to hear. For example, in some cultures it is impolite to say "no." Polite "yes" answers rather than truthful "no" answers would lead to inaccurate diagnosis and even accidental death. Only time and information can break the barriers of mistrust.

In conducting an interview with a person of another culture it must also be remembered that your own cultural characteristics may influence the responses you get in the interview. Police stations and hospitals have recently begun to realize that rape victims respond better to a person from their own female culture and therefore women police officers and health providers are utilized. Age, ethnicity, sex, educational level, and social class may greatly influence information obtainable from a respondent.

One final caution! In establishing any new relationship with persons from another culture it is important to focus at first on the similiarities rather than the differences between you and the other person. While these differences are important, as we have already indicated in this chapter, the similarities are of equal importance. A recent book on culture and communication quotes an Indian hospital administrator: "I feel you should start with a 'people' focus rather than on differences. Similiarities form a basis for relationships. Ask, 'What is common to human nature?' not 'What kind of pain does she have, a Navajo pain or an Anglo pain?'"[10]

A humorous story which reflects the necessity to listen to cues from persons of different cultural settings and to learn all you can about the person you are interviewing recently appeared in one of our campus newspapers. The story tells of a researcher who spent thirteen years compiling a dictionary of one of Papua New Guinea's 700 tribal languages. She reported her task wasn't easy. In fact, to assemble a list of verbs she had to act them out for the informant. For the word "jump" she jumped up and down in front of the village elder and recorded what he said. Six months later she found out that what he had said didn't mean "jump" at all. It meant, "Why are you acting so stupid?"

To summarize most of the information in this chapter we have adapted a short checklist which should be helpful to the professional interested in improving his or her intercultural communication.

Intercultural Check List

DOs

Know yourself.

Know your own culture.

Know your client's culture.

Treat your client's culture as equal to your own.

Be sensitive to the client's values, beliefs, attitudes, world view and social organization.

Learn the client's language whenever possible or have a translator.

Adapt your communication to the client's culture.

Do try to understand your client's nonverbal communication.

DON'Ts

Don't manipulate the client of another culture.

Don't stereotype.

Don't be ethnocentric.

Don't proselytize.

Don't use metacommunication inappropriately.

Don't be arrogant.

Don't ignore your client's customs and beliefs.[11]

Interprofessional Relationships as an Intercultural Concern

The majority of this chapter has been devoted to a discussion of the intercultural relationships that can greatly affect the health care practitioner–client relationship. In this section of the chapter we will emphasize the cultural and professional constraints that affect the interprofessional relationships between health care providers. These are:

1. *Different educational backgrounds.* Physicians generally receive more initial formal training than do other health professionals.

2. *Different career patterns.* Physicians are often self-employed while others often serve at the behest of institutions. Even in the institutional settings physicians are often not part of the organizational structure.

3. *Jargon and semantic differences.* Different words have different meanings to different professionals. For example, when physicians describe a nurse as "cooperative," they mean that she obeys orders. When a nurse talks about a "cooperative" physician she means that he is treating her as an equal.[12]

4. *Class differences.* Physicians make more money, travel with different groups of people, have more prestige and interact more often with those higher in authority.

5. *Sexual and racial differences.* Most physicians are white middle-class males, even in the 1980s. Conversely, the lower the status of the health professional, the more likely the role will be filled by a woman or a minority. Not only is there a difference in status but also a difference in pay. While over 70 percent of health care workers are female, those in high paying status positions in the health care field are male. Difficult patterns of communication that often develop between nurses and physicians are often blamed on male–female cultural differences.

6. *Value differences.* While the physician sees his or her function as curative, nurses and other health providers see their function as caring. Admitting officers see their function as being efficient, as do administrators. These conflicting goals or functions can cause confusion and conflict, both for the client and the health provider and administrator.

7. *Professional isolation.* Largely due to the factors listed above as well as to time constraints, professions are often isolated from each

other. Without different forms of informal as well as formal contact, differences and misunderstandings between the professions grow and become divisive.

Tensions that build as professionals work together can be traced to different bureaucratic and professional goals as well as divided loyalties. The hospital administrator has to be loyal to the hospital board while at the same time responding to staff and client needs. The nurse has to be concerned about peer relationships, relationships with physicians, and her concern for the individual client. Additionally, tensions are caused when every individual working in health settings brings his or her prejudices and stereotypes to the work setting. The doctor who does not respect females will have a difficult time with the nurse, who is usually female; the respiratory therapist who does not like blacks or Chicanos will have difficulty responding to orders from a minority physician.

It also must be remembered when discussing interprofessional relationships that those with "lower" positions have effective ways to combat their powerlessness in the system. In health care, as well as in other organizations, there is a tendency for those in the lower rungs of the hierarchy to keep those above them ignorant of their activities. They can refuse to share important information and insights with others or they can refuse to admit they have certain skills.

In attempting to solve interprofessional problems the solutions are very similar to the solutions given for intercultural communication. For example, spending time and listening to others is of paramount importance. Additionally, we suggest that the professionals learn problem-solving techniques which enable the parties involved to look at mutual problem areas and apply techniques which are designed to improve the decision-making process which is the major focus of the interprofessional interaction. An ethical perspective, which we will be discussing in the following section of this chapter, is also very important in interprofessional relationships.

CULTURE AND ETHICS

The different cultural groups we belong to influence our beliefs, values, and attitudes. Through the acculturation and socialization processes we are trained to recognize ethical constraints on our behavior. Right and wrong are intimately tied to the cultural groups to which we belong. Ethics play a major role in the health care delivery system, and the different cultural orientations of health professionals and consumers of health care instigate a situation where a wide range of moral and ethical positions are often in competition with one another. In the case history presented at the beginning of this chapter there are related influences of both culture and ethics. Obtaining informed consent from a client who cannot speak English is an example of a health care issue involving both cultural and ethical constraints.

Which cultural perspective should prevail within the health care system? Do legal codes of ethics take precedence? Is the Hippocratic oath the preeminent guide for ethical health care behaviors? Is the client's perspective of right and wrong of primary importance when attempting to make ethical health care decisions? The administrative hierarchy of health care delivery organizations certainly asserts a major influence on ethical standards and often conflicts with an individual's code of ethics. Religious groups are intimately involved with many health care delivery organizations and influence the ethical standards within those organizations. As you can see, ethics is a multifarious concept in health care practice. There are no easy answers to any of the questions posed about health care ethics. In the remainder of this chapter we will examine the ethical aspects of health communication.

Ethical Problem Solving in Health Care

Decisions regarding health matters that involve moral issues are called bioethical decisions and the field of study of these life-involving moral decisions is called bioethics. The term "bioethics" literally means the ethics of life. Samuel Gorovitz calls bioethics the "critical examination of the moral dimensions of decision-making in health-related contexts and in contexts involving the biological sciences."[13]

Essentially, *bioethics is the process of making moral decisions regarding health care.* The process of decision-making as well as the transmission of those ethical decisions is an important matter of study for the health communicator.

The importance of communication to ethical decision-making cannot be overemphasized. Often the health professional has the ideals and values necessary to be ethical but does not know how to translate these through the communication process into effective ethical decisions. When values collide as they often do between members of a team or between the health providers and the client or families, communication strategies such as conflict management are important. Ethics without communication becomes meaningless.

In the past bioethics has been studied from a philosophical viewpoint and the codes of the various health professions are based on these philosophical theories. Any reader interested in reviewing these theories is encouraged to do so. However, in this communication-related text we will focus on the communication part of bioethics. In order to do so, let us discuss a bioethics case, a common strategy used in teaching bioethics.

> Susie was twelve years old and in the hospital as a terminal cancer patient. Her parents asked the physician not to tell the patient she was dying. The doctor had written orders on the chart indicating that she should not be told. Late one night Susie asked the duty nurse, to whom she had become attached, if she was dying. What should the nurse say?

A perusual of this case indicates many communication-related bioethical issues such as informed consent, paternalism, rights and responsibilities in health care, the ethics of self-disclosure and the whole issue of justice and the respect for autonomy, as well as the fundamental issue of children's rights. We shall discuss some of the more communication-related issues here.

In the case just presented, informed consent is a major issue. We define *informed consent as the knowing consent of an individual or his or her legally authorized representative.* A recent national report on informed consent which emphasizes the communication process stresses these important factors among others:

1. While informed consent has substantiation in law, it is essentially an ethical imperative.
2. Ethically valid consent is a process of shared decision-making based upon mutual respect and participation and not just a required ritual.
3. Informed consent is important to all cultures. It should be required for all practitioners in their relationships with all patients. It is not a luxury for a few especially well-educated or well-informed individuals.
4. Health care providers should not ordinarily withold unpleasant information simply because it is unpleasant. Most reports on informed consent find that members of the public do not wish to have bad news withheld from them.
5. Shared decision-making based on mutual respect is ultimately the responsibility of individual health care professionals and not systems. Systems which fragment responsibility do not take the place of one individual officially charged with responsibility of seeing that informed consent takes place.
6. Patients should have access to the information they need to help them understand their conditions and make treatment decisions.

7. Techniques such as having patients express, orally or in writing, their understanding of the treatments should be explored.
8. Educators should prepare physicians and nurses to carry out the obligation of informed consent.
9. Family members should be involved in the informed consent process when that does not coerce the patient or does not violate the patient's privacy.
10. Group processes such as ethics committees should be utilized when appropriate.
11. Limits must be placed on the range of acceptable decisions that surrogates or guardians can make beyond those that apply when a person makes his or her own decisions.[14]

While these ideal generalizations apply to most groups of people, there are exceptions. Clients who are incompetent need the special guidance of surrogates acting in their behalf. Whether young children like the twelve-year old in our case, are capable of making their own decisions regarding treatment is one of the major issues in biomedical ethics today and certainly an interesting dilemma for those interested in the ethical field of children's rights as well as for communication scholars. In the case as it actually happened, the nurse did decide to tell Susie that she was very ill. She was almost fired for volunteering even that small amount of information.

The issue of whether the nurse in this case should have answered Susie's questions about death also involves the bioethical problems of rights and responsibilities as well as duties. Communication becomes an important part of this bioethical decision making as these rights and responsibilities are negotiated.

The range of bioethical decisions being negotiated privately and publicly is probably greater than at any other time in history. A surge in medical technology plus a focus on the ethical aspects of health care account in part for this emphasis. Abortion, for example, is, at this writing, one of the most heavily contested issues in the United States and the rhetoric surrounding the issue is vociferous. In abortion and other ethical debates, strategies for conflict negotiation and other communication principles and techniques can assist in effective ethical decision making even when values collide.

In addition to communication techniques, it is also important to understand the principles involved with the particular issue. Confidentiality, for example, requires that a person's right to privacy be balanced with the safety or health of others. Abortion requires the balancing of the rights of autonomy and privacy with potential rights of the fetus and of society. The right to life and the right to death involve justice, respect for life, and caring and concern for others. An understanding of the principles each culture holds dear should be an important part of the education of any professional.

The Legal and Professional Codes and Oaths

All health professionals have codes and oaths. Historically these codes and oaths have been designed to focus on values and ideals as well as to protect the professional from the infringement of others.

One of the authors of this book assigned prehealth professionals to find the code of ethics that pertained to their professions. Attempts to find these codes in local libraries or to obtain them from professionals in the community were time-consuming and largely unsuccessful, indicating the lack of emphasis placed on those codes by professionals and others.

Critics of codes indicate problems with too much generality, lack of definitional terms, and a conflict and lack of priority among values. While these codes are important in that they focus on moral principles and duties, it is clear that much more than a code is needed to ensure ethical behavior.

The law is another dimension to consider in ethical decision making. A law frequently but not always serves as a base for ethical standards. While the law often codifies society's standards, many areas of ethical concern are not covered. This makes the law important to but not definitive in ethical decision making.

Other Ethical Considerations

Stereotypes often affect ethical decision making. For example, because the elderly client is often automatically treated as incompetent, informed consent is not always requested or required. This is an example of how a cultural stereotype affects ethical decision making. Because it is often difficult and painful to tell the truth, paternalistic behavior becomes commonplace. Let us refer to an actual case.

Mr. Edwards, who had a pre-existing heart condition, was admitted to the hospital after a serious accident in which his wife was killed. Although his larynx was paralyzed, he could write on a chalkboard. He indicated that he had a living will which provided that he not be kept alive by any heroic measures in the event of any serious heart condition. The physician, however, noted on the chart that the man's son did not agree with his 85-year-old father's decision and that the son had left orders that all possible action should be taken when necessary. On the day the man's second heart attack occurred, he was resuscitated.

In this case, ethicists would see paternalism as a real issue since the client's wishes were not followed. *Paternalism* refers to an action that is seen as advocating a person's interests but which in reality limits the person's behavior, desires, or freedom of choice. Several issues are involved. The man's right to control his own life, the rights of family members, and the concern of professionals over being sued if family members or the client see their actions as incorrect are several possible areas of ethical conflicts. The issue of justice is paramount.

Truth-telling is also a vitally important ethical issue. Sissela Bok, a leading contemporary ethicist and expert on truth telling, indicates that the truth is important in most societal situations, including health-related ones. Bok expands upon this perspective in an article at the end of this chapter. An analysis of truth telling by the health communication expert can clarify truth-telling issues and make the health care professional aware that there are many communication-related variables important to this issue. The level of trust between professional and client is important to truth telling as is self-diclosure. Additionally, diplomacy or its lack can also affect the way the client receives the facts about his or her illness. It is our suggestion that difficult truth telling situations should be discussed with colleagues or others so that the right words can be used in the actual situation. Many of us who believe in the truth have a difficult time telling it!

One of the most serious day-to-day ethical issues for health professionals involves confidentiality and privacy. Computers, large bureaucratic settings with multiple records, and the many health professionals involved in a client's care are all factors that conspire to invade an individual's privacy or right to confidentiality.

It is a general rule that health professionals should not violate a client's confidentiality except when necessary to preserve the life or health of someone else. In day-to-day reality, however, the client's privacy is often violated. Many hospitals now have computers in which client records can be seen by anyone who knows how to use the computer. Doctors, nurses, and other professionals in the health setting also become hurried and careless with client information.

Solutions to this problem are complex and depend in great part upon an individual's ethical discretion. Not letting curiosity get out of bounds when a health professional is not involved with the actual case and being aware of the importance of privacy for the client's physical and mental well-being are two important ethical stances.

Advocacy is another ethical issue that involves either assisting or defending the client. An advocate pleads or defends a case supporting either action or non-action depending on the situation. Non-action takes such forms as refraining from undercutting client's decisions or refusing requests regarding clients that might not enhance overall care. Action involves doing something on behalf of the client. Both action and non-action can be ethically important, depending on the circumstances. Advocacy, or lack of it, often causes professionals to collide on what may be the best treatment. For example, nurses are often uneasy about their role in strongly encouraging clients to sign informed consents. Yet physicians can threaten to report them for refusal to follow orders in obtaining the informed consent. Nevertheless, most modern health professionals would agree that advocating (through action or nonaction) on a client's behalf is a prime ethical duty.

Many other bioethical issues are also important to the health communicator. Common to all of these ethical issues is the importance of clear and accurate communication. All the good will and philosophical intention to be ethical becomes meaningless if communication to the client is misunderstood or misconstrued. It is the argument of the authors of this book that health professionals cannot act ethically if they do not practice communication skills. Taking time to make sure the client understands instructions, medications, or the implications of treatment is of paramount importance. Learning to convey factual information without frightening clients or family is an equally important part of ethical behavior. Learning not to overstate a case is also a skill which can contribute to the conveyance of rights and responsibilities. We do not argue that being ethical or communicating accurately are easy skills to learn or maintain but we do argue that learning and maintaining them is an important part of being an ethical health practioner.

NOTES

1. Hall, 1959, Section C.
2. Deutsch, 1966, Section N.
3. Samovar, Porter, and Jain, 1981, p. 23, Section H.
4. Kalish and Collier, 1981, p. 95, Section M.
5. Samovar, Porter, and Jain, 1981, Section H.
6. Ibid, p. 47.
7. Brownlee, 1978, p. 23, Section H.
8. Sitaram and Cogdell, 1976, p. 12, Section H.

9. Hall, 1959, Section C.
10. Brownlee, 1978, p. 19, Section H.
11. Sitaram and Cogdell, 1976, pp. 235–236, Section H.
12. Barry, 1982, p. 149, Section M.
13. Gorovitz, 1977, Section M.
14. President's Commission for The Study of Ethical Problems in Medicine and Biomedical and Behaviorial Research, 1982, pp. 1–6, Section M.

READINGS

PREVIEW OF READINGS

The first article, "Communication and Gerontology: Health Communication Training for Providers of Health Services to the Elderly," deals with the growing concern about intercultural differences between the increasing elderly population and other members of society. It is Kreps' contention that health care professionals should be trained to deliver health services to the elderly as effectively and as humanely as possible through the communication process. Through communication training, health care providers can learn to use both verbal and nonverbal language more effectively with geriatric populations. Kreps places special emphasis on the needs of the dying and advocates a course in health communication for the professional who works with elderly populations. The article summarizes many important points in this book as they apply to the elderly.

"Therapy With the Terminally Ill" was written by Elizabeth Kübler-Ross; it is taken from the final chapter of her classic book, *On Death and Dying*. In this chapter she discusses the special communication needs of the dying and explores the ways communication can be used to help the terminally ill individual come to grips with his or her impending death. The cultural perspective of the terminally ill is described and the ethics of communication with the dying person is examined.

"The Ethics of Giving Placebos" by Bok examines the underlying ethical issues of honesty and information control that are part of using placebo drugs and treatments in health care. The question about what the health profession's attitude should be with regard to placebo use is addressed. What are the limitations for use of placebos? When is it unethical to prescribe placebo medications? In what situations is the use of placebos ethical? Moreover, the article raises the issue of how ethical constraints can guide health care actions. It is a classic article in the field of bioethics.

COMMUNICATION AND GERONTOLOGY: HEALTH COMMUNICATION TRAINING FOR PROVIDERS OF HEALTH SERVICES TO THE ELDERLY

Gary L. Kreps

One of the largest populations of consumers of health care services is the elderly. (Although there is a serious problem in exactly defining the population of "elderly" people since chronological age may not be the best determinant of aging, the population I am referring to here includes all of those people over the age of 65 years.)[1] As people grow older they become increasingly concerned about their physical and mental health, leading to increased seeking of health care services by the elderly. In 1977 the U.S. Department of Health, Education, and Welfare reported that age was one of the most important population characteristics in identifying the groups of people seeking health care treatment in the United States:

> Age is one of the characteristics which can be used to predict health status and judge the need for health services. In general, older people are less healthy and tend to utilize health services more frequently than younger ones. Approximately 10 percent of the U.S. population is 65 years of age or older and approximately 4 percent is 75 or older. In areas where there is high in-migration of retired persons or high out-migration of young people, these proportions may be much higher. In these areas there are likely to be higher death rates, greater prevalence of chronic conditions and greater utilization of health services, especially long-term care services.[2]

Since the elderly are a significant population of health care consumers, health care professionals should be trained to deliver health services to the elderly as effectively and as humanely as possible.

The primary tool for the delivery of health care services to people is human communication.[3] The diagnosis, education, and treatment of health problems is accomplished through the maintenance of communication relationships between the providers and consumers of health care services. There is abundant evidence that the communication between the providers and consumers of health care is in need of improvement.[4] Equally obvious is the inadequate, and often inhumane, treatment of the elderly in the health care system.[5] It is my contention that many of the problems the elderly face in receiving health care services are strongly related to problems in health care communication. These health communication problems occur between the health care provider and the consumer, as well as between members of the health care team. I advocate train-

Reprinted by permission of the author.

ing the providers of health care services in effective and sensitive methods of human communication.[6] An important aspect of communication training for health care professionals would include examination of the special communicative needs of the elderly in the delivery of health care services.

Peterson and Bolton advocate the development of educational programs in higher education that will help prepare people for occupations that deal with the problems and concerns of the elderly.[7] Since health care professionals are in occupations that deal with the problems and concerns of the elderly on an everyday basis they are an ideal population to educate about the older person. Additionally, since health care services are delivered through the use of human communication there is a need to combine gerontology education and communication education for the health care practitioner. Gerontology education will help the health care professional to better understand the elderly through acquisition of reliable information about the older individual and increased sensitization to the needs of the older population. Communication education will help the health care professional better relate his/her knowledge about the elderly and their health problems to the practice of health care delivery.

One way to combine aspects of gerontology education and communication education for the health care professional is in a college course in health communication. Health communication is a relatively new but growing area of communication education in institutions of higher education.[8] "Health communication is an area of study concerned with the role of human interaction in the health care process."[9] By focusing on the communicative demands of health care, the health care professional is motivated to recognize the importance of his/her interaction with patients and colleagues, as well as to develop effective human communication skills.

In the remainder of this paper I will describe some of the primary topics of study in health communication and relate these topics to the specific communicative needs of the elderly. There are ten primary topic areas that I concentrate on in teaching health communication. These topic areas are not exhaustive in the area of health communication; they concentrate on the human communication aspects of health care delivery, as opposed to media communication approaches to health communication. Additionally, the topics are not always mutually exclusive, but interrelate in many different ways. The common thread that holds the different topic areas together is the use of human interaction to elicit understanding between peoples, coordinate human activities, and evoke cooperation in health care.

The first topic of study in health communication is examining the relationships between health care and human communication. Human communication is established as the primary delivery system for health care services and examples of how health care professionals depend on their abilities to communicate are discussed. "For example, the doctor who interviews a new patient to establish an accurate medical history, the dentist who probes a patient's mouth to discover the source of a patient's toothache, and the pharmacist who describes the use of a prescribed drug to a customer, are all depending on their ability to communicate effectively to these health care clients to accomplish their professional tasks."[10]

Current problems in health care delivery are related to underlying problems in human communication. Many of these problems are particularly relevant to the problems in health care encountered by the elderly. Some of these problems include dehumanization of patients by health care professionals, lack of patient compliance with health care regimens and appointments, misunderstandings between patients and practitioners, cultural barriers between people in health care, and widespread dissatisfaction with the helper-helpee relationship by both patients and practitioners.[11] The development of the patient-practitioner relationship is analyzed as a possible cause for these health care problems and a potential tool for alleviating the problems. Additionally, theoretical bases of human communication and perception are examined and related to the delivery of health care services.

The second topic of study is the use of language in the delivery of health care. The functions and abuses of medical jargon are examined.[12] Public speaking and patient education skills are practiced, as well as the development of effective listening skills. Students develop the ability to explain and describe complex concepts and procedures to lay audiences. Often patients do not have the understanding of health care procedures and consequences to make informed decisions about their treatment. It is stressed that it is the responsibility of the health care practitioner to provide the patient with sufficient information to allow the patient to make a knowledgeable decision about treatment through informed consent.[13] Cultural aspects of language and language usage are discussed as well.

The third topic of discussion is the importance of nonverbal communication in health care. Sensitivity to the range of nonverbal cues being sent by both the patient and the practitioner are examined. The impact of nonverbal communication on the emotional reactions of the patient to the health care situation is emphasized.[14] Human touch has been found to be an important form of therapeutic communication in geriatric nursing.[15] Unfortunately research has also shown that those elderly residents most in need of therapeutic touches were often going untouched due to cultural barriers, sex taboos and the social structure of the health care organizations.[16]

The fourth topic of study is health care interviewing methods. The goals and responsibilities of health care interviewing are examined. The importance of establishing rapport is stressed as a crucial step to effective patient interviewing. Students are taught to become sensitive to the perspective of the patient by allowing patients to describe as fully as possible their own perceptions of their health care problem. A problem in much health care interviewing is jumping to conclusions about the patient's condition without allowing the patient to "tell his story" about why he is seeking health care.[17] Different interview questioning formats and techniques are also explored.

The fifth topic of study is therapeutic communication. Psychological and emotional aspects of illness are discussed and related to patient-practitioner communication.[18] Self-disclosure and trust are examined as crucial ingredients in the development of therapeutic relationships. Empathy is analyzed and students are encouraged to develop skills in becoming empathic helpers.[19] The

importance of establishing person-to-person rather than person-to-object relationships is stressed.

The sixth area of study is group communication in health care. The use of
health care teams in the delivery of modern medical services is examined.[20] The
family group is examined as a source of health care for members. The family is
examined in relation to placing elderly family members in long-term care centers. The extended-family model is compared to current nuclear models of family life and related to geriatric health care implications.[21] Group therapy and
problem solving is also discussed in relation to health care.

The seventh area of study is the role of conflict in health care delivery.
Intrapersonal conflict is related to the frustrations health care professionals
encounter in attempting to integrate their personal and professional roles.
Patient dissonance is also explored in relation to the powerlessness that is often
felt in relation to the treatment and control of their health care problems. Mechanisms for coping with anger and frustrations are examined and related to the
need for assertive communication in developing viable personal and interpersonal conflict strategies and tactics.[22]

The eighth topic of investigation is intercultural communication in health
care. Interprofessional relations between different members of the health care
team are examined. Male and female cultural roles are analyzed and related to
the professional roles of doctors and nurses.[23] The cultural role of the patient
is explored and related to feelings of dehumanization and stigma.[24] The elderly
are often treated as though they were children by health care practitioners, serving to alienate and dehumanize them. Problems with stereotyping people are
discussed and related to patient treatment.[25] Sensitivity to cultural differences
is fostered through discussion of the commonalities of different people seeking
health care. Carmichael comments, "The most significant intrapersonal problems of the aged may well be the effects that aging related attitudes, values, and
beliefs have on the aging process."[26] Through examination of culturally held
beliefs, values, and attitudes health professionals can begin developing awareness of cultural biases against the elderly and eliminate non-productive
stereotypes.

The ninth topic area is communication in medical organizations. Medical
organizations tend to be among the most bureaucratic, with many rules, regulations, and officials.[27] The importance of accurate and timely information in
health care organizations is stressed. Formal and informal communication networks are identified and related to the effective management of complex medical
organizations. Medical organizations and gerontology are closely related
because of the large number of older people living in health care institutions
such as geriatric centers, hospitals for the chronically ill, nursing homes and
rehabilitation hospitals. In fact, in 1974 the National Center for Health Statistics
reported that almost 1.2 million elderly people were residing in nursing home
institutions.[28] A recent study of the communication patterns of the elderly in a
retirement community has indicated that residents of the community develop
mutually therapeutic communication relationships that provide health care benefits to members of the organization.[29] Further examination of the quality and

patterns of communication in health care organizations may provide useful information for improving organizational life for long-term patients.

The final area of study is communication with the terminally ill. The communicative needs of the dying are explored.[30] Cultural perspectives on death and the dying process are examined and demystified. Problems in current health care for the terminally ill are related to communication. Students are encouraged to recognize their own mortality to help them develop empathy with the dying. The importance of allowing the dying person to prepare emotionally for death, and to die with dignity is stressed.[31] The topic area of communication with the terminally ill is, perhaps, the area of health communication that most closely interfaces with gerontology, because the older person is more acutely aware of his/her mortality. Sensitivity and respect for the dying person is crucial in establishing effective communication. Many of the topics discussed in earlier sections of the course can be applied to the communication relationship between the dying person and the health care provider. Empathy, listening skills, sensitivity to nonverbal cues, and honest communication are necessary interaction skills for the health practitioner attempting to help the dying person make a satisfying transition from life to death.

Certainly one course in health communication will not solve the variety of communication problems facing people in the health care system. By making people aware of many of these problems, however, and offering strategies for improving communication in health care, perhaps some situations that might be problematic and therefore painful to patients and practitioners will be handled more sensitively and effectively by communication trained professionals. Additionally, "As people become older and more frail, their increasing ill-health may be aggravated by problems of isolation, unsatisfactory accomodation and inadequate means. All these are likely to affect their relationship with their general practitioner."[32] The combination of communication and gerontology education in health communication courses can help the health care practitioner develop effective communication relationships with elderly patients and thereby help ease the health care problems faced by the aged.

NOTES

1. Janice Schuetz, "Lifelong Learning: Communication Education for the Elderly," *Communication Education* 29 (1980), p. 34. See also Margaret Huyck, *Growing Older* (Englewood Cliffs, N.J.: Prentice Hall, 1974), Ch. 1.
2. U.S. Department of Health, Education, and Welfare, *Papers on the National Health Guidelines: Baselines for Setting Health Goals and Standards* (Washington: DHEW Publication No. (HRA) 77–640, January, 1977), p. 53.
3. Gary L. Kreps, "Health Communication Education for Future Health Practitioners," *Health Communication Newsletter* 7 (1980), 6–8. See also Donald Cassata, "Health Communication Theory and Research: A Definitional Overview," in D. Nimmo, ed., *Communication Yearbook 4* (New Brunswick, N.J.: Transaction—International Communication Association, 1980), 583–589.

4. Harold L. Walker, "Communication and the American Health Care Problem," *Journal of Communication* 23 (1973), 349–360. See also Barbara Korsch and Vida Negrete, "Doctor-Patient Communication," *Scientific American* 227 (1972), 66–74.
5. U.S. Senate Special Committee on Aging, Subcommittee on Long Term Care, *Nursing Home Care in the United States, Failure in Public Policy: Introductory Report* (Washington: U.S. GPO, 1974). See also, U.S. Senate Special Committee on Aging, Subcommittee on Long Term Care, *Nursing Home Care in the United States, Failure in Public Policy: Introductory Report and Nine Supporting Papers* (Washington: U.S. GPO, 1975). See also M. Mendelson, *Tender Loving Greed* (New York: Knops, 1974).
6. Kreps, *op. cit.*
7. David A. Peterson and Christopher R. Bolton, *Gerontology Instruction in Higher Education* (New York: Springer Publishing Co., 1980).
8. Gary L. Kreps, "Communication Education in the Future: The Emerging Area of Health Communication," paper presented at the Central States Speech Association Convention, 1981, also in *Resources in Education* (in-press, 1981).
9. *Ibid.*, p. 7.
10. *Ibid.*
11. For a discussion of dehumanization of patients in health care see William Gaylin, *Caring* (New York: Knopf, 1976). Also, P. Langlois, "Helping Patients Cope With Hospitalization," *Nursing Outlook* 19 (1971), 334–36. Also, Anonymous, "A Consumer Speaks Out About Hospital Care," *American Journal of Nursing* 76 (1976), 1443–44. For a discussion of compliance in health care see Anthony Komaroff, "The Practitioner and the Compliant Patient," *American Journal of Public Health* 66 (1976), 833–35. Also, R. Gillum and A. Barsky, "Diagnosis and Management of Patient Noncompliance," *Journal of the American Medical Association* 228 (1974), 1563–67. Also, Joy Frelinger and Gary L. Kreps, "Patient Compliance and Personalized Physician-Patient Communication Relationships," unpublished paper, University of Southern California, 1977. For a discussion of misunderstandings in health care see J. Golden and G. Johnson, "Problems of Distortion in Doctor-Patient Communications," *Psychiatry in Medicine* 1 (1970), 127–49. Also, E. Cassell and L. Skopek, "Language as a Tool in Medicine: Methodology and Theoretical Framework," *Journal of Medical Education* 52 (1977), 197–203. Also, C. Boyle, "Difference Between Patients' and Doctors' Interpretations of Some Common Medical Terms," *British Medical Journal* 22 (1970) 286–89. For a discussion of cultural barriers in health care, see E. Friedson, "Disability as Deviance," in M. Sussman, ed., *Sociology and Rehabilitation* (Washington: American Sociological Association, 1966). Also, Dean C. Barnlund, "The Mystification of Meaning: Doctor-Patient Encounters," *Journal of Medical Education* 51 (1976), 716–25. Also, L. Lynch, ed., *The Cross Cultural Approach to Health Behavior* (Rutherford, N.J.: Farleigh Dickinson University Press, 1969). For a discussion of dissatisfaction in health care, see Korsch and Negrete, "Doctor-Patient Communication." Also, Z. Ben-Sira, "The Function of the Professional's Affective Behavior in Client Satisfaction: A Revised Approach to Social Interaction Theory," *Journal of Health and Social Behavior* 17 (1976), 3–11.
12. Nicholas C. Chriss, "Doctors Down the Logorrhea," *Los Angeles Times* (July 17, 1977), 1–3, 4. See also Barnlund, "The Mystification of Meaning . . ." Also, Golden and Johnson, "Problems of Distortion . . ."
13. R. Alfidi, "Informed Consent: A Study of Patient Reaction," *Journal of the American Medical Association* 216 (1971), 1325. Also, J. Horty, "Informed Consent: New Rule Puts Burden of Proof on Patient," *Modern Hospital* 74 (1971), 116.
14. For a discussion of the range of nonverbal behaviors and how they can be used to cause or alleviate patient fears, see Gary L. Kreps, "Nonverbal Communication in Dentistry," *Dental Assistant* 50 (1981), 18–20.

15. Wilbur A. Watson, "The Meanings of Touch: Geriatric Nursing," *Journal of Communication* 25 (1975), 104–112. Also see C. Rinck, "Interpersonal Touch Among Residents of Homes for the Elderly," *Journal of Communication* 30 (1980), 44–47.
16. Watson, "The Meanings of Touch . . ."
17. M. Wexler and L. Adler, *Help the Patient Tell His Story* (Oradel, N.J.: Medical Economics Books, 1971). Also, M. Bloom, "Interviewing the Ill Aged," *The Gerontologist* 11 (1971), 292–99. Also, A. Eustene, "Explaining to the Patient: A Therapeutic Tool and a Professional Obligation," *Journal of the American Medical Association* 165 (1957), 1110.
18. An excellent discussion of the symbolic aspects of illness appears in Barnlund, "The Mystification of Meaning . . ."
19. R. Katz, *Empathy: Its Nature and Uses* (Glencoe, Ill.: The Free Press, 1963). See also E. Stotland et al., *Empathy, Fantasy, and Helping* (Beverly Hills: Sage Publications, 1978). Also, C. Truax, "Therapist Empathy, Genuineness, and Warmth and Patient Therapeutic Outcome," *Journal of Consulting Psychology* 30 (1966), 395–401. Also, C. Truax, "The Meaning and Reliability of Accurate Empathy: A Rejoinder," *Psychological Bulletin* 77 (1972), 397–99.
20. Barbara C. Thornton, "Health Care Teams and Multimethodological Research," in B. Ruben, ed., *Communication Yearbook 2* (New Brunswick, N.J.: Transaction—International Communication Association, 1978), 538–53.
21. G. Spark and E. Brody, "The Aged as Family Members," *Family Process* 9 (1970), 195–210. Also, E. Shanas and G. Streib, eds., *Social Structure and the Family: Generational Relations* (Englewood Cliffs, N.J.: Prentice Hall, 1965). Alsom G. Streib, "Family Patterns in Retirement," *Journal of Social Issues* 14 (1958), 46–60.
22. Joyce Frost and William Wilmot, *Interpersonal Conflict* (Dubuque, Iowa: William C. Brown Company, 1978).
23. G. Corea, *The Hidden Malpractice: How American Medicine Treats Women as Patients and Professionals* (New York, William Morrow, 1977). Also see Sandra Bem and Daryl Bem, "Case Study of a Nonconscious Ideology: Training the Woman to Know Her Place," in Daryl Bem, *Beliefs, Attitudes and Human Affairs* (New York, Wadsworth, 1970), 89–90.
24. Erving Goffman, *Stigma: Notes on the Management of Spoiled Identity* (Englewood Cliffs, N.J.: Prentice Hall, 1963). Also see Friedson, "Disability as Deviance . . ."
25. Beth Hess, "Stereotype of the Aged," *Journal of Communication* 24 (1974), 74–84.
26. Carl W. Carmichael, "Communication and Gerontology: Interfacing Disciplines," *Western Speech Communication* 40 (1976), p. 123.
27. Robert House, "Role Conflict and Multiple Authority in Complex Organizations," *California Management Review* 12 (1970), 53–60. See also B. Georgopoulos, ed., *Organization Research on Health Institutions* (Ann Arbor, Mich.: Institute for Social Research, 1974). Also, B. Georgopoulos, *Hospital Organization Research: Review and Source Book* (Philadelphia: Saunders, 1975). Also, Harish C. Jain, "Supervisory Communication Effectiveness and Performance in Two Urban Hospitals," *Personnel Journal* 50 (1971), 392–95.
28. National Center for Health Statistics, *Monthly Vital Statistics* (1974). Also see Elaine Brody, *Long Term Care of Older People* (New York, Human Sciences Press, 1977), p. 35.
29. Deanne Honeyman-Goodman, "A Study of the Communication Patterns of an Aged Ethnic Population: The Old Jews of Venice, California," unpublished doctoral dissertation, University of Southern California, 1981.
30. Elizabeth Kübler Ross, *On Death and Dying* (New York: MacMillan, 1969). Also see, Austin Kutscher and Michael Goldberg, eds., *Caring for the Dying Patient and His Family* (New York: Health Sciences Publishing, 1973). Also see Larry Bugen, ed., *Death and*

Dying (Dubuque, Iowa: William C. Brown, 1979). Also see Barney Glaser and Anselm Strauss, *Awareness of Dying* (Chicago, Aldine, 1965).

31. Barney Glaser, "The Physician and the Dying Patient," *Medical Opinion and Review* 1 (1965), 108–14. See also W. Bowers, *Counseling the Dying* (New York: Thomas Nelson and Sons, 1964). Also see William Alvarez, "Care of the Dying," *Journal of the American Medical Association* 2 (1952), 86–91.

32. Ann Cartwright, *Patients and Their Doctors* (London, Routledge, 1967), p. 195.

THERAPY WITH THE TERMINALLY ILL

Elisabeth Kübler-Ross

Death belongs to life as birth does
The walk is in the raising of the foot as in the laying
of it down.

Tagore, from *Stray Birds*, CCXVII

It is evident that the terminally ill patient has very special needs which can be fulfilled if we take the time to sit and listen and find out what they are. The most important communication, perhaps, is the fact that we let him know that we are ready and willing to share some of his concerns. To work with the dying patient requires a certain maturity which only comes from experience. We have to take a good look at our own attitude toward death and dying before we can sit quietly and without anxiety next to a terminally ill patient.

The door-opening interview is a meeting of two people who can communicate without fear and anxiety. The therapist—doctor, chaplain, or whoever undertakes this role—will attempt to let the patient know in his own words or actions that he is not going to run away if the word cancer or dying is mentioned. The patient will then pick up this cue and open up, or he may let the interviewer know that he appreciates the message though the time is not right. The patient will let such a person know when he is ready to share his concerns, and the therapist will reassure him of his return at an opportune time. Many of our patients have not had more than just such a door-opening interview. They were, at times, hanging onto life because of some unfinished business; they cared for a retarded sister and had found no one to take over in case of their death, or they had not been able to make arrangements for the care of some children and needed to share this worry with someone. Others were guilt-ridden about some real or imagined "sins" and were greatly relieved when we offered them an opportunity to share them, especially in the presence of a chaplain. These patients all felt better after "confessions" or arrangements for the care of others and usually died soon after the unfinished business was taken care of.

Rarely an unrealistic fear prevents a patient from dying, as exemplified in a woman who was "too afraid to die" because she could not conceive of "being eaten up alive by the worms." She had a phobic fear of worms and at the same time was quite aware of the absurdity of it. Because it was so silly, as she herself called it, she was unable to share this with her family who had spent all their savings on her hospitalizations. After one interview this old lady was able to share her fears with us and her daughter helped her with arrangements for a cremation. This patient too died soon after she was allowed to ventilate her fears.

We are always amazed how one session can relieve a patient of a tremendous burden and wonder why it is so difficult for staff and family to elicit their needs, since it often requires nothing more but an open question.

Though Mr. E. was not terminally ill, we shall use his case as a typical example of a door-opening interview. It is relevant because Mr. E. presented himself as a dying man as a consequence of unresolved conflicts precipitated by the death of an ambivalent figure.

Mr. E., an eighty-three-year-old Jewish man, was admitted to the medical service of a private hospital because of severe weight loss, anorexia, and constipation. He complained of unbearable abdominal pains and looked haggard and tired. His general mood was depressed and he wept easily. A thorough medical work-up was negative, and the resident finally asked for a psychiatric opinion.

He was interviewed in a diagnostic-therapeutic interview with several students present in the same room. He did not mind the company and felt relieved to talk about his personal problems. He related how he had been well until four months before admission when he suddenly became "an old, sick, and lonely man." Further questioning revealed that a few weeks before the onset of all his physical complaints he lost a daughter-in-law and two weeks before the onset of his pains his estranged wife died suddenly while he was on a vacation out of town.

He was angry at his relatives for not coming to see him when he expected them. He complained about the nursing service and was generally displeased with the care he received from anybody. He was sure that his relatives would come immediately if he could promise them "a couple of thousand dollars when I die," and he elaborated at length about the housing project in which he lived with other old people and the vacation trip they all were invited to attend. It soon became evident that his anger was related to his being poor and that being poor meant that he had to take the trip when it was planned for his place of residence, i.e., he had no choice in the matter. On further questioning it became clear that he blamed himself for having been absent when his wife was hospitalized and tried to displace his guilt on the people who organized the vacation.

When we asked him if he did not feel deserted by his wife and was just unable to admit his anger at her, an avalanche of bitter feelings poured out in which he shared with us his inability to understand why she deserted him in favor of a brother (he called him a Nazi), how she raised their only son as a non-Jew, and finally how she left him alone now when he needed her the most! Since he felt extremely guilty and ashamed about his negative feelings towards the deceased, he displaced his feelings on the relatives and nursing staff. He was convinced that he had to be punished for all those bad thoughts and that he had to endure much pain and suffering to alleviate his guilt.

We simply told him that we could share his mixed feelings, that they were very human and everybody had them. We also told him bluntly that we wondered if he could not acknowledge some anger at his former wife and express it in further brief visits with us. He answered to this, "If this pain does not go away, I will have to jump out of the window." Our answer was, "Your pain may be all those swallowed feelings of anger and frustration. Get them out of your system without being ashamed and your pains will probably go away." He left with obviously mixed feelings but did ask to be visited again.

The resident who accompanied him back to his room was impressed with his slumped posture and took notice of it. He reinforced what we had said in the interview and reassured him that his reactions were very normal, after which he straightened up and returned in a more erect posture to his room.

A visit the next day revealed that he had hardly been in his room. He had spent much of the day socializing, visiting the cafetaria, and enjoying his food. His constipation and his pain was gone. After two massive bowel movements the evening of the interview, he felt "better than ever" and made plans for his discharge and resumption of some of his former activities.

On the day of discharge, he smiled and related some of the good days he had spent with his wife. He also told of the change in attitude towards the staff "whom I have given a hard time" and his relatives, especially his son whom he called to get acquainted a bit better, "since both of us may feel lonely for a while."

We reassured him of our availability should he have more problems, physical or emotional, and he smilingly replied that he had learned a good lesson and might face his own dying with more equanimity.

The example of Mr. E. shows how such interviews may be beneficial to people who are not actually ill themselves, but—due to old age or simply due to their own inability to cope with the death of an ambivalent figure—suffer a great deal and regard their physical or emotional discomforts as a means of alleviating guilt feelings for suppressed hostile wishes toward dead persons. This old man was not so much afraid to die as he was worried about dying before he had paid for his destructive wishes toward a person who had died without having given him a chance "to make up for it." He suffered agonizing pains as a means of reducing his fears of retribution and displaced much of his hostility and anger onto the nursing staff and relatives without being aware of the reasons for his resentment. It is surprising how a simple interview can reveal much of this data and a few statements of explanation, as well as reassurance that these feelings of love and hate are human and understandable and do not require a gruesome price, can alleviate much of these somatic symptoms.

For those patients who do not have a simple and single problem to solve, short-term therapy is helpful, which again does not necessarily require the help of a psychiatrist, but an understanding person, who has the time to sit and listen. I am thinking of patients like Sister I., who was visited on many occasions and who received her therapy as much from her fellow patients as she did from us. They are the patients who are fortunate enough to have time to work through some of their conflicts while they are sick and who can come to a deeper understanding and perhaps appreciation of the things they still have to enjoy. These therapy sessions, like the brief psychotherapy sessions with more terminally ill patients, are irregular in time and occurrence. They are individually arranged depending on the patient's physical condition and his ability and willingness to talk at a given time; they often include visits of just a few minutes to assure them of our presence even at times when they do not wish to talk. They continue even more frequently when the patient is in less comfort and more pain, and then take the form of silent companionship rather than a verbal communication.

We have often wondered if group therapy with a selected group of terminally ill patients is indicated, since they often share the same loneliness and isolation. Those who work on wards with terminally ill patients are quite aware of the interactions that go on between the patients and the many helpful statements that are made from one very sick patient to another. We are always amazed how much of our experiences in the seminar are communicated from one dying patient to another; we even get "referrals" of one patient from another. We have noticed patients sitting together in the lobby of the hospital who have been interviewed in the seminar, and they have continued their informal sessions like members of a fraternity. So far we have left it up to the patients how much they choose to share with others, but we are presently looking into their motivation for a more formal meeting, since this seems to be desired by at least a small group of our patients. They include those patients who have chronic illnesses and who require many rehospitalizations. They have known each other for quite a while and not only share the same illness but they also have the same memories of past hospitalizations. We have been very impressed by their almost joyful reaction when one of their "buddies" dies, which is only a confirmation of their unconscious conviction that "it shall happen to thee but not to me." This may also be a contributing factor why so many patients and their family members get some pleasure in visiting other perhaps more seriously ill patients. Sister I. used these visits as an expression of hostility, namely, to elicit patients' needs and to prove to the nursing staff that they were not efficient. By helping them as a nurse, she could not only temporarily deny her own inability to function, but she could also express her anger at those who were well and unable to serve the sick more effectively. Having such patients in a group therapy set-up would help them understand their behavior and at the same time help the nursing staff by making them more accepting of their needs.

Mrs. F. was another woman to be remembered as she started informal group therapy between herself and some very sick young patients, all of whom were hospitalized with leukemia or Hodgkin's disease, from which she had suffered for over twenty years. During the past few years she had an average of six hospitalizations a year, which finally resulted in her complete acceptance of her illness. One day a nineteen-year-old girl, Ann, was admitted, frightened of her illness and its outcome and unable to share this fear with anyone. Her parents had refused to talk about it, and Mrs. F. then became the unofficial counselor for her. She told her of her sons, her husband, and the house she had taken care of for so many years in spite of the many hospitalizations, and finally enabled Ann to ventilate her concerns and ask questions relevant to her. When Ann was discharged, she sent another young patient to Mrs. F. and so a chain reaction of referrals began to take place, quite comparable to group therapy in which one patient replaces another. The group rarely consisted of more than two or three people and remained together as long as the individual members were in the hospital.

The Silence that Goes Beyond Words

There is a time in a patient's life when the pain ceases to be, when the mind slips off into a dreamless state, when the need for food becomes minimal and the awareness of the environment all but disappears into darkness. This is the time when the relatives walk up and down the hospital hallways, tormented by the waiting, not knowing if they should leave to attend the living or stay to be around for the moment of death. This is the time when it is too late for words, and yet the time when the relatives cry the loudest for help—with or without words. It is too late for medical interventions (and too cruel, though well meant, when they do occur), but it is also too early for a final separation from the dying. It is the hardest time for the next of kin as he either wishes to take off, to get it over with; or he desperately clings to something that he is in the process of losing forever. It is the time for the therapy of silence with the patient and availability for the relatives.

The doctor, nurse, social worker, or chaplain can be of great help during these final moments if they can understand the family's conflicts at this time and help select the one person who feels most comfortable staying with the dying patient. This person then becomes in effect the patient's therapist. Those who feel too uncomfortable can be assisted by alleviating their guilt and by the reassurance that someone will stay with the dying until his death has occurred. They can then return home knowing that the patient did not die alone, yet not feeling ashamed or guilty for having avoided this moment which for many people is so difficult to face.

Those who have the strength and the love to sit with a dying patient in the *silence that goes beyond words* will know that this moment is neither frightening nor painful, but a peaceful cessation of the functioning of the body. Watching a peaceful death of a human being reminds us of a falling star; one of the million lights in a vast sky that flares up for a brief moment only to disappear into the endless night forever. To be a therapist to a dying patient makes us aware of the uniqueness of each individual in this vast sea of humanity. It makes us aware of our finiteness, our limited lifespan. Few of us live beyond our three score and ten years and yet in that brief time most of us create and live a unique biography and weave ourselves into the fabric of human history.

The water in a vessel is sparkling; the water in the sea is dark.
The small truth has words that are clear; the great truth has great silence.

Tagore, from *Stray Birds*, CLXXVI

THE ETHICS OF GIVING PLACEBOS

Sissela Bok

In 1971 a number of Mexican-American women applied to a family-planning clinic for contraceptives. Some of them were given oral contraceptives and others were given placebos, or dummy pills that looked like the real thing. Without knowing it the women were involved in an investigation of the side effects of various contraceptive pills. Those who were given placebos suffered from a predictable side effect: 10 of them became pregnant. Needless to say, the physician in charge did not assume financial responsibility for the babies. Nor did he indicate any concern about having bypassed the "informed consent" that is required in ethical experiments with human beings. He contented himself with the observation that if only the law had permitted it, he could have aborted the pregnant women!

The physician was not unusually thoughtless or hardhearted. The fact is that placebos are so widely prescribed for therapeutic reasons or administered to control groups in experiments, and are considered so harmless, that the fundamental issues they raise are seldom confronted. It appears to me, however, that physicians prescribing placebos cannot consider only the presumed benefit to an individual patient or to an experiment at a particular time. They must also take into account the potential risks, both to the patient or the experimental subject and to the medical profession. And the ethical dilemmas that are inherent in the various uses of placebos are central to such an estimate of possible benefits and risks.

The derivation of "placebo," from the Latin for "I shall please," gives the word a benevolent ring, somehow placing placebos beyond moral criticism and conjuring up images of hypochondriacs whose vague ailments are dispelled through adroit prescriptions of beneficent sugar pills. Physicians often give a humorous tinge to instructions for prescribing these substances, which helps

Reprinted by permission of *Scientific American* 231 (1974): 17–23.

to remove them from serious ethical concern. One authority wrote in a pharmacological journal that the placebo should be given a name previously unknown to the patient and preferably Latin and polysyllabic, and "it is wise. if it be prescribed with some assurance and emphasis for psychotherapeutic effect. The older physicians each had his favorite placebic prescriptions—one chose tincture of Condurango, another the Fluid-extract of *Cimicifuga nigra*." After all, are not placebos far less dangerous than some genuine drugs? As another physician asked in a letter to *The Lancet*: "Whenever pain can be relieved with two milliliters of saline, why should we inject an opiate? Do anxieties or discomforts that are allayed with starch capsules require administration of a barbiturate, diazepam or propoxyphene?"

Before the 1960's placebos were commonly defined as just such pharmacologically inactive medications as salt water or starch, given primarily to satisfy patients that something is being done for them. It has only gradually become clear that any medical procedure has an implicit placebo effect and, whether it is active or inactive, can serve as a placebo whenever it has no specific effect on the condition for which it is prescribed. Nowadays fewer sugar pills are prescribed, but X-rays, vitamin preparations, antibiotics and even surgery can function as placebos. Arthur K. Shapiro defines a placebo as "any therapy (or component of therapy) that is deliberately or knowingly used for its nonspecific, psychologic or psycho-physiologic effect, or that . . ., unknown to the patient or therapist, is without specific activity for the condition being treated."

Clearly the prescription of placebos is intentionally deceptive only when the physician himself knows they are without specific effect but keeps the patient in the dark. In considering the ethical issues attending deception with placebos I shall exclude the many procedures in which physicians have had— or still have—misplaced faith; that includes most of the treatments prescribed until this century and a great many still in use but of unproved or even disproved value.

Considering that in the past more therapies had little or no specific effect (yet sometimes succeeded thanks to faith on the part of healers and sufferers) and that we now have more effective remedies, it might be thought that the need to resort to placebos would have decreased. Improved treatment and diagnosis, however, have raised the expectations of patients and health professionals alike and consequently the incidence of reliance of placebos has risen. This is true of placebos given both in experiments and for therapeutic effect.

Modern techniques of experimentation with humans have vastly expanded the role of placebos as controls. New drugs, for example, are compared with placebos in order to distinguish the effects of the drug from chance events or effects associated with the mere administration of the drug. They can be tested in "blind" studies, in which the subjects do not know whether they are receiving the experimental drug or the placebo, and in "double-blind" studies, in which neither the subjects nor the investigators know.

Experiments involving humans are now subjected to increasingly careful safeguards for the people at risk, but it will be a long time before the practice of deceiving experimental subjects with respect to placebos is eradicated. In all the studies of the placebo effect that I surveyed in a study initiated as a fellow of the Interfaculty Program in Medical Ethics at Harvard University, only one indicated that those subjected to the experiment were informed that they would receive placebos; indeed, there was frequent mention of intentional deception. For example, a study titled "An Analysis of the Placebo Effect in Hospitalized Hypertensive Patients" reports that "six patients . . . were asked to accept hospitalization for approximately six weeks . . . to have their hypertension evaluated and to undertake a treatment with a new blood pressure drug . . . No medication was given for the first five to seven days in the hospital. Placebo was then started."

As for therapeutic administration, there is no doubt that studies conducted in recent decades show placebos can be effective. Henry K. Beecher studied the effects of placebos on patients suffering from conditions including postoperative pain, angina pectoris and the common cold. He estimated that placebos achieved satisfactory relief for about 35 percent of the patients surveyed. Alan Leslie points out, moreover, that "some people are temperamentally impatient and demand results before they normally would be forthcoming. Occasionally, during a period of diagnostic observation or testing, a placebo will provide a gentle sop to their impatience and keep them under control while the important business is being conducted."

A number of other reasons are advanced to explain the continued practice of prescribing placebos. Physicians are acutely aware of the uncertainties of their profession and of how hard it is to give meaningful and correct answers to patients. They also know that disclosing uncertainty or a pessimistic prognosis can diminish benefits that depend on faith and the placebo effect. They dislike being the bearers of uncertain or bad news as much as anyone else. Sitting down to discuss an illness with a patient truthfully and sensitively may take much-needed time away from other patients. Finally, the patient who demands unneeded medication or operations may threaten to go to a more cooperative doctor or to resort to self-medication; such patient pressure is one of the most potent forces perpetuating and increasing the resort to placebos.

There are no conclusive figures for the extent to which placebos are prescribed, but clearly their use is widespread. Thorough studies have estimated that as many as 35 to 45 percent of all prescriptions are for substances that are incapable of having an effect on the condition for which they are prescribed. Kenneth L. Melmon and Howard F. Morrelli, in their textbook *Clinical Pharmacology*, cite a study of treatment for the common cold as indicating that 31 percent of the patients received a prescription for a broad-spectrum or medium-spectrum antibiotic, 22 percent received penicillin and 6 percent received sulfonamides—"none of which could possibly have any beneficial specific pharmacological effect on the viral infection per se." They point out further that thousands of doses of vitamin B-12 are administered every year "at considerable expense to patients without pernicious anemia," the only condition for which the vitamin is specifically indicated.

In view of all of this it is remarkable that medical textbooks provide little analysis of placebo treatment. In a sample of 19 popular recent textbooks in medicines, pediatrics, surgery, anaesthesia, obstetrics and gynecology only three even mention placebos, and none of them deal with either the medical or the ethical dilemmas placebos present. Four out of six textbooks on pharmacology consider placebos, but with the exception of the book by Melmon and Morrelli were distorted. Often the two are mingled. Consider the intertwining of distortion, mystification and failure to inform in the following statement, made to unsuspecting recipients of placebos in an experiment performed in a psychiatric outpatient clinic: "You are to receive a test that all patients receive as part of their evaluation. The test medication is a nonspecific autonomous nervous system stimulant."

Even those who recognize that placebos are deceptive often dispel any misgivings with the thought that they involve no serious deception. Placebos are regarded as being analogous to the innocent white lies of everyday life, so trivial as to be quite outside the realm of ethical evaluation. Such liberties with language as telling someone that his necktie is beautiful or that a visit has been a pleasure, when neither statement reflects the speaker's honest opinion, are commonly accepted as being so trivial that to evaluate them morally would seem unduly fastidious and, from a utilitarian point of view, unjustified. Placebos are not trivial, however. Spending for them runs into millions of dollars. Patients incur greater risks of discomfort and harm than is commonly understood. Finally, any placebo uses that are in fact trivial and harmless in themselves may combine to form nontrivial practices, so that repeated reliance on placebos can do serious harm in the long run to the medical profession and the general public.

Consider first the cost to patients. A number of the procedures undertaken for their placebo effect are extremely costly in terms of available resources and of expense, discomfort and risk of harm to patients. Many temporarily successful new surgical procedures owe their success to the placebo effect alone. In such cases there is no intention to deceive the patient; physician and patient alike are deceived. On occasion, however, surgery is deliberately performed as a placebo measure. Children may undergo appendectomies or tonsillectomies that are known to be unnecessary simply to give the impression that powerful measures are being taken or because parents press for the operation. Hysterectomies and other operations may be performed on adults for analogous reasons. A great many diagnostic procedures that are known to be unnecessary are undertaken to give patients a sense that efforts are being made on their behalf. Some of these carry risks; many involve discomfort and the expenditure of time and money. The potential for damage by an active drug given as a placebo is similarly clear-cut. Calvin M. Kunin, T. Tupasi and W. Craig have described the ill effects—including death—suffered by hospital patients as a result of excessive prescription of antibiotics, more than half of which they found had been unneeded, inappropriately selected or given in incorrect dosages.

Even inactive placebos can have toxic effects in a substantial proportion of cases; nausea, dermatitis, hearing loss, headache, diarrhea and other symptoms have been cited. Stewart Wolf reported on a double-blind experiment to test the effects of the drug mephenesin and a placebo on disorders associated with anxiety and tension. Depending on the symptom studied, roughly 20 to 30 percent of the patients were better while taking the pills and 50 to 70 percent were unchanged, but 10 to 20 percent were worse—"whether the patient was taking mephenesin or placebo." A particularly serious possible side effect of even a harmless substance is dependency. In one case a psychotic patient was given placebo pills and told they were a "new major tranquilizer without any side effects." After four years she was taking 12 tablets a day and complaining of insomnia and anxiety. After the self-medication reached 25 pills a day and a crisis had occurred, the physician intervened, talked over the addictive problem (but not the deception) with the patient and succeeded in reducing the dose to two a day, a level that was still being maintained a year later. Other cases have been reported of patients' becoming addicted or habituated to these substances to the point of not being able to function without them, at times even requiring that they be stepped up to very high dosages.

Most obvious, of course, is the damage done when placebos are given in place of a well-established therapy that is clearly indicated for the patient's condition. The Mexican-American women I mentioned at the outset, for example, were actually harmed by being given placebo pills in the guise of contraceptive pills. In 1966 Beecher, in an article on the ethics of experiments with human subjects, documented a case in which 109 servicemen with streptococcal respiratory infections were given injections of a placebo instead of injections of penicillin, which was already known to prevent the development of rheumatic fever in such patients and which was being given to a larger group of patients. Two of the placebo subjects developed rheumatic fever and one developed an acute kidney infection, whereas such complications did not occur in the penicillin-treated group.

There have been a number of other experiments in which patients suffering from illnesses with known cures have been given placebos in order to study the course of the illness when it is untreated or to determine the precise effectiveness of the known therapy in another group of patients. Because of the very nature of their aims the investigators have failed to ask subjects for their informed consent. The subjects have tended to be those least able to object or defend themselves: members of minority groups, the poor, the institutionalized and the very young.

A final type of harm to patients given placebos stems not so much from the placebo itself as from the manipulation and deception that accompany its prescription. Inevitably some patients find out that they have been duped. They may then lose confidence in physicians and in bona fide medication, which they may need in the future. They may even resort on their own to more harmful drugs or other supposed cures. That is a danger associated with all deception: its discovery leads to a failure of trust when trust may be most needed. Alternatively, some people who do not discover the deception and are left believing that a placebic remedy works may continue to rely on it under the wrong circumstances. This is particularly true with respect to drugs, such as antibiotics, that are used sometimes for their specific action and sometimes as placebos. Many parents, for example, come to believe they must ask for the prescription of antibiotics every time their child has a fever.

The major costs associated with placebos may not be the costs to patients themselves that I have discussed up to this point. Rather they may be costs to new categories of patients in the future, to physicians who do not abuse placebo treatment and to society in general.

Deceptive practices, by their very nature, tend to escape the normal restraints of accountability and so can spread more easily. There are many instances in which an innocuous-seeming practice has grown to become a large-scale and more dangerous one; warnings against "the entering wedge" are often rhetorical devices but may sometimes be justified when there are great pressures to move along the undesirable path and when the safeguards against undesirable developments are insufficient. In this perspective there is reason for concern about placebos. The safeguards are few or nonexistent against a practice that is secretive by its very nature. And there are ever stronger pressures—from drug companies, patients eager for cures and busy physicians—for more medication, whether it is needed or not. Given such pressures the use of placebos can spread along a number of dimensions.

The clearest danger lies in the gradual shift from pharmacologically inert placebos to more active ones. It is not always easy to distinguish completely inert substances from somewhat active ones and these in turn from more active ones. It may be hard to distinguish between a quantity of an active substance so low that it has little or no effect and quantities that have some effect. It is not always clear to physicians whether patients require an inert placebo or possibly a more active one, and there can be the temptation to resort to an active one just in case it might also have a specific effect. It is also much easier to deceive a patient with a medication that is known to be "real" and to have power. One recent textbook in medicine goes so far as to advocate the use of small doses of effective compounds as placebos rather than inert substances— because it is important for both the doctor and the patient to believe in the treatment! The fact that the dangers and side effects of active agents are not always known or considered important by the physician is yet another factor contributing to the shift from innocuous placebos to active ones.

Meanwhile the number of patients receiving placebos increases as more and more people seek and receive medical care and as their desire for instant, push-button alleviation of symptoms is stimulated by drug advertising and by rising expectations of what "science" can do. Reliance on placebic therapy in turn strengthens the belief that there really is a pill or some other kind of remedy for every ailment. As long ago as 1909 Richard C. Cabot wrote, in a perceptive paper on the subject of truth and deception in medicine. The majority of placebos are given because we believe the patient ... has learned to expect medicine for every symptom, and without it he simply won't get well. True, but who taught him to expect a medicine for every symptom? He was not born with that expectation . . . It is we physicians who are responsible for perpetuating false ideas about disease and its cure . . . With every placebo that we give we do our part in perpetuating error, and harmful error at that."

A particularly troubling aspect of the spread of placebos is that it now affects so many children. Parents increasingly demand pills, such as powerful stimulants, to modify their children's behavior with a minimum of effort on their part; there are some children who may need such medication but many receive it without proper diagnosis. As I have mentioned, parents demand antibiotics even when told they are unneccessary, and physicians may give in to the demands. In these cases the very meaning of "placebo" has shifted subtly from "I shall please the patient" to "I shall please the patient's parents."

Deception by placebo can also spread from therapy and diagnosis to experimental applications. Although placebos can be given nondeceptively in experimentation, someone who is accustomed to prescribing placebos therapeutically without consent may not take the precaution of obtaining such consent when he undertakes an experiment on human subjects. Yet therapeutic deception is at least thought to be for the patient's own good, whereas experimental deception may not benefit the subject and may actually harm him; even the paternalistic excuse that the investigator is deceiving the patient for his own good then becomes inapplicable.

Finally, acceptance of placebos can encourage other kinds of deception in medicine such as failure to reveal to a patient the risks connected with an operation, or lying to terminally ill patients. Medicine lends itself with particular ease to deception for benevolent reasons because physicians are so clearly more knowledgeable than their patients and the patients are so often in a weakened or even irrational state. As Melvin Levine has put it, "the medical profession has practiced as if the truth is, in fact, a kind of therapeutic instrument [that] . . . can be altered or given in small doses . . . [or] not used at all when deemed detrimental to the patients . . . Many physicians have utilized truth distortion as a kind of anesthetic to promote comfort and ease treatment." Such practices are presumably for the good of patients. No matter how cogent and benevolent the reasons for resorting to deception may seem, when those reasons are considered in secret, without the consent of the doctored, they tend to be reinforced by less benevolent pressures, self-deception begins to blur nice distinctions and occasions for giving misleading information multiply.

Because of all these ways in which placebo usage can spread it is impossible to look at each incident of manipulation in isolation. There are no watertight compartments in medicine. When the costs and benefits of any therapeutic, diagnostic or experimental procedure are weighed, not only the individual consequences but also the cumulative ones must be taken into account. Reports of deceptive practices inevitably filter out, and the resulting suspicion is heightened by the anxiety that threats to health always create. And so even the health professionals who do not mislead their patients are injured by those who do and the entire institution of medicine is threatened by practices lacking in candor, however harmless the results may appear to be in some individual cases.

What should be the profession's attitude with regard to placebos? In the case of most experimental applications there are ways of avoiding deception without abandoning placebo controls. Subjects can be informed of the nature of the experiment and of the fact that placebos will be administered; if they then consent to the experiment, the use of placebos cannot be considered surreptitious. Although the subjects in a blind or double-blind experiment will not know exactly when they are receiving placebos or even whether they are receiving them, the initial consent to the experimental design, including placebos, removes the ethical problems having to do with deception. If, on the other hand, there are experiments of such a nature that asking subjects for their informed consent to the use of placebos would invalidate the results or cause too many subjects to decline, then the experiment ought not to be performed and the desired knowledge should be sought by means of a different research design.

As for the diagnostic and therapeutic use of placebos, we must start with the presumption that it is undesirable. By and large, given the principle of informed consent as well as concern for human integrity, no measures that affect someone's health should be undertaken without explanation and permission. Placebos are not so trivial as to be unworthy of ethical evaluation; they carry a definite possibility of harm and discomfort to patients as well as high collective costs; as a result placebo prescriptions present a more serious inroad on patient decision making than has been appreciated up to now. Surreptitious diagnostic and therapeutic administration of placebos should therefore be ruled out whenever possible.

The prohibition should not be absolute, however. In some cases the balance of benefit over cost is so overwhelming that reasonable people would choose to be deceived. There is no clear formula that will quickly reveal in each case whether the benefits will greatly outweigh the possible harm. Much of the problem can be avoided if care is taken to avoid placebos if possible and to observe the following principles in the remaining cases: (1) Placebos should be used only after a careful diagnosis; (2) no active placebos should be employed, merely inert ones; (3) no outright lie should be told and questions should be answered honestly; (4) placebos should never be given to patients who have asked not to receive them; (5) placebos should never be used when other treatment is clearly called for or all possible alternatives have not been weighed.

If placebo medicine is to be thus limited, the information provided to both medical personnel and patients will have to change radically. Placebos, so often resorted to and yet so rarely mentioned, will have to be discussed from scientific as well as ethical points of view during medical training. Textbooks will have to confront the medical and ethical dilemmas analytically and exhaustively. Similarly, much education must be provided for the public. There must be greater stress on the autonomy of the patient and on his right to consent to treatment or to refuse treatment after being informed of its nature. Understanding of the normal courses of illnesses should be stressed, including the fact that most minor conditions clear up by themselves rather quickly. The great pressure patients exert for more medication must be countered by limitations on drug advertising and by information concerning the side effects and dangers of drugs.

I have tried to show that the benevolent deception exemplified by placebos is widespread, that it carries risks not usually taken into account, that it represents an inroad on informed consent, that it damages the institution of medicine and contributes to the erosion of confidence in medical personnel.

Honesty may not be the highest social value; at exceptional times, when survival is at stake, it may have to be set aside. To permit a widespread practice of deception, however, is to set the stage for abuses and growing mistrust. Augustine, considering the possibility of giving official sanction, to white lies, pointed out that "little by little and bit by bit this will grow and by gradual accessions will slowly increase until it becomes such a mass of wicked lies that it will be utterly impossible to find any means of resisting such a plague grown to huge proportions through small additions."

EPILOGUE

THE COMPETENT HEALTH COMMUNICATOR

In this epilogue, we will review and summarize the primary health communication skills we have presented in this book. Development of these skills enable members of the health care team to become competent health communicators.

In the final analysis the quality of health care depends on the quality of human communication between interdependent health care providers and consumers. Effective communication allows health care professionals to gather full and accurate information from their clients, dispense clear and persuasive information to health care consumers, and elicit cooperation from their peers and co-workers. Similarly, effective communication enables consumers of health care services to request the specific information and help they need from health care providers, accurately interpret the wide range of messages that are part of health care treatment, and participate more fully in the health care process. Moreover, effective communication in health care facilitates the development of productive interpersonal relationships between members of the health care team (including health care consumers), and enables them to behave ethically.

One of the primary purposes of this book is to help convince people of the importance of human communication in the delivery of health care services. As well as attempting to promote increased awareness of the importance of communication in health and health care, this book attempts to identify some of the major functions and settings for communication in health care. Yet, even if we are successful in achieving these goals in this book, simply developing knowledge about why communication is important and how it functions in the health care system is not enough to begin to improve communication in the health care system. To improve communication, knowledge must be augmented by improved communication strategies and skills. Knowledge of communication in health care provides people with understanding, but when knowledge is combined with skills real change and improvement can begin, due to the emergence of competent health communicators.

Development of Communication Competencies

Several strategies and competencies for human communication in health care can be derived from the chapters and readings in this book. Although we have purposefully avoided easy answers or golden rules for every communication situation because we feel that to identify oversimplistic panaceas for complex communication problems would be counterproductive, there are several general principles of communication that take into account the multivariate (transactional) nature of human communication. Rather than telling you specifically what to do in any given situation, we will promote several communication strategies you may employ to help you adapt to the health communication situations you encounter.

Competent health communicators possess the following six communication skills: *awareness, compassion, descriptiveness, receptiveness, adaptiveness,* and *ethics*. These six general communication skills will allow the health communicator to interact strategically in health care situations. These six communication skills are not discrete competencies, but interact in a wholistic way to encompass the complex and idiosyncratic demands of effective communication. Effective communication encompasses not only the specific teleological, goal-oriented outcomes of communicative interactions, but also the qualitative perceptions of interaction satisfaction held by communicators within the health care system.

The first of the communication skills, communication awareness, deals with the health communicator's ability to recognize and accurately interpret the wide range of message cues available to him or her in health care settings. These message cues derive from intrapersonal as well as interpersonal levels, refer to verbal and nonverbal messages, and encompass messages emanating from the communication environment as well as from communicators. As we discussed earlier in the book in Chapter 2, we are unable to perceive everything there is to perceive in any given situation due to sensory and cognitive space limitations. Therefore, the key to communicative awareness is not to try to perceive everything in a communication situation, but to focus on the most important messages in each situation, utilizing past experiences in interpreting these messages, and updating our perceptions of reality by focusing on different communication cues available to us in the situation. Sherlock Holmes is a symbol of an individual who demonstrates the communication competancy of awareness. He always seems to pick up on key cues about people and the environment, interpreting these cues to develop a full and clear understanding of the communication situation.

Communicator compassion refers to the level of sensitivity and caring an individual has and can demonstrate for others. In Chapter 5 we examined empathy and caring as two of the communication characteristics leading to therapeutic communication. Empathy enables people to fully understand and relate to others, while caring refers to the expression of empathy and concern for the well being of others. By developing the characteristics of empathy and caring health communicators can demonstrate compassion for others. This enables health communicators to establish effective interpersonal relationships, encourages the sharing of relevant information, and improves their ability to influence and cooperate with others. Moreover, compassion humanizes communication in health care, helping to relieve much of the fear, trauma, and stigma that so often surrounds the "sick role" and health care. In a recent book on the physician–client relationship, Preston (1981) emphasizes that most problems in health care arise out of the physician's lack of balance between emphasis on *curing* and emphasis on *caring*. Preston contends that physicians often emphasize curing the client, without much concern for exhibiting caring for the client. He further suggests that this lack of caring in modern medicine is partly responsible for driving health consumers to quackery and avoiding medical care.[1]

Descriptiveness in communication refers to the ability to express ideas and information clearly and concisely to others. In modern health care it becomes increasingly difficult to understand the many advanced technologies and complexities of the delivery system, let alone describe these complexities vividly and precisely to lay audiences. Moreover, there has been such an overwhelming growth of different specialty areas in health care that health care specialists often find it difficult to explain the intricacies of their own area of expertise to other health care specialists. Yet, since health care demands the interdependent cooperation and understanding of many specialists and lay people it is crucial that health communicators develop their abilities to communicate descriptively. Some of the message strategies descriptive health communicators use to convey precise information are explaining complex terms and processes, giving examples that the people they are talking to can relate to and understand, restating difficult concepts creating redundancy, and seeking feedback. Explanations describe why things are the way they are and why you are planning to behave in certain ways. Examples illustrate the ideas and concepts you are trying to convey. Redundancy refers to repetition of message and repetition of communication channel; by expressng your ideas in different ways (using different words), and through different means (for example, through writing, through interpersonal contact, using diagrams, or televised media programs), you can increase the chance that others will understand the information you are trying to convey. Feedback allows you to check on the accuracy of your attempts to explain a complex concept to others. Asking someone to describe what they have understood based upon what you have told them will provide you with feedback about the descriptiveness of your communication technique. Additionally, using commonly shared words and other symbols when communicating with others will improve the descriptiveness of health communication.

Communication receptiveness refers to the inclusion of others in interaction. Receptive communicators are able to encourage true dialogue between people; rather than talking *at* people they talk *with* people. Receptiveness also refers to the communicator's ability to accept information from others, rather than dogmatically holding on to their own preconceived notions about reality. In Chapter 2 we discussed the differences between personal and object communication. By treating a person with respect and really listening to what they say, allowing what they say to affect you, you communicate personally. Personal communication is a key aspect of becoming a receptive communicator. Communication receptiveness also involves conviviality and accessibility. Conviviality is communicating in an affable and hospitable manner, while accessibility refers to being open and approachable to communication from others. Receptiveness encourages interaction between people and helps to elicit true cooperation between communicators. In the first chapter we discussed the importance of cooperation between health care providers and consumers in coping with many of the health care issues related to compliance. In Chapter 6 on group communication and Chapter 7 on organizational communication in health care we also stressed cooperation between members of the health care team and system in providing high quality health care services. Receptiveness in communication encourages the development of effective relationships in health care settings.

Adaptive health communicators can adjust their communication strategies and behaviors to the specific individual and specific situation they find themselves in. The adaptative health communicator creates messages that speak to the individuality of the person they are communicating with, as well as to the individuality of the communication setting that exists. Each person has their own intricate backgrounds, and to the extent you can meet the other person's needs with your communication the more effective your interaction with them will be. In the fifth chapter we described meeting the other person's needs as the development of implicit contracts between communicators in interpersonal relationships, where each communicator attempts to adapt their behaviors to fit the expectations of the other. In Chapter 8 we discussed the affects of cultural differences among people on their communication.

To a certain extent we all have cultural differences. Sometimes these differences are slight, while at other times the differences are dramatic. The more we are able to recognize these differences and adapt our communication accordingly, the more likely it is that we will be able to achieve our goals through communication. The setting where communication occurs also affects interaction. By taking into consideration the place where communication occurs, the other people present, the time communication occurs, and the past experiences communicators have had with one another, we can recognize the influence of setting on communication. Adaptive communicators attempt to communicate appropriately in the setting they are in, as well as communicating appropriately with the person they are interacting with.

Ethical health communicators are aware of the moral and social standards for their actions, and utilize these standards to guide their health care behaviors. In Chapter 8 we described some of the health communication aspects of ethics, including the establishment of equal relationships, sharing of timely and accurate information, sensitivity in communication to the needs of others, and honesty in communicating with others. Ethical standards are established through dialogue between members of a professional community. As issues are discussed and different actions are considered the members of the profession can judge the ethics of alternative courses of actions. Being a health professional implies behaving and communicating in a professional manner. By assessing the ethics of health care decisions and actions the health practitioner can truly be a professional, for communication ethics are the standards that direct professional behavior.

NOTES

1. Preston, 1981, Section A.

BIBLIOGRAPHY

Content Theme Key

A	Health Care and Human Communication
B	Verbal Communication In Health Care
C	Nonverbal Communication In Health Care
D	Health Care Interviewing
E	Therapeutic Communication
F	Group Communication In Health Care
G	Conflict In Health Care
H	Intercultural Communication In Health Care
J	Communication In Health Care Organizations
K	Communication With the Terminally Ill
L	Media and Technology In Health Care
M	Ethical Aspects Of Health Care
N	General Communication Literature

A. Health Care and Human Communication

Adler, H. "The Doctor–Patient Relationship." *Annals of Internal Medicine* 78 (1973): 595–98.

Adler, K. "Doctor–Patient Communication: A Shift to Problem Oriented Research." *Human Communication Research* 3 (1977): 179–90.

Alexander, F, *Psychosomatic Medicine*. New York: W. W. Norton, 1950.

Alpert, J. "Broken Appointments." *Pediatrics*, 34 (1964): 127–32.

Ambuel, J. et al. "Urgency As A Factor In Clinical Attendance." *American Journal of Diseases of Children* 108 (1964): 394–98.

Anonymous. "A Consumer Speaks Out About Hospital Care." *American Journal of Nursing* 76 (1976): 1443–44.

Anonymous. "I am Your Patient and I am Afraid." *Coverage* (Karser Hospitals Newsletter), December 16, 1977.

Anthony, W, "The Relationship Between Human Relationship Skills and an Index of Psychological Adjustment." *Journal of Counseling Psychology* 20 (1973): 489–90.

Archer, J. et al. "New Methods For Education, Treatment and Research In Human Interaction." *Journal of Counseling Psychology* 19 (1972): 275–81.

Arnold, R. et al. "Comprehension and Compliance With Medical Instructions In A Suburban Pediatric Practice." *Clinical Pediatrics* 9 (1970): 48–51.

Arntson, P. et al. "Pediatrician–Patient Communication, Final Report." In B. Ruben ed. *Communication Yearbook 2.* New Brunswick, N.J.: Transaction-International Communication Association, 1978, 504–22.

Artiss, K. *The Symptom as Communication in Schizophrenia.* New York: Grune and Stratton, 1959.

Artiss, K. and Levine, A. "Doctor–Patient Relation In Severe Illness". *New Eng-*

land Journal of Medicine, 288 (1973): 1210–14.

Ascione, F. and Rarim, R. "Physician's Attitudes Regarding Patients' Knowledge of Prescribed Medications." *Journal of the American Pharmacy Association* 15 (1975): 386–90.

Atman, N. "Understanding Your Patient's Emotional Response." *Journal of Practical Nursing* 22 (1972): 22–5.

Babbie, S, *Medical Communication Requirements*. Springfield, Va: US Pacific, 1973.

Balint, M. *The Doctor, His Patient and the Illness*. London: Pittman Medical Publishing Co., 1960.

Balint, M. "The Doctor's Therapeutic Function." *The Lancet 1 (1965): 1177–80.*

Bandler, R, and Grinder, J. The Structure of Magic I: A Book About Language and Therapy. Palo Alto, Ca: Science and Behavior Books, 1975.

Banks, S, and Vastyan, E. "Humanistic Studies In Medical Education." *Journal of Medical Education* 48 (1973): 248–57.

Barach, A. "Extramedical Influence of the Physician." *Journal of the American Medical Association* 181, 5 (1962): 393–95.

Barber, B. "Compassion in Medicine: Toward New Definitions and New Institution." *New England Journal of Medicine.* 295 (1976): 939–43.

Barber, G. "Communications in Medicine" *Practitioner*, 196 (1966): 134–38.

Barnlund, D, "The Mystification of Meaning: Doctor Patient Encounters." *Journal of Medical Education* 51 (1976): 716–25.

Barnlund, D. "Therapeutic Communication." In D. Barnlund, ed., *Interpersonal Communication*. Boston: Houghton-Mifflin, 1968: 613–45.

Barofsky, I. *Medication Compliance: A Behavorial Management Approach*. Thorofare, N.J.: Charles B. Slack, 1977.

Bateson, G. *Steps to An Ecology of the Mind*. New York: Ballantine Books, 1972.

Batey, M. "The Process Recording—A Method of Teaching Interpersonal Relationship Skills." *Nursing Forum* 2 (1963): 65.

Beavers, W. et al. "Communication Patterns of Mothers of Schizophrenics." *Family Process* 4 (1965): 95–104.

Becker, M. "The Health Belief Model and Personal Health Behavior: Introduction." *Health Education Monographs* 2 (1974a): 326–27.

Becker, M. "The Health Belief Model and Sick Role Behavior" *Health Education Monographs* 2 (1974b): 409–19.

Becker, M. et al. "The Health Belief Model and Prediction of Dietary Compliance: A Field Experiment." *Journal of Health and Social Behavior* 18 (1977): 348–66.

Becker, M. and Maiman, L. "Sociobehavior Determinants of Compliance With Health and Medical Care Recommendations." *Medical Care* 13 (1975): 10–24.

Beecher, H. "Evidence for Increased Effectiveness of Placebos With Increased Stress." *American Journal of Phsyiology* 187 (1956).

Beecher, H. "Nonspecific Forces Surrounding Disease and the Treatment of Disease." *Journal of the American Medical Association* 179 (1962): 437–40.

Beecher, H. "Surgery as Placebo: A Quantitative Study of Bias." *Journal of the American Medical Association* 176 (1961): 1102–07.

Beecher, H. "The Powerful Placebo." *Journal of the American Medical Association* 159 (1955): 1602–06.

Beisser, A. and Glasser, N. "The Precipitating Stress Leading to Psychiatric Hospitalization." *Comprehensive Psychiatry* 9 (1968):50–61.

Belsky, M. and Gross, L. *Beyond the Medical Mystique: How to Choose and Use Your Doctor*. Greenwich, Conn: Fawcett Publishing Co., 1975.

Benson, H. *The Relaxation Response*. New York: Avon Books, 1975.

Bergeron, J. "Tell Me, I Need to Know." *American Journal of Nursing* 71 (1971): 1573–74.

Bienvenu, M. "Measurement of Marital Communication." *Family Coordinator* 1 (1970): 26–33.

Blackwell, B. "Patient Compliance." *New England Journal of Medicine* 289 (1973): 249–52.

Blackwell, B. "Upper Middle Class Adult Expectations About Entering the Sick-role For Physical and Psychiatric Dysfunctions." *Journal of Health and Social Behavior* 8 (1967): 83–95.

Bloom, S. *The Doctor and His Patient: A Sociological Interpretation.* New York: International Universities Press, 1975.

Bloom, S. and Wilson, R. "Patient Practitioner Relationships." In H. Freeman, et al. eds. *Handbook of Medical Sociology.* Englewood Cliffs, N.J: Prentice-Hall, 1972, 315–42.

Bloom, S. et al. "Physician–Patient Expectations in Primary Care." *Bulletin of the New York Academy of Medicine* 53 (1977): 75–82.

Bloor, M. and Horobin, G. "Conflict and Conflict Resolution in Doctor–Patient Interaction." In C. Cox and A. Mead, eds. *A Sociology of Medical Practice.* London: Collier-MacMillen, 1975, 271–83.

Blum, L. *Reading Between the Lines: Doctor–Patient Communication.* New York: International Universities Press, 1972.

Blum, R. *The Management of the Doctor–Patient Relationship.* New York: MacGraw-Hill, 1960.

Bochner, A. "Conceptual Frontiers In the Study of Communication In Families: An Introduction to the Literature." *Human Communication Research* 2 (1976): 381–97.

Bolton, B. and Sommer, P. "Mode of Address and Patient Satisfaction in Rehabilitation: An Experimental Study." *Journal of Health and Social Behavior* 11 (1970):215–19.

Bothamy, V. "Communication and the Ventilated Patient." *Nursing Times* 71 (1975): 628–30.

Bowden, C. and Burstein, A. *Psychosocial Basis of Medical Practice: An Introduction to Human Behavior.* Baltimore: William and Wilkes, 1974.

Bowers, W. *Interpersonal Relations In the Hospital.* Springfield, Ill: Charles C. Thomas Publishers, 1960.

Bowers, W. *Techniques In Medical Care.* Springfield, Ill: Charles C. Thomas Publishers, 1962.

Brodie, D. et al. "Expanded Roles for the Pharmacist." *American Journal of Pharmacy Education* 37 (1973): 591.

Brown, E. *Newer Dimensions In Patient Care.* New York: Russell Sage, 1965.

Browne, K. and Freeling, P. *The Doctor–Patient Relationship.* Edingurgh, E. and S. Livingstone (1967).

Buehler, R. and Richmond J., "Interpersonal Communication Behavior Analysis: A Research Method." *Journal of Communication* 13 (1963): 146–55.

Burg, F. et al. "A Method for Defining Competency in Pediatrics." *Journal of Medical Education* 51 (1976): 824–28.

Calnan, M. "Patient-Centered Communication." *Supervisor Nurse* 2 (1971): 67–71.

Campbell, A. "Subjective Measures of Well-Being." *American Psychologist* (1976): 117–24.

Cannon, W. *The Wisdom of the Body.* New York: W. W. Norton, 1963.

Carmichael, C. "Communication and Gerontology: Interfacing Disciplines." *Western Speech* 40 (1976): 121–29.

Caron, H. "Patients' Cooperation With A Medical Regimen." *Journal of the American Medical Association* 203, (1968): 922–26.

Cartwright, A. *Human Relations and Hospital Care.* London: Routledge and Kegan Paul, 1964.

Casella, C. *Training Exercises To Improve Interpersonal Relations in Health Care Organizations.* Greenvale, N.Y.: Panel Publishers, 1977.

Cassata, D. "Health Communication Theory and Research: A Definitional Overview." In D. Nimmo, ed., *Communication Yearbook 4.* New Brunswick, N.J: Transaction-International Communication Association, 1980, 583–89.

Cassata, D. "Health Communication Theory and Research: An Overview of the

Communication Specialist Interface." In B. Ruben, ed. *Communication Yearbook 2*. New Brunswick, N.J: Transaction-International Communication Association, 1978, 495–504.

Chesler, J. "The Medical Student and Human Relations." *Journal of Medical Education*. 34 (1959): 1101–05.

Clyne, M. "The Doctor–Patient Relationship As A Diagnostic Tool." *Psychiatry in Medicine*. 3 (1972): 343–55.

Coe, R. *Sociology of Medicine*. New York: McGraw Hill, 1970.

Collins, Mattie. *Communication in Health Care*. St. Louis: C. V. Mosby, 1983.

Costello, D. "Health Communication Theory and Research: An Overview." In D. Nimmo, ed., *Communication Yearbook 1*. New Brunswick, N.J., Transaction-International Communication Association (1977): 555–67.

Costello, D. and Pettegrew, L. "Health Communication Theory and Research: An Overview of Health Organisations." In D. Nimmo, ed., *Communication Yearbook 3*. New Brunswick, N.J., Transaction-International Communication Association, 1979: 607–23.

Costely, D. "Basis for Effective Communication." *Supervisor Nurse* 4 (1973): 19–22.

Coulthard, M. and Ashby, M. "Talking With the Doctor, 1." *Journal of Communication* 25 (1975): 140–47.

Counte, Michael and Christman, Luther. *Interpersonal Behavior and Health Care*. Boulder, Co.: Westview Press, 1981.

Cousins, N. *Anatomy of An Illness as Perceived by the Patient*. New York: W. W. Norton, 1979.

Crown, S. "Failures of Communication." *Lancet* 2 (1971): 1021–22.

Cumming, J. "Communication: An Approach to Chronic Schizophrenia." In L. Appleby, J. Scher, and J. Cumming, eds., *Chronic Schizophrenia: Exploration in Theory and Treatment*. Glencoe, Ill.: The Free Press, 1960, 106–19.

Dacey, M. and Wintrols, R. "Human Behavior: The Teaching of Social and Behavioral Sciences In Medical Schools." *Social Science and Medicine 7* (1973): 943–57.

Daly, M. and Hulka, B. "Talking With the Doctor, 2." *Journal of Communication* 25 (1975): 148–52.

Dance, F. "The Communication of Health." *The Ohio Speech Journal* 8 (1970): 28–30.

David, M. "Variations in Patients" Compliance With Doctors' Advice: An Empirical Analysis of Patterns of Communication." *American Public Health Association 58 (1968): 274–88*.

Davis, F. "Uncertainty in Medical Prognosis, Clinical and Functional." *American Journal of Pharmacy* 66 (1960): 41–47.

Davis, G. "Pharmacist–Patient Communication: Its Effect on Pharmacy's Image." *American Journal of Pharmacy* (1976): 168–79.

Davis, M. "Physiological, Psychological, and Demographic Factors in Patient Compliance With Doctor's Orders." *Medical Care* 6 (1968): 115–22.

Davis, M. "Variations in Patients' Compliance With Doctor's Orders: Analysis of Congruence Between Survey Responses and Results of Empirical Investigations." *Journal of Medical Education* 41 (1966): 1037–48.

Davis, M. "Variations in Patients' Compliance With Doctor's Advice: An Empirical Analysis of Patterns of Communication." *American Journal of Public Health* 58 (1966): 274–88.

Davis, M. "Variations in Patients' Compliance With Doctor's Orders: Medical Practice and Doctor Patient Interaction." *Psychiatry in Medicine* 2 (1971): 31–54.

Davis, M. "Predicting Non-Compliant Behavior." *Journal of Health and Social Behavior* 8 (1967): 265–71.

Davis, M. and Eichorn, R. "Compliance With Medical Regimens: A Panel Study." *Journal of Health and Human Behavior* 4 (1963): 240–49.

Davis, M. and Von DerLippe, R. "Discharge from Hospital Without Medical Advice: A Study of Reciprocity in the Doctor–Patient Relationship." *Social Science and Medicine* 1 (1967): 336–44.

Davis, R. "Communication With the Stroke Patient." *Bedside Nurse* 3 (1970): 24–26.

Davitz, L. *Interpersonal Processes in Nursing-Case Histories.* New York: Springer Publishing Company, 1970.

Davitz, L and Pendleton, S. "Nurses' Inferences of Suffering." *Nursing Research* 18 (1969): 100–07.

Decastro, F. "Doctor–Patient Communication: Exploring the Effectiveness of Care In A Primary Care Clinic." *Clinical Pediatrics.* 11 (1972): 86–87.

Dennert, J. "On Humanizing Medical Education: Toward Personal Responsibility." In *Humanizing the Process of Medical Education: Winning Essays of the Medical Student and Housestaff Essay Contest.* Philadelphia: Society for Health and Human Values (1976): 17–29.

Dervin, B. et al. "The Human Side of Information: An Exploration In a Health Communication Context." In D. Nimmo, ed., *Communication Yearbook 4.* New Brunswick, N.J.: Transaction-International Communication Association, 1980.

Dichter, E. "A Psychological Study of the Hospital-Patient Relationship—The Patient's Greatest Need is Security." *Modern Hospital* 83 (1954): 56–68.

Diers, D, et al. "The Effect of Nursing Interaction on Patients in Pain." *Nursing Research* 15 (1966): 225–28.

DiMatteo, M. "A Social Psychological Analysis of Physician–Patient Rapport: Toward a Science of the Art of Medicine." *Journal of Social Issues* 35 (1979): 12–33.

DiMatteo, M. and Friedman, H. *Social Psychology and Medicine.* Cambridge, Mass.: Oelgeschlager, Gunn, and Hain, 1982.

Dingle, J. "The Ills of Man." *Scientific American* 229 (1973): 77–82.

Donabedian, A. "Promoting Quality Through Evaluating the Process of Patient Care." *Medical Care* 6 (1968): 181–82.

Dorroh, T. *Between Patient and Health Worker.* New York: MacGraw-Hill, 1974.

Dubos, R. *Man, Medicine, and Environment.* New York: Mentor Books, 1969.

Dubos, R. *The Mirage of Health.* New York: Harper and Row, 1968.

Dye, M. "Validating a Theory of Nursing Practice; Clarifying Patients' Communication." *The American Journal of Nursing* 63 (1963): 56–59.

Elder, J. *Transactional Analysis In Health Care.* Menlo Park, Ca.: Addison-Wesley, 1968.

Elstein, A. et al. "Methods and Theory In the Study of Medical Inquiry." *Journal of Medical Education* 47 (1972): 85–92.

Engel, G. "Are Medical Schools Neglecting Clinical Skills?" *Journal of the American Medical Association* 236 (1976): 861–63.

Entralgo, P. *Doctor and Patient,* New York: McGraw Hill, 1969.

Filep, R. "The ATS-6 Experiments in Health and Education: An Overview." *Journal of Communication* 27 (1977): 159–65.

Fish, D. "Support for Social Science Research in Medicine in Canada." *Milbank Memorial Fund Quarterly.* 49 (1971): 194–216.

Fletcher, C. *Communication in Medicine.* London: Nuffield Provincial Hospitals Trust, 1973.

Francis, U. et al. "Gaps in Doctor–Patient Communication: Patients' Responses to Medical Advice." *New England Journal of Medicine* 280 (1969): 5351–60.

Frank, J. *Persuasion and Healing,* rev. ed. Baltimore: Johns Hopkins University Press, 1973.

Frank, J. "The Faith that Heals", *Johns Hopkins Medical Journal* 137 (1975): 127–31.

Freedman, C. "Communication Between Mother, Doctor, and Nurse, In Hospital Obstetrics." *Hospital Topics* 44 (1966): 102–07.

Freeman, B. et al. "Gaps in Doctor–Patient Communication: Doctor–Patient Interaction Analysis." *Pediatrics Research* 5 (1971): 298–311.

Freidson, E. *Patient's View of Medical Practice.* New York: Russell Sage, 1961.

Friedman, H. and DiMatteo, M. "Health Care as an Interpersonal Process." *Journal of Social Issues* 35 (1979): 12–33.

Freymann, J. "Medicine's Great Schism: Prevention vs. Cure: An Historical Interpretation." *Medical Care* 13 (1975): 525–36.

Friedman, H. and DiMatteo, M. "Health Care as an Interpersonal Process," Journal of Social Issues 35 (1975): 12–33.

Fuchs, V. *Who Shall Live? Health Economics and Social Choice.* New York: Basic Books, 1974.

Fuller, D. and Quesada, G. "Communication in Medical Therapeutics." *Journal of Communication* 23 (1973):361–70.

Gadd, A. "Educational Aspects of Integrating Social Sciences in the Medical Curriculum." *Social Sciences and Medicine* 7 (1973): 975–84.

Galton, L. "How to Communicate With Your Doctor." *Parade* (Feb. 1978): 20.

Gazda, G. et al. *Interpersonal Communication: A Handbook for Health Professionals.* Rockville, Md.: Aspen Systems Corp., 1982.

Gerrard, B. et al., *Interpersonal Skills for Health Professionals.* Reston, Va.: Reston Publishing Co., 1980.

Gibb, J. "Defensive Communication." *Journal of Communication* 11 (1961): 141–48.

Gillon, R. and Barsky, A. "Diagnosis and Management of Patient Compliance." *Journal of the American Medical Association.* 228 (1974): 1563–67.

Glowgo, B. "Effects of Health Methods on Appointment Breaking." *Public Health Reports* 85 (1970): 41–50.

Gochman, D. "Measuring Health-Relevant Expectancies." *Psychological Reports* 24 (1969): 880.

Gochman, D. "The Development of Health Beliefs." *Psychological Reports* 31 (1972a): 259–66.

Gochman, D. "The Organizing Role of Motivation in Health Beliefs and Intentions." *Journal of Health and Social Behavior* 13 (1972b). 285–93.

Goldberg, J. and Goldberg, A. "Family Communication." *Western Speech* 40 (1976): 104–10.

Goldsmith, J. and McFall, R. "Development and Evaluation of An Interpersonal Skill Training Program for Psychiatric Inpatients." *Journal of Abnormal Psychology* 84 (1975): 51–58.

Gorovitz, S. and MacIntyre, A. "Toward a Theory of Medical Fallibility." *Journal of Medicine and Philosophy* 1 (1976): 51–71.

Gorton, J. *Behavioral Components of Patient Care.* New York: MacMillan, 1970.

Goss, M. "Influence and Authority Among Physicians In Outpatient Clinics." *American Sociological Review* 26 (1961): 39–50.

Gosset, J. "Communication Between the Physician and His Patient." *World Medical Journal* 15 (1968): 86–89.

Gozzi, E. "Gaps in Doctor–Patient Communication: Implications for Nursing Practice." *American Journal of Nursing* 69 (1969): 529–33.

Grayson, H. et al. "A Systematic and Comprehensive Approach to Teaching and Evaluating Interpersonal Skills." *Journal of Medical Education* 52 (1977): 906–13.

Green, W. "Some Perspectives for Observing and Interpreting Biopsychological Relations and Doctor-Patient Relations." *Perspectives in Biology and Medicine* 2 (1959): 453–73.

Grissenger, S. et al. "Protocol for Consultation With Discharged Patients About Their Medications." *Hospital Pharmacy* 8 (1973): 175–83.

Gruen, W. "Communication Problems as a Possible Contribution to Chronicity in Mental Patients." *Social Science and Medicine* 4 (1970): 307–26.

Guerney, B. *Relationship Enhancement* Washington, D.C.: Jossey-Bass Publishers, 1977.

Guthrie, D. "Communication: One Path to A Better Health." *Bedside Nurse* 4 (1971): 22–24.

Haggerty, R. and Roghmann, K. "Noncompliance and Self-Medication. Two Neglected Aspects of Pediatric Pharmacology." *Pediatric Clinics of North America.* 19 (1972): 101–15.

Hall, B. "Human Relations in the Hospital Setting." *Nursing Outlook* 16 (1964): 44.

Handkins, R. and Munz, D. "Essential Hypertention and Self-Disclosure." *Journal of Clinical Psychology* 34 (1978): 870–75.

Harlem, O. *Communication in Medicine.* Paris: S. Karger, 1977.

Hart, R. and Burks, D. "Rhetorical Sensitivity and Social Interaction." *Speech Monographs* 39 (1972): 75–91.

Hart, R. et al. "Attitudes Toward Communication and the Assessment of Rhetorical Sensitivity." *Communication Monographs* 47 (1980): 1–22.

Harper, D. "Patient Follow-up of Medical Advice. A Literature Review." *Journal of the Kansas Medical Society.* 72 (1971): 265–71.

Harris, B. et al. "Quantitative Study of Doctor-Patient Communication in Rheumatic Diseases." *Arizona Medicine* 30 (1973): 262–63.

Hays, J. "Analysis of Nurse-Patient Communication." *American Journal of Nursing* 69 (1969): 1928–30.

Hein, E. "Listening." *Nursing '75* 5 (1975): 93–104.

Herlicky, C. "Physican–Patient Rapport: A Vital Relationship." *Journal of the Medical Association of Alabama* 40 (1970): 181.

Hertz, P. and Stamps, P. "Appointment-Keeping Behavior Re-evaluated." *American Journal of Public Health* 67 (1977): 1033–36.

Hess, J. "A Comparison of Methods for Evaluating Medical Student Skill In Relation to Patients." *Journal of Medical Education* 89 (1969): 934–38.

Hodgins, E. "Listen: The Patient." *The New England Journal of Medicine* 274 (1966): 657–61.

Hoekelman, R. "Nurse-Physician Relationships." *American Journal of Nursing* 75 (1975): 1150–52.

Hofer, H. "Learning the Physician-Patient Relationship." *Journal of American Medical Association* 12 (1960): 1301–04.

Holder, L. "Effects of Source, Message, and Audience on Health Behavior Compliance." *Health Service Reports* 87 (1972): 343–50.

Hooper, L. and McWilliams, P. *Care of the Nursing Home Patient.* Boston, Little, Brown (1967).

Horn, D. "A Model for the Study of Personal Choice Health Behavior." *International Journal of Health Education* 19 (1976): 89.

Hornsby, J. "Interpersonal Skills Development: A Model for Dentistry." *Journal of Dental Education* 39 (1975): 728–31.

Hopkins. P. and Wolff, H. *Principles and Psychosomatic Disorders.* Oxford: Pergamon Press, 1965.

Hubbard, J. et al. "An Objective Evaluation of Clinical Competence." *New England Journal of Medicine* 272 (1965): 1321–28.

Hudson, J. and Giacalone, J. "Current Issues in Primary Care Education: Review and Commentary." *Journal of Medical Education* 50 (1975): 211–33.

Hulka, B et al. "Communication Compliance, and Concordance Between Physicians and Patients With Prescribed Medications." *American Journal of Public Health* 66 (1976): 847–53.

Hulka, B., et al. "Doctor-Patient Communication and Outcomes Among Diabetic Patients." *Journal of Community Health* 1 (1975a): 15.

Hulka, B. et al. "Medication Use and Misuse: Physician-Patient Discrepancies." *Journal of Chronic Diseases* 28 (1975b): 7–21.

Hunter, D. and Bomford, R. *Hutchinson's Clinical Methods* (15th ed.) Philadelphia: J. B. Lippincott Company, 1968.

Hurtado, A. et al. "Determinants of Medical Care Utilization: Failure to Keep Appointments." *Medical Care* 11 (1973): 189–98.

Hussar, D. "Pharmacy Practice—The Importance of Effective Communications." *American Journal of Pharmacy* 148 (1976): 136–47.

Jaccord, J. "A Theoretical Analysis of Selected Factors Important to Health Education Strategies." *Health Education Monographs* 3 (1975): 152–67.

Jackson, D., (ed), *Communication, Family and Marriage: Human Communication*

Vol 1, Palo Alto, Ca.: Science and Behavior Books, 1968a.

Jackson, D. *Therapy, Communication and Change: Human Communication* Vol 2, Palo Alto, Ca.: Science and Behavior Books, 1968b.

Janis, I. and Feshback, S. "Effects of Fear Arousing Communications." *Journal of Abnormal and Social Psychology* 48 (1953): 788–92.

Jason, H. "The Relevance of Medical Education to Medical Practice." *Journal; of the American Medical Association.* 212 (1970): 2092–95.

Johannse, W. et al. "On Accepting Medical Recommendations." *Archives of Environmental Health.* 12 (1966): 63–69.

Johnson, D. *Reaching Out: Interpersonal Effectiveness and Self-Actualization.* Englewood Cliffs, N.J.: Prentice-Hall, 1972.

Johnson, D. *Total Patient Care: Foundations and Practice*, 2nd ed. St. Louis: C. V. Mosby, 1968.

Johnson, J. "Effects of Structuring Patient's Expectations on Their Reactions to Threatening Events." *Nursing Research* 21 (1972): 449–503.

Jonas, S. "Appointment Breaking In a General Medical Clinic." *Medical Care* 9 (1971): 82–88.

Joyce, C. et al. "Quantitative Study of Doctor–Patient Communication." *Quarterly Journal of Medicine* 38 (1969): 183–94.

Kane, R. and Deuschle, K. "Problems in Doctor–Patient Communication." *Medical Care* 5 (1967): 260–71.

Katz, E. et al. "Doctor–Patient Exchanges: A Diagnostic Approach to Organizations and Professions." *Human Relations* 22 (1969): 309–24.

Kemper, T. et al. "Social Science in Schools of Medicine: Problems, Prospects, and A Program." *The Milbank Memorial Fund Quarterly* 49 (1971): 244–73.

Kerksz, R. "Research on Doctor–Patient Relationship in a General Hospital Setting." *Psychotherapy and Psychosomatics* 18 (1970): 50–55.

Kindig, D. "Interdisciplinary Education For Primary Health Care Team Delivery." *Journal of Medical Education* 50 (1975): 97–110.

King, M. et al. *Irresistable Communication: Creative Skills For Health Professionals.* Philadelphia: W. B. Saunders Company, 1983.

Kirch, A. "The Health Care System and Health: Some Thoughts on a Famous Misalliance." *Inquiry* (1974): 269–75.

Kirscht, J. et al. "Public Responses to Various Written Appeals to Participate in Health Screening." *Public Health Reports* 90 (1975): 539–43.

Kline, R. et al. "Communication Issues in Different Public Health Areas." *Advances in Consumer Research* 3 (1976): 290–94.

Knowles, J. ed. *Doing Better and Feeling Worse: Health Care in the U.S.* New York: W, W. Norton, 1977.

Kogler-Hill, S. "Health Communication: Focus on Interprofessional Relationships." *Communication Administration Bulletin* 25 (1978): 31–36.

Komaroff, A. "The Practitioner and the Compliant Patient." *American Journal of Public Health* 66 (1976): 833–35.

Korsch, B. M. and Negrete, V. "Doctor–Patient Communication." *Scientific American* 227 (1972): 66–74.

Korsch, B. M. et al. "Gaps In Doctor–Patient Communication." *Pediatrics* 42 (1968): 855–71.

Korsch, B. M. et al. "Practical Implications of Doctor–Patient Interaction Analysis for Pediatric Practice." *American Journal of Diseases of Children* 121 (1971): 109–14.

Kosa, J. "Entrepreneurship And Charisma In The Medical Profession." *Social Science and Medicine* 4 (1970):25–40.

Kreps, G. "Communication Training for Health Care Employees: Implications for Higher Education and the Health Care Industry," *Issues in Higher Education* 12, (1983, in-press).

Kreps, G. "Pharmacists As Communicators." *Indiana Pharmacist* 63 (1982a): 59–66.

Kreps, G. "Design for a Communication

Course for Health Professionals." *Resources in Education* 17 (1982b), available from the ERIC Clearinghouse on Reading and Communication Skills # ED-210-752.

Kreps, G. "Communication and Gerontology: Health Communication Training for Providers of Health Services to the Elderly." *Resources in Education* 17 (1982c), available from the ERIC Clearinghouse on Reading and Communication Skills # ED-209-702.

Kreps, G. "Communication Training for Health Care Professionals." *Resources in Education* 17 (1982d), available from the ERIC Clearinghouse on Reading and Communication Skills # ED-210-755.

Kreps, G. *Health Communication: A Selected Annotated Bibliography.* Annandale, Va.: ERIC-Speech Communication Module, 1982e.

Kreps, G. "Communication Education in the Future: The Emerging Area of Health Communication." *Indiana Speech Journal* 16 (1981): 30–39.

Kreps, G. "The Application of Health Communication Knowledge." *Health Communication Issues* 8 (1981): 3.

Kreps, G. "Health Communication Education For Future Health Practitioners." *Health Communication Newsletter* 7 (1980): 6–8.

Kron, T. *Communication in Nursing.* Philadelphia: W. B. Saunders Company, 1972.

Kutner, B. "Physician–Patient Relationships: A Theoretical Framework." In J. Pealman and E. Hartley, eds. *Frestschrift for Gardner Murphy* New York: Harper and Row, 1960, 1–16.

Lambert, E. *Modern Medical Mistakes.* Bloomington, Ind.: Indiana University Press, 1978.

Lander, L. *Defective Medicine.* New York: Farrar, Straus and Giroux, 1978.

Lapinsoh, L. "The Iatrogenic State and the Physician–Patient Relationship." *Journal of the Albert Einstein Medical Center* 7 (1959): 286–88.

Larson, D. and Rootman, I. "Physician

Role Performance and Patient Satisfaction." *Journal of Communication* 19 (1969): 308–16.

Levine, H. and McGuire, C. "The Use of Role-Playing to Evaluate Affective Skills in Medicine." *Journal of Medical Education* 45 (1970): 700–05.

Ley, P. and Spelman, M. *Communication With the Patient.* St. Louis: Warren H. Green, 1967.

Lineiian, D. "What Does the Patient Want to Know?" *American Journal of Nursing* 66 (1966): 1066–70.

Lockerby, F. *Communication for Nurses.* St. Louis: C. V. Mosby Company, 1968.

Loomis, H. and Horsley, J. *A Behavioral Approach to Nursing Practice.* New York: McGraw-Hill, 1974.

Lum, J. "Interaction Patterns of Nursing Personnel." *Nursing Research* 19 (1970): 324–30.

MacBryde, C. *Signs and Symptoms,* (4th ed.). Philadelphia: J. B. Lippincott, 1964.

Malaphy, B. "The Effect of Instruction and Labeling on the Number of Medication Errors Made by Patients at Home." *American Journal of Hospital Pharmacy* 23 (1966): 282.

Marston, M. "Compliance With Medical Requimens: A Review of the Literature." *Nursing Research* 19 (1970): 312–23.

Maslow, A. *Toward A Psychology of Being,* 2nd ed. New York: Van Nostrand Reinhold Company, 1968.

Matthews, D. and Hingson, R. "Improving Patient Compliance: A Guide for the Physician." *Medical Clinic of North America* 61 (1977): 879–89.

Maward, B. "Relation of Student Learning to Physician Performance." *Journal of American Medical Association* 198 (1966): 767–69.

Mazzulla, J. et al. "Variations In Interpretation of Prescription Instructions." *Journal of the American Medical Association* 227 (1974): 929.

McIntosh, J. "Process of Communication, Information Seeking Control Associated With Cancer: A Selected Review of the Literature." *Social Science and Medicine* 8 (1974): 167–87.

McKegney, F. and Krupp, P. "A Useful Coordination Between Gross Anatomy and Human Behavior Courses." *Journal of Medical Education* 52 (1977): 425–26.

Mechanic, D. "Response Factors in Illness: The Study of Illness Behavior." *Social Psychiatry* 1 (1966): 11–20.

Mendelsohn, R. *Confessions of A Medical Heretic*. Chicago: Contemporary Books, Inc., 1979.

Mendelsohn, R. *Male Practice: How Doctors Manipulate Women*. Chicago: Contemporary Books, Inc., 1981.

Menninger, R. "Psychiatry 1976: Time for a Holistic Medicine." *Annals of Internal Medicine* 84 (1976): 603–04.

Mercer, L. "Beware of 'I Just Shot My Grandmother' Kind of Talk," a ditto prepared at Texas Womens University, Houston, Texas (undated).

Meyer, A. and Otle, H. "The Semantic Differential As A Measure of the Patients' Image of Their Therapist." *Knokke* 18 (1970): 56–60.

Milgram, S. "Some Conditions of Obedience and Disobedience to Authority." *Human Relations* 18 (1965): 57–76.

Miller, J. "Information Input Overload and Psychopathology." *American Journal of Psychiatry* 116 (1960): 695–704.

Million, T., ed. *Medical Behavioral Science*. Philadelphia: W. B. Saunders Company, 1975.

Mohammed, M. "Patients' Understanding of Written Health Information." *Nursing Research* 13 (1964): 101–08.

Moriwaki, S. "Self-Disclosure, Significant Others and Psychological Well-Being in Old Age." *Journal of Health and Social Behavior* 14 (1973): 226–32.

Morse, B. and Van Den Berg, E. "Interpersonal Relationships in Nursing Practice: An Interdisciplinary Approach." *Communication Education* 27 (1978): 158–62.

Munn, H. and Metzger, N. *Effective Communication in Health Care*. Rockville, Md.: Aspen Systems Corporation, 1981.

Murphy, E. *The Logic of Medicine*. Baltimore: Johns Hopkins University Press, 1976.

Nash, J. "Frontiers in the Communication Curriculum: Health Communication." *Communication Administration Bulletin* 21 (1977): 69–73.

Neal, H. *Better Communications For Better Health*. New York: Columbia University Press, 1962.

Nehren, J. and Batey, M. "The Process Recording." *Nursing Forum* 2 (1963): 65–73.

Nelson, B. "Study Indicates Which Patients Nurses Don't Like: The Unpleasant, The Long Term, The Mentally Ill, The Hypochondriacs, and The Dying." *Modern Hospital* 119 (1973): 70–72.

Nemiah, J. "Introduction to the Discussion on Doctor/Patient Relationship." *Knokke* 18 (1970): 103–16.

Noxarian, L. et al. "Effects of a Mailed Reminder on Appointment-Keeping." *Pediatrics* 53 (1974): 349–52.

O'Brien, M. *Communication and Relationships in Nursing*, 2nd ed. St. Louis: C. V. Mosby, 1978.

Oken, D. "What to Tell Cancer Patients." *Journal of the American Medical Association* 175 (1961): 1120–28.

Orlando, I. *Dynamic Nurse–Patient Relationship*. New York: Putman, 1969.

Ort, R. et al. "The Doctor–Patient Relationship as Described by Physicians and Medical Students." *Journal of Health and Human Behavior* 5 (1964): 25–33.

Ostwald, P. "How the Patient Communicates About Disease With the Doctor." In Seabeok, T. et al. (eds), *Approaches To Semiotics*. The Hague: Mouton and Company, 1964.

Ostwald, P. "Symptoms, Diagnosis, and Concepts of Disease: Some Comments on the Semiotics of Physician–Patient Communication." *Social Science Information* 7 (1968): 95–106.

Page, W. "Rhetoritherapy vs. Behavior Therapy: Issues and Evidence." *Communication Education* 29 (1980): 95–104.

Palmer, J. "Staff–Patient Communications in a Chest Hospital." *Clinical Epidemology and Social Medicine* 20 (1966): 195–201.

Parkes, C. "Communication and Cancer: A Social Psychiatrist's View." *Social Science and Medicine* 8 (1974): 189–90.

Patrick, D. et al. "Toward an Operational Definition of Health." *Journal of Health and Social Behavior* 14 (1973): 6–23.

Pellegrino, E. "What's Wrong With Nurse Physician Relationships In Today's Hospitals?" *Journal of American Medical Association* 40 (1966): 70–80.

Perls, F. *Gestalt Therapy Verbatim.* Moab, Utah: Real People Press, 1969.

Peterson, J. "Consumers' Knowledge of and Attitudes Toward Medical Malpractice." *In Appendix, Report of the Secretary's Commission on Medical Malpractice* Washington: U.S. Department of Health, Education and Welfare, 1973.

Pettegrew, L. et al., eds., *Straight Talk: Explorations in Provider and Patient Interaction* Louisville, Ky.: Humana/I.C.A., 1982.

Phillips, G. "Reticence: Pathology of the Normal Speaker." *Speech Monographs* 35 (1968): 39–49.

Phillips, G. "Rhetoritherapy Versus the Medical Model." *Communication Education* 26 (1977): 34–43.

Phillips, G. and Metzger, N. "The Reticence Syndrome: Some Theoretical Considerations about Etiology and Treatment." *Speech Monographs* 40 (1973): 220–30.

Pierce, R. and Drasgow, J. "Teaching Facilitative Interpersonal Functioning to Psychiatric Impatients." *Journal of Counseling Psychology* 16 (1969): 295–99.

Pluckham, M. *Human Communication: The Matrix of Nursing.* New York: McGraw-Hill, 1978.

Pogge, R. "The Toxic Placebo." *Medical Times* 91 (1963): 778–81.

Polgar, S. "Health and Human Behavior: Areas of Interest Common to the Social and Medical Sciences." *Current Anthropology* 3 (1962): 159–205.

Pollack, S. and Manning, P. "An Experience in Teaching The Doctor Patient Relationship to First-Year Medical Students." *Journal of Medical Education* 42 (1967): 770–74.

Pratt, L. et al. "Physicians' View on the Level of Medical Information Among Patients." *American Journal of Public Health* 47 (1957): 1277–83.

Preston, T. *The Clay Pedestal: A Reexamination of the Doctor-Patient Relationship.* Seattle: Madrona Publishers, 1981.

Purtilo, R. *The Allied Health Professional and the Patient.* Philadelphia: W. B. Saunders, 1973.

Quint, J. "Communications Problems Affecting Patient Care in Hospitals." *Journal of the American Medical Association* 195 (1966): 126–217.

Reeder, L. "The Patient-Client As A Consumer: Some Observations On the Changing Professional-Client Relationship." *Journal of Health and Social Behavior* 13 (1972): 406–12.

Regan, L. "Physician and Patient." *The Journal of the American Medical Association* 58 (1955): 255–57.

Rhee, S. "Factors Determining the Quality of Physician Performance." *Medical Care* 14 (1976): 733–50.

Rhee, S. "Relative Importance of Physicians' Personal and Situational Characteristics for the Quality of Patient Care." *Journal of Health and Social Behavior* 18 (1977): 10–15.

Rioch, D. "Communication in the Laboratory and Communication in the Clinic." *Psychiatry* 26 (1963): 2090–221.

Roberts, C. "Blueprint for Improved Physician–Patient Relations." *The Journal of the American Medical Association* 149 (1952): 1194–96.

Robinson, A. "Communicating With Schizophrenic Patients." *American Journal of Nursing* 60 (1960): 1120–23.

Robinson, A. *Working With the Mentally Ill,* 4th ed. Philadelphia: J. B. Lippincott Company, 1971.

Robinson, L. "Patients' Information Base: A Key to Care." *Canadian Nurse* 70 (1974): 34–36.

Rogers, E. *Communication Strategies For Family Planning.* New York: Free Press, 1973.

Rose, S. et al. "Measuring Interpersonal Competence." *Social Work* 22 (1977): 125–29.

Rosenberg, M. *From Now On*. St. Louis: Community Psychological Consultants, 1976.

Ross, C. *Personal and Vocational Relationships in Practical Nursing*, 3rd ed. Philadelphia: J. B. Lippincott Company, 1969.

Rossiter, C. and Pearce, N. *Communicating Personally*. Indianapolis: Bobbs-Merrill, 1975.

Samora, J. et al. "Knowledge About Specific Diseases in Four Selected Samples." *Health and Human Behavior* 3 (1962): 176.

Sanazaro, P. and Williamson, J. "Research in Medical Education. A Classification of Physician Performance In Internal Medicine." *Journal of Medical Education* 43 (1968): 389–97.

Schallen, W. "Communication and the School Health Program." *Journal of Scholastic Health* 47 (1977): 415–17.

Scheff, T. "Decision Rules, Types of Error and Their Consequences in Medical Diagnosis." *Behavioral Science* 8 (1963): 97–107.

Scheflen, A. "Human Communication: Behavioral Programs and Their Integration In Interaction." *Behavioral Science* 13 (1968): 44–55.

Schimmel, E. "Hazards of Hospitalization." *Annals of Internal Medicine* 60 (1964): 100–16.

Schlegel, R. "The Role of Persuasive Communications in Drug Disvasion." *Journal of Drug Education* 7 (1977–78): 279–90.

Schlesinger, R. et al. "Out-Patient Care— The Influence of Interrelated Needs." *American Journal of Public Health* 52 (1962): 1844–52.

Schuetz, J. "Lifelong Learning: Communication Education for the Elderly." *Communication Education* 29 (1980): 33–41.

Schutz, W. *The Interpersonal Underworld*. Palo Alto, Ca: Science and Behavior Books, 1966.

Schutz, W. *A Three Dimensional Theory of Interpersonal Behavior*. New York: Holt, Rinehart, Winston, 1958.

Scoggins, J. "Communicate Damn It." *RN* 39 (1976): 38–41.

Scott, N. et al. "Interaction Analysis As a Method For Assessing Skill in Relating to Patients: Studies on Validity." *British Journal of Medical Education* 7 (1973): 174–78.

Seligmann, A. et al. "Level of Medical Information Among Clinic Patients." *Journal of Chronic Disorders* 6 (1957): 497–509.

Sethee, U. "Verbal Responses of Nurses to Patients in Emotion-Laden Situations in Public Health Nursing." *Nursing Research* 16 (1967): 365–68.

Shapiro, A. "Factors Contributing to the Placebo Effect: Their Implications For Psychotherapy." *American Journal of Psychotherapy* 18 (1964): 73–88.

Shenkin, B. and Warner, D. "Open Information and Medical Care: A Proposal for Reform." *Connecticut Medicine* 39 (1975): 33–34.

Simons, R. and Pardes, H., eds. *Understanding Human Behavior In Health and Illness*. New York: Williams and Wilkins, 1977.

Singer, M. and Wynee, L. "Principles for Scoring Communication Defects and Deviances in Parents of Schizophrenics: Rorschach and TAT Scoring Manuals." *Psychiatry* 29 (1966): 260–88.

Skipper, J. and Leonard, R. *Social Interaction and Patient Care*. Philadelphia: J. B. Lippincott Co., 1965.

Sojit, C. "Dyadic Interaction in a Double Bind Situations." *Family Process* 8 (1969): 235–59.

Spelman, M. et al. "How Do We Improve Doctor–Patient Communications In Our Hospitals." *World Hospitals* 2 (1966): 126–34.

Spiegel, A. "Educating Patients, Having Patience and Testing New Approaches." *Medical Times* 92 (1964): 969–74.

Stergachis, A. *A Person-Orientation in Pharmacy* Minneapolis: University of Minnesota Press, 1970.

Stimson, G. "Obeying Doctor's Orders: A View From the Other Side." *Social Science and Medicine* 8 (1974): 97–104.

Stimson, G. and Webb, B. *Going to See the Doctor: The Consultation Process in Gen-*

eral Practice. London: Routledge and Kegan Paul, 1975

Stoeckle, J. et al. "Going to See the Doctor: The Contributions of the Patient to the Decision to Seek Medical Aid." *Journal of Chronic Disease* 16 (1963): 975–89.

Sullivan, H. *The Interpersonal Theory of Psychiatry.* New York: W. W. Norton, 1953.

Travelbee, J. *Interpersonal Aspects of Nursing.* Philadelphia: F. A. Davis, 1966.

Truax, C. and Mitchell, R. "Research on Certain Therapist Interpersonal Skills in Relation to Process and Outcome." In A. Bergin, and S. Garfield, eds., *Handbook of Psychotherapy and Behavior Change.* New York: Wiley, 1971, 299–344.

Tubesing, D. "The Wholistic Health Center Project: An action Research Model for Providing Preventative, Whole-Person Health Care at a Primary Level." *Medical Care* 15 (1977): 217–27.

Tubesing, D. *Wholistic Health: A Whole-Person Approach to Primary Health Care.* New York: Human Sciences Press, 1979.

Underward, P. "Communication Thru Role Playing." *American Journal of Nursing* 71 (1971): 1184–86.

Véron, E. "Communication, Client, Community and Agency." *Social Work* 9 (1974): 12–17.

Véron, E. and Sluzki, C. "Communication and Neurosis: Semantic Components in Neurotic Verbal Communications." *Social Science and Medicine* 4 (1970): 75–94.

Vincent, P. "Factors Influencing Patient Noncompliance: A Theoretical Approach." *Nursing Research* 20 (1971): 509–16.

Von Wright, G. *Explanation and Understanding.* New York: Cornell University Press, 1971.

Vorhaus, M. *The Changing Doctor–Patient Relationship.* New York: Horizon Press, 1957.

Vuori, H. et al. "Doctor–Patient Relationship in the Light of Patient's Experiences." *Social Science and Medicine* 6 (1972):723–30.

Waitzkin, H. and Stoekle, J. "The Communication of Information About Illness." *Advances in Psychosomatic Medicine* 8 (1972): 180–215.

Waitzkin, H. and Stoekle, J. "Information Control and the Micropolitics of Health Care: Summary of an Ongoing Research Project." *Social Science and Medicine* 10 (1976): 263–76.

Walker, H. "Communication and the American Health Care Problem." *Journal of Communication* 23 (1973): 349–60.

Walker, S. *Psychiatric Signs and Symptoms Due to Medical Problems.* Springfield, Ill.: Charles C. Thomas Publishers, 1967.

Wallace, R. and Benson, H. "The physiology of Meditation." *Scientific American* 226 (1972): 84–90.

Waltzlawick, P. "A Review of the Double Bind Theory." *Family Process* 2 (1963):132–53.

Waltzlawick, P., Beavin, J. and Jackson, D. *Pragmatics of Human Communication.* New York: W. W. Norton, 1967.

Webb, R. "Fear and Communication." *Journal of Drug Education* 4 (1974): 979–1103.

Welford, W. "Closing the Communication Gap." *Nursing Times* 71 (1975): 114–17.

Werner, A. and Schneider, J. "Teaching Medical Students Interactional Skills: A Research-Based Course In the Doctor-Patient Relationship." *New England Journal of Medicine* 22 (1974): 1232–37.

Whitehorn, J. "Orienting Medical Students Toward the Whole Patient." *Journal of the American Medical Association* 164 (1957): 538–41.

Wilden, A. *System and Structure: Essays in Communication and Change.* London: Tavistock, 1972b.

Wiley, L. "Communications." *Nursing 76* (1976):1412–15.

Wilson, J. "Doctor and Patient Today." *Lancet* 2 (1961): 201–02.

Wittenborn, J. et al. *Communication and Drug Abuse.* Springfield, Ill.: Charles C. Thomas, 1970.

Wolf, S. "Effects of Suggestion and Conditioning on the action of Chemical Agents in Human Subjects: The Pharmacology of Placebos." *Journal of Clinical Investigation* 29 (1950): 100–09.

Woods, D. "Talking to People is a Doctor Game That Doctors Don't Play." *Canadian Medical Association Journal* 113 (1975): 1105–06.

Wylie, E. and Morris, A. "Pitfalls of Emotional Involvement." *Nursing '76* 6 (1976): 42–47.

Zborowski, M. *People in Pain.* San Francisco: Jossey-Bass Inc., 1969.

Zola, I. "Problems of Communication, Diagnosis, and Patient Care: The Interplay of Patient, Physician Clinic Organization." *Journal of Medical Education* 38 (1963): 829–38.

B. Verbal Communication In Health Care

Aguilera, D. "Relationship Between Physical Contact and Verbal Interaction Between Nurses and Patients." *Journal of Psychiatric Nursing* 11 (1967): 13–17.

Ascione, F. and Rarim, R. (1975): See Section A.

Bandler, R. and Grinder, J. (1975): See Section A.

Bateson, G. "The Message, 'This is Play.'" In B. Schaffner ed., *Group Processes, II.* Madison, N.J.: Madison Printing Co., 1955.

Beavers, W. et al. (1965): See Section A.

Bird, B. *Talking With Patients.* Philadelphia: J.B. Lippincott, 1955.

Bolton, B. and Sommer, P. (1972): See Section A.

Boyle, C. "Difference Between Patient's and Doctors' Interpretations of Some Common Medical Terms." *British Medical Journal* 22 (1970): 286–89.

Bugental, D. et al. "Verbal-Nonverbal Conflict in Parental Message to Normal and Disturbed Children." *Journal of Abnormal Psychology* 77 (1971): 6–10.

Calnan, J. and Barabas, A. *Speaking At Medical Meetings.* London: William Heinemann Medical Books, Ltd., 1972.

Cassell, E. and Skopek, L. "Language As A Tool in Medicine: Methodology and Theoretical Framework." *Journal of Medical Education* 52 (1977): 197–203.

Chriss, N. "Doctors Down the Logorrhea," *Los Angeles Times,* July 17, 1977.

David, M. (1968): See Section A.

Davis, L. "A System Approach to Medical Information." *Method of Information in Medicine* 12 (1973): 1–6.

Davitz, J. and Davitz, L. "The Communication of Feeling by Content-Free Speech." *Journal of Communication* 9 (1958): 6–13.

Day, S *Communication of Scientific Information.* New York: Karger, 1975.

Dervin, B. et al, (1980): See Section A.

Detmer, D. and Conrad, H. "Reflections Upon Directive Language in Health Care." *Social Science and Medicine* 9 (1975): 553–58.

Diers, D. and Leonard, R. "Interaction Analysis in Nursing Research." *Nursing Research* 21 (1972): 419–28.

Dinoff, M. et al. "Conditioning Verbal Behavior of a Psychiatric Population in a Group Therapylike Situation." *Journal of Clinical Psychology* 16 (1960): 371–72.

Dirckx, J. *The Language of Medicine.* New York: Harper and Row, 1976.

Ekman, P. "Body Position, Fasial Expression, and Verbal Behavior During Interviews." *Journal of Abnormal and Social Psychology* 68 (1964) 295–301.

Endler, N. "The Effects of Verbal Reinforcement on Conformity and Deviant Behavior." *Journal of Social Psychology* 66 (1965): 147–54.

Fair, E. "So You Have to Make a Speech?" *Supervisor Nurse* 2 (1971): 58–59.

Gladstein, G. "Nonverbal Communication and Counseling Psychotherapy." *The Counseling Psychologist* 4 (1974): 34–57.

Goffman, E. *Stigma: Notes on the Management of Spoiled Identity.* Englewood Cliffs, N.J.: Spectrum, 1963.

Golden, J. and Johnson, G. "Problems of Distortion in Doctor–Patient Communications." *Psychiatry In Medicine* 1 (1970): 127–49.

Hawkins, C. *Speaking and Writing in Medicine.* Springfield, III: Charles C. Thomas Publishers, 1967.

Hein, E. (1975): See Section A.

Hodgins, E. (1966): See Section A.

Holder, L. (1972): See Section A.

Illardo, J. "Ambiguity Tolerance and Disordered Communication: Therapeutic Aspects." *Journal of Communication* 23 (1973): 361–70.

Jaffe, J. "The Study of Language In Psychiatry: Psycholinguistics and Computational Linguistics." In S. Arieti, ed., *American Handbook of Psychiatry*, Vol. 3. New York: Basic Books, 1966, 689–704.

Jones, S. "Directivity vs. Nondirectivity: Implications for the Examination of Witnesses in Law for the Fact-Finding Interview." *Journal of Communication* 19 (1969): 64–75.

Kelly, F. "Paralinguistic Indicators of Patient's Affect: Attitudinal Significance of Length of Communication." *Psychological Reports* 32 (1973): 1223–26.

Kirscht, J. et al. (1975): See Section A.

Kreps, G. "Nonverbal Communication in Dentistry." *The Dental Assistant* 50 (1981) 18–20.

Labov, W. and Fanshel, D. *Therapeutic Discourse: Psychotherapy as Conversation.* New York: Academic Press, 1977.

Lacon, J. and Wilden, A. *The Language of the Self.* New York: Delta, 1975.

Langer, E. and Abelson, R. "A Patient By Another Name . . . Clinician Group Difference in Labeling Bias." *Journal of Consulting and Clinical Psychology* 42 (1974): 4–9.

Ley, P. "Primary, Rated Importance and the Retall of Medical Statements." *Journal of Health and Social Behavior* 13 (1972): 311–17.

Ley, P. et al. "A Method of Increasing Patients' Recall of Information Presented by Doctors." *Psychological Medicine* 3 (1973): 217–20.

Mabry, E. "Sequential Structure of Interaction in Encounter Groups." *Human Communication Research* 1 (1975): 302–07.

MacBryde, C. (1964): See Section A.

Matarazzo, J. and Wiens, A. "Influence on Durations of Interviewee Silence." *Journal of Experimental Research in Personality* 2 (1967): 56–69.

Miller, J. (1960): See Section A.

Mohammed, M. (1964): See Section A.

Morris, L. et al. "Drug Name Familiarity and the Placebo Effect." *Journal of Clinical Psychology* 30 (1974): 280–82.

Ostwald, P. (1964): See Section A.

Ostwald, P. (1968): See Section A.

Quint, J. "Institution Practices of Information Control." *Psychiatry* 28 (1965): 119–28.

Reik, T. *Listening With the Third Ear.* New York: Farrar, Straus, and Giroux, 1977.

Roland, C. and Cox, B. "A Mandatory Course In Scientific Writing for Undergraduate Medical Students." *Journal of Medical Education* 51 (1976): 89–93.

Samora, J. et al. "Medical Volcabulary Knowledge Among Hospital Patients." *Journal of Health and Human Behavior* 2 (1961): 91–99.

Scott, N. et al. (1973): See Section A.

Seay, T. and Altekruse, M. "Verbal and Nonverbal Behavior In Judgements of Facilitative Conditions." *Journal of Counseling Psychology* 26 (1979): 108–19.

Seligmann, A. et al. (1957): See Section A.

Sethee, U. (1967): See Section A.

Shands, H. *Semiotic Approaches to Psychiatry.* The Hague: Mouton, 1970.

Sluzki, C. and Veron, E. "Interpersonal Effects of Semantic Patterns." In S. Arieti, ed., *The World Biennial of Psychiatry and Psychotherapy*, Vol. 2. New York: Basic Books, 1973.

Tring, F. and Hayes-Allen, M. "Understanding and Misunderstanding of Some Medical Terms." *British Journal of Medical Education* 7 (1973): 53–59.

Tuckman, B. "Interpersonal Probing and Revealing and Systems of Integrative Complexity." *Journal of Personality and Social Psychology* 3 (1966): 655–64.

Veron, E. and Sluzki, C. (1970): See Section A.

Vetter, H. *Language Behavior and Psychopathology.* Chicago: Rand McNally, 1969.

Von Wright, G. (1971): See Section A.

Wagner, M. "Reinforcement of the Verbal Productivity in Group Therapy." *Psychological Reports* 19 (1966): 1217–18.

Williams, R. and Blanton, R. "Verbal Conditioning in a Psychotherapeutic Situation." *Behaviour Research and Therapy* 6 (1968): 97–103.

C. Nonverbal Communication In Health Care

Aguilera, D. (1967): See Section B.

Barnett, K. "A Survey of the Current Utilization of Touch by Health Team Personnel with Hospitalized Patients." *International Journal of Nursing Studies* 9 (1972a): 195–209.

Barnett, K. "A Theoretical Construct of the Concept of Touch as They Relate to Nursing." *Nursing Research* 21 (1972b): 102–10.

Beier, E. *The Silent Language of Psychotherapy*. Chicago: Aldine, 1966.

Berger, M. "Nonverbal Communications in Group Psychotherapy." *International Journal of Group Psychotherapy* 8 (1958): 161–78.

Birdwhistell, R. "Contributions of Linguistic-Kinesic Studies to the Understanding of Schizophrenia." In A. Auerback, ed., *Schizophrenia: An Intergrated Approach*. New York: Ronald, 1959.

Bugental, D. et al. (1971): See Section B.

Cash, T. et al. "When Counselors are Heard But Not Seen: Initial Impact of Physical Attractiveness." *Journal of Counseling Psychology* 22 (1975): 273–79.

Charny, E. "Postural Configurations in Psychotherapy." *Psychosomatic Medicine* 28 (1966): 305–15.

Davitz, J. and Davitz, L. (1958): See Section B.

Day, F. "The Patient's Perception of Touch." In E. Anderson, et al., eds. *Current Concepts In Clinical Nursing*. St. Louis: C. V. Mosby, 1973, 266–75.

Diers, D. and Leonard, R. (1972): See Section B.

Dittman, A. "The Relationship Between Body Movement and Moods in Interviews." *Journal of Consultant Psychology* 26 (1962): 480.

Eisler, R. et al. "Effects of Videotape and Instructional Feedback on Nonverbal Marital Interactions: An Analogue Study." *Behavior Therapy* 5 (1973): 551–58.

Ekman, P. (1964): See Section B.

Ekman, P. "Nonverbal Behavior in Psychotherapy Research." In J. Shlien, ed. *Research in Psychotherapy*. Chicago: American Psychological Association, 1967.

Goffman, E. "On Face-Work: An Analysis of Ritual Elements in Social Interaction." *Psychiatry* 18 (1955): 213–31.

Goffman, E. (1963): See Section B.

Haggard, E. and Isaacs, K. "Micromomentary Social Expression as Indictors of Ego Mechanisms in Psychotherapy." In L. Gottschalk and A. Auerbach, eds., *Methods of Research in Psychotherapy*. New York: Appleton Century Crofts, 1966.

Hall, E. *Beyond Culture*. Garden City, N.Y.: Doubleday, 1977.

Hall, E. *The Hidden Dimension*. Garden City, N.Y.: Doubleday, 1966.

Hall, E. *The Silent Language* Garden City, N.Y.: Doubleday, 1959.

Hampe, W. "Territory Defense and Fear of the Therapist." *Voices* 3 (1966): 47–52.

Hein, E. (1975): See Section A.

Kahn, M. "Nonverbal Communication and Marital Satisfaction." *Family Process* 9 (1970): 449–56.

Kelly, F. (1973): See Section B.

Knapp, M. *Nonverbal Communication in Human Interaction*, 2nd ed. New York: Holt, Rinehart, and Winston, 1978.

Kreps, G. (1981): See Section B.

Lacrosse, M. "Nonverbal Behavior and Perceived Counsel or Attractiveness and Persuasiveness." *Journal of Counseling Psychology* 22 (1975): 563–66.

Lassen, C. "Effect of Proximity on Anxiety and Communication in the Initial Psychiatric Interview." *Journal of Abnormal Psychology* 81 (1973) 220–32.

Loeb, F. "The Microscopic Film Analyses of the Function of a Recurrent Behaviorial Pattern in a Psychotherapy Session." *Journal of Nervous and Mental Disorders* 147 (1968): 605–17.

MacBryde, C. (1964): See Section A.

Maltz, M. *Psycho-cybernetics*. New York: Pocket Books, Inc., 1973.

Mehrabian, A. and Ferris, S. "Inference of Attitude From Nonverbal Communication in Two Channels." *Journal of Consulting Clinical Psychology* 31 (1967): 248–52.

Mehrabian, A. and Wiener, M. "Decoding of Inconsistent Communications." *Journal of Personnel Social Psychology* 6 (1967): 109–114.

Milmoe, S. et al. "The Doctor's Voice: Postdictor of Successful Referral of Alcohlic Patients." *Journal of Abnormal Psychology* 72 (1967): 78–84.

Montagu, A. *Touching: The Human Significance of Skin*. New York: Columbia University Press, 1971.

Nguyen, T. et al. "The Meanings of Touch: Sex Differences," *Journal of Communication* 25 (1975): 92–103.

Piliavin, J. and Piliavin, I. "The Effects of Blood on Reactions to a Victim." *Journal of Personality and Social Psychology* 23 (1972): 235–61.

Rinck, C. et al. "Interpersonal Touch Among Residents of Homes for the Elderly." *Journal of Communication* 30 (1980): 44–47.

Scheflen, A. "Communication and Regulations in Psychotherapy Transaction." *Psychiatry* 26 (1963): 126–36.

Scheflen, A. *Communicational Structure: Analysis of A Psychotherapy Transaction*. Bloomington, Ind.: Indiana University Press, 1973.

Scheflen, A. "Quasi-Courtship Behavior in Psychotherapy." *Psychiatry* 28 (1965): 245–57.

Scheflen, A. "The Significance of Posture in Communication Systems." *Psychiatry* 27 (1964): 316–31.

Schmidt, L. and Strong, S. "Attractiveness and Influence in Counseling." *Journal of Counseling Psychology* 18 (1971): 348–51.

Seay, T. and Altekruse, M. (1979): See Section B.

Strong, S. and Dixon, D. "Expertness, Attractiveness, and Influence in Counseling. *Journal of Counceling Psychology* 18 (1971): 562–70.

Strong, S. et al. "Nonverbal Behavior and Perceived Counselor Characteristics." *Journal of Counseling Psychology* 18 (1971): 554–61.

Watson, W. "Body Image and Staff-to-Resident Deportment In a Home for the Aged." *Aging and Human Development* 1 (1970): 345–59.

Watson, W. "The Meanings of Touch: Geriatric Nursing." *Journal of Communication* 25 (1975): 104–12.

Zuk, G. et al. "Some Dynamics of Laughter During Family Therapy." *Family Process* 2 (1963): 302–13.

D. Health Care Interviewing

Adler, L. and Enelow, A. "An Instrument to Measure Skill in Diagnosing Interviewing: A Teaching and Evaluation Tool." *Journal of Medical Education* 41 (1966): 281–88.

Adler, L. et al. "Changes In Medical Interviewing Style After Instruction With Two Closed-Circuit Television Techniques." *Journal of Medical Education* 45 (1970): 21–28.

Alfidi, R. "Informed Consent: A study of Patient Reaction." *Journal of the American Medical Association* 216 (1971): 1325–29.

Alger, I. and Hogan, P. "Enduring Effects of Videotape Playback Experience on Family and Marital Relationships." *American Journal of Orthospsychiatry* 39 (1969): 86–98.

Arntson, P. et al. (1978): See Section A.

Balint, E. and Norell, J. *Six Minutes For the Patient*. London: Pitman Medical Publishing Company, 1964.

Barbee, R. et al. "The Quantitativve Evaluation of Student Performance In the Medical Interview." *Journal of Medical Education* 42 (1967) 238–43.

Barbee, R. and Feldman, S. "A Three-Year Longitudinal Study of the Medical Interview and Its Relationship to Student Performance in Clinical Medicine." *Journal of Medical Education* 45 (1970): 770–76.

Barrows, H. *Simulated Patients (Programmed Patients)*. Springfield, Ill.: Charles C. Thomas Publishers, 1971.

Beers, T. and Foreman, M. "Intervention Patterns in Crisis Interviews." *Journal of Counseling Psychology* 23 (1976): 87–91.

Belsky, M. and Gross, L. (1975): See Section A.

Benjamin, A. *The Helping Interview*, 3rd ed. Boston: Houghton Mifflin Company, 1981.

Bergeron, J. (1971): See Section A.

Bermosk, L. "Interviewing." *Supervisor Nurse* 4 (1973): 46–56.

Bernstein, L. et al. *Interviewing: A Guide for Health Professionals*. New York: Appleton-Century-Crofts, 1974.

Bernstein, L. and Dana, R. *Interviewing and the Health Professionals*. New York: Appleton-Century-Crofts, 1970.

Bird, B. (1955): See Section B.

Blaxter, M. "Diagnosis as Category and Process: The Case of Alcoholism." *Social Science and Medicine* 12 (1978): 9–18.

Bloom, M. et al. "Interviewing the Ill Aged." *The Gerontologist* 11 (1971): 292–99.

Bolte, G. "A Communications Approach to Marital Counseling." *The Family Coordinator* 19 (1970): 32–40.

Bowers, W. (1962): See Section A.

Brown, E. (1965): See Section A.

Browne, K. and Freeling, P. (1967): See Section A.

Calnan, M. (1971): See Section A.

Carkhuff, R. *The Art of Helping*. Amherst, Mass.: Human Resource Development Press, 1972.

Carroll, J. and Monroe, J. "Teaching Medical Interviewing: A Critique of Educational Research and Practice. *Journal of Medical Education* 54 (1979): 498–500.

Carroll, J. and Monroe, J. "Teaching Clinical Interviewing In the Health Professions: A Review of Empirical Research." *Evaluation and the Health Professions* 3 (1980): 21–45.

Carter, G. "History Taking and Interviewing Technique." *Journal of Medical Education* 30 (1955): 315–26.

Cash, T. et al. (1975): See Section C.

Cassata, D. et al. "A Program For Enhancing Medical Interviewing Using Videotape Feedback In the Family Practice Residency." *Journal of Family Practice* 4 (1977): 673–77.

Cassata, D. et al. "An Advanced Medical School Interviewing Course Using Videotape Feedback: A Systematic Approach." *Journal of Medical Education* 55 (1976): 939–42.

Cassata, D. and Clements, P. "Teaching Communication Skills Through Videotape Feedback: A Rural Health Program." *Biosciences Communications* 4 (1978): 39–50.

Cline, D. and Garrard, J. "A Medical Interviewing Course: Objectives, Techniques, and Assessment." *American Journal of Psychiatry* 130 (1973): 574–78

Clyne, M. (1972): See Section A.

Cole, P. et al. "Drug Consultation: Its Significance to the Discharged Patient and Its Relevance to the Role For the Pharmacist." *American Journal of Hospital Pharmacy* 28 (1971): 954.

Collins, E. "Do We Really Advise the Patient?" *Journal of the Florida Medical Association* 42 (1955): 111–15.

Davis, R. (1970): See Section A.

Davitz, L. (1970): See Section A.

DeBlassie, R. *Counseling With Mexican-American Youth: Preconceptions and Processes*. Austin, Tx.: Learning Concept, 1976.

Dittman, A. (1962): See Section C.

Dobbs, H. and Carek, D. "The Conceptualization and Teaching of Medical Interviewing." *Journal of Medical Education* 47 (1972): 272–76.

Easson, E. "Reactions of Cancer Patients on Being Told Their Diagnosis." *British Medical Journal* (1959): 779–83.

Egbert, L. et al. "Reduction of Postoperative Pain by Encouragement and Instruction of Patients." *New England Journal of Medicine* 270 (1964): 825–27.

Elstein, A. et al. (1972): See Section A.

Enelow, A. and Swisher, S. *Interviewing and Patient Care*. New York: Oxford University Press, 1972.

Enelow, A. et al. "Programmed Instruction In Interviewing: An Experiment In Medical Education." *Journal of the American Medical Association* 212 (1970): 1843–46.

Engel, G. (1976): See Section A.

Engel, G. and Morgan, W. *Interviewing The Patient*. London: London: W. B. Saunders Company, 1973.

Eustene, A. "Explaining to The Patient: A Therapeutic Tool and a Professional Obligation." *Journal of the American Medical Association* 165 (1957): 1110–13.

Farsad, P. et al. "Teaching Interviewing Skills to Pediatric House Officers." *Pediatrics* 61 (1978): 384–88.

Fisher, H. "Interviewing Cross-Culturally." In H. Prosser, ed., *Intercommunication Among Nations and Peoples*. New York: Harper and Row, 1973.

Foley, R. and Sharf, B. "The Five Interviewing Techniques Most Frequently Overlooked By Primary Care Physicians." *Behavioral Medicine* 11 (1981): 26–31.

Freedman, C. (1966): See Section A.

Freidman, R. "A Computer Program for Simulating the Patient–Physician Encounter." *Journal of Medical Education* 48 (1963): 610–25.

Fritzen, R. and Mazer, G. "The Effects of Fear Appeal and Communication Upon Attitudes Toward Alcohol Consumption." *Journal of Drug Education* (1975): 171–81.

Froelich, R. "A Course In Medical Interviewing." *Journal of Drug Education* 44 (1969): 1165–69.

Garland, L. *Nurse–Patient Communication*. Dubuque, Iowa: McMillan, 1967.

Grissinger, S. (1973): See Section A.

Hawes, L. "Development and Application of an Interview Coding System." *Central States Speech Journal* 23 (1972): 92–99.

Hawes, L. "The Effects of Interviewer Style on Patterns of Dyadic Communication." *Speech Monographs* 39 (1972): 114–23.

Hawes, L. and Foley, J. "A Markov Analysis of Interviewe Communication." *Speech Monographs* 40 (1973): 208–19.

Hayes, D. et al. "Preparation of Medical Students for Patient Interviewing ." *Journal of Medical Education* 46 (1971): 863–68.

Hays, E. and Mandel, J. "Interviewing: A Definition and Description."*Central States Speech Journal* 21 (1970): 126–29.

Helfer, R. "An Objective Comparison of the Pediatric Interviewing Skills of Freshman and Senior Medical Students." *Pediatrics* 45 (1970): 623–27.

Helfer, R. and Ealy, K. "Observation of Pediatric Interviewing Skills: A Longitudinal and Cross-Sectional Study." *American Journal of Diseases of Children* 123 (1972): 556–60.

Helfer, R. et al. "Pediatric Interviewing Skills Taught by Non-Physicians." *American Journal of Diseases of Children* 129 (1975): 1053–57.

Helfer, R. and Hess, J. "An Experimental Model for Making Objective Measurements of Interviewing Skills." *Journal of Clinical Psychology* 26 (1970): 327–31.

Helfer, R. and Levin, S. "The Use of Videotape In Teaching Clinical Pediatrics." *Journal of Medical Education* 42 (1967): 367.

Heller, K. et al. "The Effects of Interviewer Style in a Standardized Interview." *Journal of Consulting Psychology* 30 (1966): 501–08.

Hess, J. (1969): See Section A.

Hollingford, G. et al. "A Method of Evaluating Student–Patient Interviews." *Journal of Medical Education* 32 (1957): 853–58.

Hubbard, J. et al. (1965): See Section A.

Hunter, D. and Bomford, R. (1968): See Section A.

Hutter, M. et al. "Interviewing Skills: A Comprehensive Approach to Teaching and Evaluation." *Journal of Medical Education* 52 (1977): 328–33.

Ivey, A. *Microcounseling: Innovations In Interview Training*. Springfield, Ill.: Charles C. Thomas, 1971.

Jackson, D. et al. "A Method of Analysis of a Family Interview." *Archives of General Psychiatry* 5 (1961): 321–39.

Jason, H. et al. "New Approaches to Teaching Basic Interviewing Skills to Medical Students." *American Journal of Psychiatry* 127 (1971): 1404–07.

Jones, S. (1969): See Section B.

Kahn, G. et al. "Teaching Interpersonal

Skills in Family Practice." *The Journal of Family Practice* 8 (1979): 309–16.

Kimball, C. "Techniques of Interviewing: Interviewing and the Meaning of the Symptom." *Annals of Internal Medicine* 71 (1969): 147–53.

Kimball, C. "Techniques of Interviewing: Setting Up an Interviewing Course." *Psychiatry In Medicine* I (1970): 167–70.

Klemer, R. "Talking With Patients About Sexual Problems." *Post-Graduate Medicine* 40 (1966): 160–66.

Korsch, B. and Aley, E. "Pediatric Interviewing Techniques." *Current Problems in Pediatrics* (1973): 1–42.

Kounin, J. et al. "Experimental Studies of Clients' Reactions to Initial Interviews." *Human Relations* 9 (1956): 265–93.

Lassen, C. (1973): See Section B.

Loesch, L. and Loesch, N. "What Do You Say After You Say Mm-Hmm?" *American Journal of Nursing* 75 (1975): 807–09.

MacKinnon, R. and Michels, R. *The Psychiatric Interview In Clinical Practice.* Philadelphia: W. B. Saunders, 1971.

Maguire, P. "The Use of Patient Simulation In Training Medical Students In History-Taking Skills." *Medical and Biological Illustration* 26 (1976): 91–95.

Matarazzo, R. et al. "Learning the Art of Interviewing: A Study of What Beginning Students Do and Their Patterns of Change." *Psychotherapy: Therapy, Research and Practice* 2 (1965): 49–60.

McQuown, N. et al. *The Natural History of An Interview.* Chicago: University of Chicago Library, 1971.

Meadow, R. and Hewitt, C. "Teaching Communication Skills With the Help of Actresses and Video-tape Stimulation." *British Journal of Medical Education* 6 (1972): 317–322.

Meares, A. *The Medical Interview: A Study of Clinically Significant Interpersonal Reactions.* Springfield, Ill: Charles C. Thomas Publisher, 1957.

Molode, D. and Wiens, A. "Interview Interaction Behavior of Nurses with Task Versus Person Orientation." *Nursing Research* 17 (1968): 45–57.

Moreland, J. et al. "An Evaluation of Microcounseling as an Interviewer Training Tool." *Journal of Consulting Clinical Psychology* 41 (1973): 294–300.

Morgan, W. and Engel, G. *The Clinical Approach to the Patient.* Philadelphia: W. B. Saunders Company, 1969.

Oken, D. (1961): See Section A.

Rasche, L. et al. "Evaluation of a Systematic Approach to Teaching Interviewing." *Journal of Medical Education* 49 (1974): 589–95.

Sapira, J. "Reassurance Therapy: What to Say to Symptomatic Patients With Benign Diseases." *Annals of Internal Medicine* (1972): 603–04.

Scheff, T. (1963): See Section A.

Schmitt, F. and Wooldridge, P. "Psychological Preparation of Surgical Patients." *Nursing Research* 22 (1973): 108–15.

Schubert, M. *Interviewing In Social Work Practice.* New York: Council on Social Work Education, 1971.

Schwartz, W. "Decision Analysis: A Look at the Chief Complaints." *New England Journal of Medicine* 300 (1975): 556–59.

Scott, N. et al. "Changes in Interviewing Styles of Medical Students." *Journal of Medical Education* 50 (1975): 1124–26.

Stevenson, I. *Medical History Taking.* New York: Paul B. Hoeber, Inc., 1960.

Stevenson, I. *The Diagnostic Interview,* 2nd ed. New York: Harper & Row 1971.

Stewart, C. and Cash, W. *Interviewing Principles and Practices,* 2nd ed. Dubuque, Iowa: William C. Brown, 1978.

Stillman, P. et al. "The Use of Paraprofessionals to Teach Interviewing Skills." *Pediatrics* 57 (1976): 769–74.

Stimson, G. and Webb, B. (1975): See Section A.

Tuckman, B. (1966): See Section B.

Watzlawick, P. "A Structured Family Interview." *Family Process* 5 (1966): 256–71.

Wexler, M. and Adler, L. *Help the Patient Tell His Story.* Oradel, N.J.: Medical Economics Book Division, 1971.

Zakus, G. et al. "Teaching Interviewing for Pediatrics." *Journal of Medical Education* 51 (1976): 325–31.

E. Therapeutic Communication

Aderman, D. and Berkowits, L. "Observational Set, Empathy, and Helping." *Journal of Personality and Social Psychology* 14 (1970): 141–48.

Adler, H. (1973) See Section A.

Anthony, W. (1973): See Section A.

Archer, J. et al. (1972): See Section A.

Artiss, K. and Levine, A. (1973): See Section A.

Ashby, W. "The Application of Cybernetics to Psychiatry." *British Journal of Psychiatry* 100 (1954): 114–24.

Atman, N. (1972): See Section A.

Bakan, D. *Disease, Pain and Sacrifice: Toward a Psychology of Suffering.* Boston: Beacon Press, 1968.

Balint, M. (1965): See Section A.

Bandler, R. and Grinder, J. (1975): See Section A.

Barber, B. (1976): See Section A.

Barnlund, D. (1968): See Section A.

Barrett-Hennard, G. "Dimensions of Therapist Response as Causal Factors in Therapeutic Change." *Psychological Monographs* 76 (1962): 562.

Bateson, G. (1955): See Section B.

Bateson, G. (1972): See Section A.

Beier, E. (1966): See Section C.

Bennett, P. and Maley, R. "Modification of Interactive Behaviors in Chronic Mental Patients." *Journal of Applied Behavior Analysis* 6 (1973): 609–20.

Ben-Sira, Z. "Involvement With A Disease and Health Promoting Behaviors." *Social Science and Medicine* (1977): 165–73.

Ben-Sira, Z. "The Function of the Professional's Affective Behavior in Client Satisfaction: A Revised Approach to Social Interaction Theory." *Journal of Health and Social Behavior* 17 (1976): 3–11.

Berenson, B. and Mitchell, K. "Therapeutic Conditions After Therapist-Intiated Confrontation." *Journal of Clinical Psychology* 24 (1968): 363–64.

Berger, M. (1958): See Section C.

Bergin, A. and Jasker, L. "Correlates of Empathy in Psychotherapy: A Replication." *Journal of Abnormal Psychology* 74 (1969): 477–81.

Bergin, A. and Soilomin, S. "Personality and Performance Correlates of Empathic Understanding in Psychotherapy." In J. Hart and T. Tomlinson, eds. *New Directions in Client Centered Therapy.* Boston: Houghton Mifflin, 1970, 233–36.

Bicket, W. "Auto Therapy: The Future is Now." *Journal of the American Pharmaceutical Association* NS 12 (1975): 560–62, 564.

Bolte, G. (1970): See Section D.

Bromberg, W. "An Analysis of Therapeutic Artfulness." *American Journal of Psychiatry* 114 (1958): 719–26.

Bundza, K. and Simonson, N. "Therapist Self-Disclosure: Its Effects On Impressions of Therapist and Willingness to Disclose." *Psychotherapy: Theory, Research, and Practice* 10 (1973): 215–17.

Burke, R. et al. "Informal Helping Relationships in Work Organizations." *Academy of Management Journal* 19 (1976): 370–77.

Carkhuff, R. (1972): See Section D.

Carkhuff, R. *Helping and Human Relations* (2 Vols.). New York: Holt, Rinehart and Winston, 1971.

Carkhuff, R. *The Development of Human Resources.* New York: Holt, Rinehart and Winston, 1971.

Carkhuff, R. "Toward a Comprehensive Model of Facilitative Interpersonal Processes." *Journal of Counseling Psychology* 14 (1967): 67–72.

Cartwright, R. and Lerner, B. "Empathy, Need to Change and Improvement in Psychotherapy." In G. Stollak et al. eds. *Psychotherapy Research: Selected Readings.* Chicago: Rand McNally, 1966, 537–45.

Cohen, R. "The Effects of Group Interaction and Progressive Hierarchy Presentation on Desensitization of Test Anxiety." *Behaviour Research and Therapy* 7 (1969): 15–26.

Colm, H. "Healing as Participation: Comments Based on Paul Tillich's Existential Philosophy." *Psychiatry* 16 (1953): 99–111.

Combs, A. *Helping Relationships.* Boston: Allyn and Bacon, 1972.

Costello, D. "Therapeutic Transactions: An Approach to Human Communications." In R. Budd and B. Ruben, eds. *Approaches to Human Communication.* New York: Spartan, 1972.

Crisp, A. "Therapeutic Aspects of the Doctor-Patient Relationship." *Psychotherapy and Psychosomatics* 18 (1970): 12–33.

Cumming, J. (1960): See Section A.

Dichter, E. (1954): See Section A.

Dinoff, M. et al. (1960): See Section B.

Dymond, R. "A Scale For the Measurement of Empathetic Ability." *Journal of Consulting Psychology* 14 (1949): 127–33.

Easson, E. (1959): See Section D.

Egbert, L. et al. (1964): See Section D.

Ehrlich, H. and Bauer, M. "Therapists' Feelings Toward Patients and Patient Treatment and Outcome." *Social Science and Medicine* I (1967): 283–91.

Eustene, A. (1957): See Section D.

Ewin, D. "Relieving Suffering and Pain With Hypnosis." *Geriatrics* 33 (1978):

Fiedler, F. "The Concept of An Ideal Therapeutic Relationship." *Journal of consulting Psychology* 14 (1950): 239–45.

Fiedler, F. "The Concept of An Ideal Therapeutic Relationship." *Journal of Consulting Psychology* 14 (1950): 239–45.

Fiedler, F. "A Comparison of Therapeutic Relationship in Psychoanalytic Nondirective and Adlerian Therapy." *Journal of Counsulting Psychology* 14 (1950): 436–45.

Fiedler, F. "Quantitative Studies on the Role of Therapists' Feelings Toward Their Patients." In O. Mowrer, ed. *Psychotherapy Theory and Research.* New York: Ronald Press, 1953, 296–315.

Friedman, C. "Making Abortion Consultants Therapeutic." *American Journal of Psychiatry* 130 (1973): 1257–61.

Fuller, D. and Quesada, G. (1973): See Section A.

Gaylin, W. *Caring.* New York: Alfred A. Knopf, Inc., 1976.

Gibb, J. (1961): See Section A.

Gillis, J. "Social Influence Therapy: The Therapist As Manipulator." *Psychology Today* 8 (1974): 90–95.

Gladstein, G. (1974): See Section B.

Goldsmith, J. and McFall, R. (1975): See Section A.

Greenberg, S. *The Quality of Mercy.* New York: Atheneum Publishers, 1971.

Guerney, B. (1977): See Section A.

Haley, J. "The Family of the Schizophrenic: A Model System." *Journal of Nervous and Mental Disorders* 129 (1966): 357–374.

Haley, J. *Problem-Solving Therapy.* San Francisco: Jossey-Bass, Inc., 1976.

Haley, J. "Research on Family Patterns: An Instrument Measurement." *Family Process* 3 (1964): 41–65.

Hampe, W. (1966): See Section B.

Handkins, R. and Munz, D. (1978): See Section A.

Hargreaves, W. and Runyon, N. "Patterns of Psychiatric Nursing Role Differences In Nurse-Patient Interaction." *Nursing Research* 18 (1969): 300–07.

Hart, R. and Burks, D. (1972): See Section A.

Hart, R. et al. (1980): See Section A.

Hinterkopf, E. and Brunswick, L. "Teaching Therapeutic Skills to Mental Patients," *Psychotherapy: Theory, Research and Practice* 12 (1975): 8–12.

Hunt, R. *Interpersonal Strategies For System Management: Applications of Counseling and Participative Principles.* Monterey, Ca.: Brooks/Cole, 1974.

Illardo, J. (1973): See Section B.

Jackson, D. (1968a): See Section A.

Jackson, D. (1968b); See Section A.

Jackson, D. ed. *Therapy, Communication and Change: Human Communication, Volume 2.* Palo Alto, Ca: Science and Behavior Books, 1968.

Jackson, D. et al. "Family Interaction, Family Homeostasis, and Some Implications For Conjoint Family Psychotherapy." In J. Masserman, ed. *Individual and Familial Dynamics.* New York: Grune and Stratton, Inc., 1959: 122–41.

Jackson, D. et al. (1961): See Section D.

Jaffe, J. (1966): See Section B.

Johnson, D. (1972): See Section A.

Johnson, D. "The Effects of Warmth of Interaction, Accuracy of Understanding, and the Proposals of Compromises on the Listener's Behavior." *Journal of counseling Psychology* 18 (1971): 207–16.

Johnson, D. "The Effects of Expressing Warmth and Anger Upon the Actor and the Listener." *Journal of Counseling Psychology* 18 (1971): 571–78.

Julian, J. et al. "Quasi-Therapeutic Effects of Intergroup Competition." *Journal of Personality and Social Psychology* 3 (1966): 321–27.

Katz, R. *Empathy: Its Nature and Uses.* Glencoe, Ill: Free Press, 1963.

Kurtz, R. and Grummon, D. "Different Approaches to the Measurement of Therapist Empathy and Their Relationship to Therapy Outcomes." *Journal of Consulting Clinical Psychology* 39 (1972): 106–15.

Labov, W. and Fanshel, D. (1977): See Section B.

Lair, C. et al. "Keeping The Patient In Therapy." *Medical Times* 93 (1964): 1127–34.

Lesser, M. "Perception of Illness At A Therapeutic Community for Ex-Drug Addicts: 'Legitimate Deviancy' or Escape?" *Social Science and Medicine* 8 (1974): 483–87.

Liebhart, E. "Empathy and Emergency Helping: The Effects of Personality, Self-Concern and Acquaintance." *Journal of Experimental Social Psychology* 8 (1972): 404–11.

Loeb, F. (1968): See Section C.

Macaulay, J. and Berkawitz, L. eds. *Altruism and Helping Behavior.* New York: Academic Press, 1970.

MacKinnon, R. and Michels, R. (1971): See Section D.

Martin, J. et al. "Process Variables and Psychotherapy: A Study of Conseling and Friendship." *Journal of Counseling Psychology* 13 (1966): 356–59.

Matarazzo, R. "Reasearch on the Teaching and Learning Of Psychotherapeutic Skills." In A. Bergin and S. Garfield, eds. *Handbook of Psychotherapy and Behavior Change.* New York: Wiley, 1971.

Mayeroff, M. *On Caring.* New York: Perennial Library (Harper and Row), 1971.

McNamara, E. "The Caring Employer Helps the Troubled Employee." *Hospital Progress* 50 (1976): 93–96.

Mehrabian, A. and Epstein, N. "A Measure of Emotional Empathy." *Journal of Personality* 40 (1972): 425–543.

Miller, L. "Short Term Therapy With Adolescents." In H. Parad, ed. *Crisis Intervention: Selected Readings.* New York: Family Service Association, 1965.

Moore, B. "Cultural Differences and Counseling Perspectives." *Texas Personnel and Guidance Association Journal* 3 (1974): 39–44.

Morris, D. *Intimate Behavior.* New York: Random House, 1971.

Mullen, J. and Abeles, N. "Relationship of Liking, Empathy and Therapists' Experience to Outcome of Therapy." In *Psychotherapy 1971*, Chicago: Aldine-Atherton, 1972, 256–60.

Naegele, K. *Health and Healing.* San Francisco: Jossey-Bass Publishers, 1970.

Northouse, P. "Predictors of Empathic Ability in an Organizational Setting." *Human Communication Research* 3 (1977): 176–78.

Olson, D., ed. *Treating Relationships.* Lake Mills, Iowa: Graphic Publishing, 1976.

Pederson, P. et al. *Counseling Across Cultures.* Honolulu: East-West Center Press, 1976.

Peitchinis, J. "Therapeutic Effectiveness of Counseling by Nursing Personnel." *Nursing Research* 21 (1972): 138–48.

Perls, F. (1969): See Section A.

Pettegrew, L. "An Investigation of Therapeutic Communicator Style." In B. Ruben, ed. *Communication Yearbook 1.* New Brunswick, N.J.: Transaction-International Communication Association, 1977, 593–604.

Pettegrew, L. and Thomas, R. "Communication Style Differences In Formal Versus Informal Therapeutic Relationships." In B. Ruben, ed., *Communication Yearbook 2.* New Brunswick, N.J.: Transaction-International Communication Association, 1978, 523–37.

Phillips, G. and Metzger, N. *Intimate Com-*

munication. Boston: Allyn and Bacon, 1976.

Porter, E. *Therapeutic Counseling*. Boston: Houghton Mifflin Company, 1950.

Poser, E. "The Effect of Therapists' Training on Group Therapeutic Outcome." *Journal of Consulting Psychology* 30 (1966): 283–89.

Quinn, R. "Psychotherapists' Expressions As An Index to the Quality of Early Therapeutic Relationships Established by Representatives of the Non-Directive Alderian and Psychoanalytic Schools" In O. Mowrer, ed. *Psychotherapy Theory and Research*. New York: Ronald Press, 1953, 301.

Rappaport, J. and Chinsky, J. "Accurate Empathy: Confusion of A Construct." *Psychological Bulletin* 77 (1972): 400–04.

Reik, T. (1977): See Section B.

Reisman, J. and Yamokoski, T. "Psychotherapy and Friendship: An Analysis of The Communication of Friends." *Journal of Counseling Psychology* 21 (1974): 269–73.

Rice, L. "Therapists' Style of Participation and Case Outcome." *Journal of Consulting Psychology* 29 (1965): 155–60.

Reiff, P. *Triumph of the Therapeutic: Uses of Faith After Freud*. New York: Harper Torchbook, 1968.

Rogers, C. R. *Client-Centered Therapy*. Boston: Houghton Mifflin, 1951.

Rogers, C. R. "Empathic: An Unappreciated Way of Being." *The Counseliling Psychologist* 12 (1975): 2–10.

Rogers, C. R. *On Becoming a Person*. Boston: Houghton Mifflin, 1961.

Rogers, C. R. *On Personal Power*. New York: Delacorte Press, 1977.

Rogers, C. R. "The Interpersonal Relationship: The Core of Guidance." *Harvard Educational Review* 32 (1962): 415–29.

Rogers, C. R. "The Necessary and Sufficient Conditions of Therapeutic Personality Change." *Journal of Consulting Psychology* 21 (1957): 95–103.

Rogers, C. R., ed. *The Therapeutic Relationship and Its Impact*. Madison, Wis.: University of Wisconsin Press, 1967.

Rogers, C. R. "The Therapeutic Relationship: Recent Theory and Research."

Australian Journal of Psychology 17 (1965): 95–108.

Rose, S. et al. (1977): See Section A.

Rossiter, C. "Defining Therapeutic Communication." *Journal of Communication* 25 (1975): 127–30.

Rossiter, C. and Pearce, N. (1975): See Section A.

Ruesch, J. *Disturbed Communication*. New York: W. W. Norton and Co. Inc., 1957.

Ruesch, J. "General Theory of Communication In Psychiatry." In S. Arieti, ed. *American Handbook of Psychiatry*, Vol I. New York: Basic Books, 1959, 895–908.

Ruesch, J. *Therapeutic Communication*. New York: W. W. Norton and Co. Inc., 1961.

Ruesch, J. "The Role of Communication in Therapeutic Transactions." *Journal of Communication* 13 (1963): 132–39.

Ruesch, J. and Bateson, G. *Communication: The Social Matrix of Psychiatry*. New York: W. W. Norton and Co. Inc., 1951.

Ruesch, J. and Brodsky, C. "The Concept of Social Disability." *Archives of General Psychology* (1968): 394–403.

Satir, V. *Conjoint Family Therapy*. Palo Alto, Ca.: Science and Behavior Books, Inc., 1964.

Satir, V. *Peoplemaking*. Palo Alto, Ca.: Science and Behavior Books, 1972.

Scheflen, A. (1963): See Section C.

Scheflen, A. (1973): See Section C.

Scheflen, A. "Natural History Method in Psychotherapy: Communication Research." In L. A. Gottschalk and A. Auerback, eds. *Methods of Research in Psychotherapy*. New York: Appleton-Century-Crofts, 1966.

Scheflen, A. (1965): See Section C.

Scheflen, A. "Regressive One-to-One Relationships." *Psychiatric Quarterly* 23 (1960): 692–709.

Schmidt, L. and Strong, S. (1971): See Section B.

Searles, H. "The Effort to Drive The Other Person Crazy—An Element in the Etiology and Psychotherapy of Schizophrenia." *British Journal of Medical Psychology* 32 (1959): 1–18.

Seay, T. and Altekruse, M. (1979): See Section B.

Shands, H. (1970): See Section B.

Shapiro, A. (1964): See Section A.

Shapiro, D. "Empathy, Warmth and Genuineness in Psychotherapy." *British Journal of Social and Clinical Psychology* 8 (1969): 350–61.

Shapiro, J. et al. "Therapeutic Conditions and Disclosure Beyond the Therapeutic Encounter." *Journal of Consulting Psychology* (1969): 290–94.

Shave, D. *The Therapeutic Listener.* Huntington, N.Y.: Krieger, 1974.

Silverman, S. *Psychologic Cues in Forecasting Physical Illness.* New York: Appleton-Century-Crofts, 1970.

Simonson, N. and Bahr, S. "Self-Disclosure by the Professional and Para-Professional Therapist." *Journal of Consulting and Clinical Psychology* 42 (1972): 359–63.

Skydell, B. and Crowder, A. *Diagnostic Procedures: A Reference for Health Practitioners and a Guide for Patient Counseling* Boston: Little Brown and Co., 1975.

Sluzki, C. and Ransom, D., eds. *Double Bind: The Foundation of the Communicational Approach to the Family.* New York: Grune and Stratton, 1976.

Sluzki, C. and Veron, E. "The Double Bind As A Universal Pathogenic Situation." *Family Process* 10 (1971): 397–410.

Sluzki, C. and Veron, E. (1973): See Section B.

Sojit, C. (1969): See Section A.

Spiegal, J. "The Social Roles of Doctor and Patient in Psychoanalysis and Psychotherapy." *Psychiatry* 17 (1954): 369–76.

Spiegal, R. "Specific Problems of Communication In Psychiatric Conditions." In S. Arieti, ed. *American Handbook of Psychiatry,* Vol I. New York: Basic Books, 1959, 909–49.

Stergachis, A. (1970): See Section A.

Stotland, E. et al. *Empathy, Fantasy and Helping.* Beverly Hills, Ca.: Sage Publications, 1978.

Stratton, J. "Cross-Cultural Counseling: A Problem in Communication." *Psychiatric Forum* 5 (1975): 15–19.

Strong, S. and Dixon, D. (1971): See Section B.

Strupp, H. "The Interpersonal Relationship as a Vehicle For Therapeutic Learning." *Journal of Consulting and Clinical Psychology* 41 (1973): 113–15.

Thornton, B., et al. "Communication with Patients Regarding Pain and Anxiety." *The Dental Assistant* 51 (1982): 22–23.

Truax, C. "Effective Ingredients in Psychotherapy: An Approach to Unraveling the Patient-Therapist Interaction." In G. Stollak, et al., eds *Psychotherapy Research: Selected Readings.* Chicago: Rand McNally, 1966, 586–94.

Truax, C. "Therapist Empathy, Genuineness, and Warmth and Patient Therapeutic Outcome." *Journal of Consulting Psychology* 30 (1966): 395–401.

Truax, C. "The Meaning and Reliability of Accurate Empathy: A Rejoinder." *Psychological Bulletin* 77 (1972): 397–99.

Truax, C. and Carkhuff, R. "Client and Therapist Transparency in the Psychotherapeutic Encounter." *Journal of Counseling Psychologyg* 12 (1965): 3–9.

Truax, C. and Carkhuff, R. *Toward Effective Counseling and Psychotherapy: Training and Practice.* Chicago: Aldine Publishing Company, 1967.

Truax, C. and Mitchell, R. (1971): See Section A.

VanDerVeen, F. "Client Perception of Therapist Conditions as a Factor in Psychotherapy." In J. Hart and T. Tomlinsin, eds. *New Directions in Client-Centered Therapy.* Boston: Houghton Mifflin, 1970, 214–22.

Vaughn, D. and Burgoon, M. "Interpersonal Communication In the Therapeutic Setting: Mariah or Messiah." In G. Miller, ed. *Explorations in Interpersonal Communication.* Beverly Hills, Ca.: Sage Publications, 1974.

Watzlawick, P. and Weakland, J., eds., *The Interactional View: Studies at the Mental Research Institute, Palo Alto, 1965–1974.* New York: W. W. Norton, 1977.

Weakland, J. "Communication and Behavior: An Introduction." *American Behavioral Scientists* 10 (1967): 1–3.

Whitehorn, J. "Psychiatric Implications of the Placebo Effect." *American Journal of Psychiatry* 114 (1958): 662–64.

Williams, R. and Blanton, R. (1968): See Section B.

Wynne, L. "Communication Disorders and the Quest for Relatedness in Families of Schizophrenics." *American Journal of Psychoanalysis* 30 (1971): 100–14.

Zimmer, J. and Anderson, S. "Dimensions of Positive Regard and Empathy." *Journal of Consulting Psychology* 15 (1968): 417–26.

F. Group Communication In Health Care

Babcock, D. "An Introduction to Some Basic Concepts of TA and Its Usefulness to Nurses." *American Journal of Nursing* 76 (1976): 1153–55.

Baldwin, D. et al. *Interdisciplinary Health Care Teams In Teaching and Practice* Reno: University of Nevada/New Health Perspectives Inc. 1980.

Baldwin, D. et al. "A Study of Patient Response to Student Interdisciplinary Health Care Teams." In Baldwin et al., eds., *Interdisciplinary Health Care Teams In Teaching and Practice*. Reno: University of Nevada/New Health Perspectives Inc., 1980.

Bates, B. "Doctor and Nurse: Changing Role Relations." *New England Journal of Medicine* 194 (1970): 129–34.

Bates, B. "Nurse/Physician Teamwork." *International Nursing Review* 13 (1966): 43–54.

Bates, B. "Physician and Nurse Practitioner: Conflict and Reward." *Annals of Internal Medicine* 82 (1975): 702–06.

Ben-David, J. "The Professional Role of the Physician in Bureaucratized Medicine: A Study In Role Conflict." *Human Relations* 11 (1958): 255–57.

Bion, W. "Group Dynamics: A Re-View." *The International Journal of Psycho-Analysis* 33 (1952): 235–47.

Bloch, R. "The Nurses' Ombudsman." *American Journal of Nursing* 76 (1976): 1631–33.

Bloomfield, H. "Assertive Training in an Outpatient Group of Chronic Schizo-phrenics: A Preliminary Report." *Behavior Therapy* 4 (1973): 277–81.

Bochner, A. (1976): See Section A.

Boyer, L. et al. "A Student-Run Course In Interprofessional Relations." *Journal of Medical Education* 52 (1977): 183–89.

Braunwald, E. "Future Shock in Academic Medicine." *The New England Journal of Medicine* 19 (1972): 1031–35.

Brunetto, E. and Birk, P. "The Primary Call Nurse—The Generalist In A Structured Health Care Team." *American Journal of Public Health* 62 (1972): 785–94.

Calnan, J. and Barabas, A. (1972): See Section B.

Calnan, M. and Hanron, J. "The Team Conference." *Supervisor Nurse* 2 (1971): 83–89.

Charns, M. "Breaking The Tradition Barrier: Managing Integration In Health Care Facilities." *Health Care Management Review* 1 (1976): 55–67.

Christman, L. P. "Nurse-Physician Communications In the Hospital." *International Nursing Review* 13 (1966): 49–57.

Churchill, S. and Glasser, P. "Small Group in the Mental Hospital." In P. Glasser et al., eds. *Individual Change Through Small Groups*. New York: The Free Press, 1974.

Cooper, S. "Committees That Work." *The Journal of Nursing Administration* 3 (1973): 30–35.

Costello, D. "Communication Patterns in Family Systems." *Nursing Clinics of North America* 4 (1969): 721–29.

Dyer W. *Team Building: Issues and Alternatives*. Reading, Mass: Addison-Wesley, 1977.

Frank, L. "Interprofessional Communication," *American Journal of Public Health*. 51 (1961): 1798–1804.

Freidson, E. *Professional Dominance: The Social Structure of Medical Care*. Chicago: Aldine Publications, 1970.

Geyman, J. "Is There a Difference Between Nursing Practice and Medical Practice." *Journal of Family Practice* 5 (1977): 935–36.

Given, B. and Simmons, S. "The Interdisciplinary Health Care Team." *Nursing Forum* 16 (1977): 165–84.

Grissenger, S. et al. (1973): See Section A.

Hayes, S. and Patterson, M. "Interaction Between Students in Multidisciplinary Health Teams." *Journal of Medical Education* 50 (1975): 473–75.

Holton, S. "The Woman Physician: A Study of Role Conflict." *Journal of American Medical Women's Association* 24 (1969): 638–45.

House, R. "Role Conflict and Multiple Authority in a Complex Organizations." *California Management Review* 12 (1970): 53–60.

Johnson, T. *Professions and Power.* London: MacMillan, 1972.

Katz, E. et al. (1969): See Section A.

Kindig, D. (1975): See Section A.

Kosa, J. (1970): See Section A.

Kubala S. and Clever, L. "Acceptance of the Nurse Practitioner." *American Journal of Nursing Research* 74 (1974): 451–52.

Lashoff, J. "The Health Care Team in the Mile Square Arena, Chicago." *Bulletin New York Academy of Medicine* 444 (1968): 1363–69.

Levin, P. and Berne, E. "Games Nurses Play." *American Journal of Nursing* 72 (1972): 483–87.

Long, A. and Atkins, J. "Communication Between General Practitioners and Consultants." *British Medical Journal* (1974): 456–59.

Loomis, M. *Group Process for Nurses* St. Louis: C. V. Mosby Company, 1979.

MacDonald, M. et al. "Social Skills Training: The Effects of Behavior Rehearsal In Groups in Dating Skills." *Journal of Counseling Psychology* 22 (1975): 224–30.

Nagi, S., "Teamwork In Health Care In the United States: A Sociological Perspective." In *The Milbank Quarterly.* New York: Health and Society Press, 1975.

Pratt, H. "The Doctor's View of the Nurse-Physician Relationship." *Journal of Medical Education* 40 (1965): 767–71.

"Psychiatry By Teamwork." *Frontiers of Psychiatry* 12 (1982): 1–13.

Purtilo, R. (1973): See Section A.

Riley, A. and Martin, B. "We Took the

Strain Out of Nursing and Lab Relations." *RN* 38 (1975): 45–46.

Rockoff, M. "Interactions Between Medical Students and Nursing Personnel." *Journal of Medical Education* 48 (1973): 725–31.

Rogers, E. (1973): See Section A.

Schaefer, J. "The Interrelatedness of Decision Making and The Nursing Process." *American Journal of Nursing* 74 (1974): 1852–55.

Seward, J. "Role of the Nurse: Perceptions of Nursing Students and Auxiliary Nursing Personnel." *Nursing Research* 18 (1969): 164–69.

Slocum, J. et al. "An Analysis of Need Satisfaction and Job Performance Among Professional and Paraprofessional Hospital Personnel." *Nursing Research* 21 (1972): 338–41.

Stephens, L. "Staff Communications on the Medical and Surgical Services: A Research Note." *Journal of Health and Social Behavior* 8 (1967): 148–53.

Talland, G. and Clark, D. "Evaluation of Topics in Therapy Group Discussion." *Journal of Clinical Psychology* 10 (1954): 131–37.

Thornton, B. "Health Care Teams and Multimethodological Research." In B. Ruben, ed. *Communication Yearbook 2.* New Brunswick, N.J.: Transaction-International Communication Association, 1978, 538–53.

Thornton, B., et al. "Interaction on Health Care Teams." In Baldwin, et al., eds., *Interdisciplinary Health Care Teams in Teaching and Practice.* Reno, Nevada: University of Nevada/New Health Perspectives, Inc., 1980a.

Thornton, B., et al. "Role Relationships On Interdisciplinary Health Care Teams." In Baldwin, et al., eds., *Interdisciplinary Health Care Teams In Teaching and Practice.* Reno, Nevada: University of Nevada/New Health Perspectives, Inc., 1980b.

Thornton, B., et al. "The Team Approach To Research On Interdisciplinary Health Care Teams." In Baldwin, et al., eds., *Interdisciplinary Health Care Teams In Teaching and Practice.* Reno,

Nevada: University of Nevada/New Health Perspectives, Inc., 1980c.

Valadez, A. and Anderson, E. "Rehabilitation Workshops, Change in Attitudes of Nurses." *Nursing Research* 21 (1972): 132–37.

Wagner, M. (1968): See Section B.

Wagner, M. "Reinforcement of the Expression of Anger Through Role-Planning." *Behavior Research and Therapy* 6 (1968): 91–94.

Watson, W. (1975): See Section B.

Wessen, A. "Hospital Ideology and Communication Between Ward Personnel." In E. Jaco, ed. *Patients, Physicians and Illness* Glencoe, Ill: Free Press, 1958.

Wise, H. et al. *Making Health Teams Work.* Cambridge, Mass: Ballinger, 1974.

Wise, H. "The Primary Care Health Team." *Archives of Internal Medicine* 130 (1972): 438–44.

Wynne, L. (1971): See Section E.

Yanda, R. *Doctors as Managers of Health Care Teams.* New York: AMACOM, 1977.

Zola, I. (1963): See Section A.

Zuk, G. et al. (1963): See Section C.

G. Conflict in Health Care

Antley, M. and Antley, R. "Obsolescence: The Physician or the Diagnostician Role." *Journal of Medical Education* 47 (1972): 737–38.

Arndt, C. and Laeger, E. "Role Strain In a Diversified Role Set, Parts I and II." *Nursing Research* 19 (1970): 253–59, 495–501.

Bates, B. (1975): See Section F.

Bates, E. and Moore, B. "Stress in Hospital Personnel." *The Medical Journal of Australia.* 2 (1975): 765–67.

Beecher, H. (1956): See Section A.

Beisser, A. and Glasser, N. (1968): See Section A.

Berenson, B. and Mitchell, K. (1968): See Section E.

Bishop, R. "Anxiety and Readership of Health Information." *Journalism Quarterly* 51 (1974): 40–46

Bloch, R. (1976): See Section F.

Bloomfield, H. (1973): See Section F.

Bloor, M. and Horobin, G. (1975): See Section A.

Bothamy, V. (1975): See Section A.

Bowman, R., and Culpepper, R. "Power for Change." *American Journal of Nursing* 74 (1974): 1054–56.

Dodge, D. and Martin, W. *Social Stress and Illness.* Notre Dame, Ind.: University of Notre Dame Press, 1970.

Holton, S. (1969): See Section F.

Koestenbaum, P. *Managing Anxiety.* Englewood Cliffs, N.J.: Prentice-Hall, 1974.

Kosa, J. and Coker, R. "The Female Physician in Public Health: Conflict and Reconciliation of the Sex and Professional Roles." *Sociology and Social Research* 49 (1965): 294–305.

Lazarus, R. *Psychological Stress and the Coping Process.* New York: McGraw Hill, 1966.

Margolis, B. et al. "Job Stress: An Unlisted Occupational Hazard." *Journal of Occupational Medicine* 16 (1974): 659–61.

McCroskey, J. "Measures of Communication Bound Anxiety." *Speech Monographs* 37 (1970): 269–77.

Mendelsohn, J. and Berklehamer, J. "Bridging One Gap Between Doctor and Patient: The Role of the Patient Advocate." *Clinical Pediatrics* 13 (1974): 1017–18.

Meyer, M. "The Effect of Types of Communication of Patients' Reaction to Stress." *Nursing Research* 13 (1964): 126–31.

Pettegrew, L. et al. "Job Related Stress In a Medical Center Organization: Management of Communication Issues." In D. Nimmo, ed., *Communication Yearbook 4.* New Brunswick, N.J.: Transaction-International Communication Association, 1980, 626–52.

Ravich, R. et al. "Hospital Ombudsman Smooths the Flow of Services and Communication." *Journal of American Medical Association* 43 (1969): 150–66.

Riley, A. and Martin, B. (1975): See Section F.

Skipper, J. and Leonard, R. "Children, Stress and Hospitalization: A Field Experiment." *Journal of Health and*

Social Behavior 9 (1968): 275–87.

Valadez, A. and Anderson, E. (1972): See Section F.

Wagner, M. (1968): See Section F.

H. Intercultural Communication in Health Care

Aletky, P. et al. "Sex Differences and Placebo Effects: Motivation as an Intervening Variable." *Journal of Consulting and Clinical Psychology* 43 (1975): 278.

Anderson, O. *Health Care: Can There Be Equity? The United States, Sweden, and England.* New York: Wiley, 1972.

Antley, M. and Antley, R. (1972): See Section G.

Apostle, D. and Oder, F. "Factors That Influence the Public's View of Medical Care." *Journal of the American Medical Association* 202 (1967): 592–98.

Arndt, C. and Laeger, E. (1970): See Section G.

Atkyns, R. et al. "Sources of Drug Information Among Adults." *Journal of Drug Education* 5 (1975): 161–69.

Barach, A. (1962): See Section A.

Bates, B. (1970): See Section F.

Bates, B. (1966): See Section F.

Bates, B. (1975): See Section F.

Becker, H. *Outsiders: Studies in the Sociology of Deviance.* New York: The Free Press, 1963.

Becker, M. (1974a): See Section A.

Becker, M. (1974b): See Section A.

Becker, M. et al. (1977): See Section A.

Becker, M. and Maiman, L. (1975): See Section A.

Beckman, B. "Life Stress and Psychological Well-Being." *Journal of Health and Social Behavior* 12 (1971): 35–45.

Beecher, H. (1956): See Section A.

Ben-Sira, Z. (1977): See Section E.

Bienvenu, M. (1970): See Section A.

Blackwell, B. (1967): See Section A.

Bloom, S. (1975): See Section A.

Bond, M. "Psychological and Psychiatric Aspects of Pain." *Anaesthesia* 33 (1978): 355–61.

Bowden, C. and Burstein, A. (1974): See Section A.

Boyer, L. et al. (1977): See Section F.

Brinton, D. "Value Differences Between Nurses and Low-Income Families." *Nursing Research* 21 (1972): 46–52.

Brodie, D. et al. (1973): See Section A.

Brownlee, A. *Community, Culture, and Care: A Cross Cultural Guide For Health Workers.* St. Louis: C.V. Mosby Company, 1978.

Bullough, B. "Poverty, Ethnic Identity and Preventive Health Care." *Journal of Health and Social Behavior* 13 (1974): 347–59.

Chamberlin, R. and Rodenbaugh, J. "Delivery of Primary Health Care: Union Style." *New England Journal of Medicine* 294 (1976): 641–45.

Charns, M. (1976): See Section F.

Chen, P. "Medical Systems in Malaysia: Cultural Bases and Differential Use." *Social Science and Medicine* 9 (1975): 171–80.

Chesler, P. *Women and Madness.* New York: Avon Books, 1972.

Christman, L. P. (1966): See Section F.

Colm, H. (1953): See Section E.

Cooley, C. *Social Aspects of Illness.* Philadelphia: W. B. Saunders, 1951.

Coombs, R. and Vincent, C., eds. *Psychosocial Aspects of Medical Training.* Springfield, Ill.: Charles C. Thomas, 1971.

Corea, G. *The Hidden Malpractice: How American Medicine Treats Women as Patients and Professionals.* New York: William Morrow, 1977.

Cousins, N. (1979): See Section A.

Cox, C. and Mead, A. *A Sociology of Medicine Practice.* London: Collier-MacMillian, 1975.

Crane, A. "The Social Potential of the Patient: An Alternative to the Sick Role." *Journal of Communication* 25 (1975): 131–39.

Dodge, J. "Nurses' Sense of Adequacy and Attitudes Toward Keeping Patients Informed. *Journal of Health and Human Behavior* 2 (1961): 213.

Dubos, R. (1969): See Section A.

Dubos, R. (1971): See Section A.

Duff, R. and Hollingshead, A. *Sickness and Society.* New York: Harper and Row, 1968.

Ehrlich, H. and Bauer, M. (1967): See Section E.

Eisler, J. et al. "Relationship Between Need for Social Approval and Post Operative Recovery and Welfare." *Nursing Research* 21 (1972): 520–25.

Endler, N. (1965): See Section B.

Enelow, A. and Adler, L. "Diseases of the Nervous System: An Instrument for Studying Role-Perception in Physicians." *A practical Journal on Psychiatry and Neurology* 16 (1965): 4.

Enelow, A. and Adler, L. "An Instrument for Studying Role-Perception in Physicians." *Modern Hospital* 118 (1972): 68–71.

Fabrega, H. *Disease and Social Behavior: An Interdisciplinary Perspective.* Cambridge, Mass.: MIT, 1974.

Farquaar, J. and Maccoby, N. "Community Education for Cardio-Vascular Health." *The Lancet*, June 4 (1977): 1192–94.

Fejer, D. et al. "Sources of Information About Drugs Among High School Students." *Public Opinion Quarterly* 35 (1971) 235–41.

Fish, D. (1971): See Section A.

Freimuth, V. and Jamieson, K. *Communicating with the Elderly: Shattering Stereotypes.* Urbana, Ill.: ERIC/SCA, 1979.

Glittenberg, J. "Adapting Health Care to a Cultural Setting." *American Journal of Nursing* 74 (1974): 2218–21.

Gochman, D. (1972a): See Section A.

Gochman, D. (1972b): See Section A.

Gochman, D. "Preventative Encounters and Their Psychological Correlates." *American Journal of Public Health* 64 (1974): 1096–98.

Goffman, E. *Asylums: Essays on the Social Situations of Mental Patients and Other Inmates.* New York: Doubleday-Anchor, 1961.

Goffman, E. (1955): See Section C.

Goffman, E. *Stigma: Notes on the Management of Spoiled Identity.* Englewood Cliffs, N.J.: Spectrum, 1963.

Goffman, E. (1960): See Section B.

Goosey, R. "Communications In Health Education and The Asian in the U.K." *Journal of Human Nutrition* 31 (1977): 249–50.

Gouldner, A. "The Norm of Reciprocity: A Preliminary Statement." *American Sociological Review* 25 (1960): 161–78.

Green, L. "The Health Belief Model and Personal Health Behavior: Editorial." *Health Education Monographs* 2 (1974): 324–25.

Haefner, D. "The Health Belief Model and Preventative Dental Behavior." *Health Education Monographs* 2 (1974): 421–31.

Haney, C. "Illness Behavior and Psychosocial Correlates of Cancer." *Social Science and Medicine* 11 (1977): 223–28.

Hanneman, G. "Communicating Drug-Abuse Information Among College Students." *Public Opinion Quarterly* 37 (1973): 171–91.

Hanson, R. "Communicating Health Arguments Across Cultures." *Nursing Research* 12 (1963): 237–41.

Henderson, L. "Physician and Patient as a Social System." *New England Journal of Medicine* 212 (1935): 819–23.

Henry, J. *Pathways to Madness.* New York: Random House, 1971.

Holton, S. (1969): See Section F.

Hoppe, S. and Heller, P. "Alienation, Familism, and the Utilization of Health Services by Mexican-Americans." *Journal of Health and Social Behavior* 16 (1975): 304–14.

House, R. (1970): See Section F.

Hulka, B. et al. "Satisfaction with Medical Care In a Low Income Population." *Journal of Chronic Diseases* 24 (1971): 661.

Isguith, R. "Health-Related Services Audiovisual Aids for Spanish-Speaking Audiences." *Health Services Reports* 89 (1974): 188–202.

Jaco, E. "Medical Care: Its Social and Organizational Aspects." *New England Journal of Medicine* 269 (1963): 18–22.

Jaco, E. *Patients, Physicians, and Illnesses.* New York: The Free Press, 1972.

Jain, H. *Understanding Intercultural Communication.* Belmont, Ca.: Wadsworth Publishing Co, 1981.

Johnson, J. (1972): See Section A.

Johnson, T. (1972): See Section F.

Kaiser, B. and Kaiser, I. "The Challenge of the Women's Movement to American

Gynocology." *American Journal of Obstetrics and Gynocology* 120 (1974): 652–65.

Kasl, S. "The Health Belief Model and Behavior Related to Chronic Illness." *Health Education Monographs* 2 (1974): 433–53.

Kasl, S. and Cobb, S. "Health Behavior, Illness Behavior and Sick Role Behavior." *Archives of Environmental Health* 12 (1966): 246–66, 531–41.

King, S. *Perception of Illness and Medical Practice.* New York: Russell Sage, 1962.

Kirscht, J. "Public Response to Various Written Appeals to Participants in Health Screening The Health Belief Model and Illness Behavior." *Health Education Monographs* 2 (1974): 387–408.

Kirscht, J. et al. "Psychological and Social Factors as Predictors of Medical Behavior. *Medical Care* 14 (1976): 422–31.

Kirscht, J. "Research Related to the Modification of Health Beliefs." *Health Education Monographs* 2 (1974): 455–69.

Kleinman, A. et al. "Culture, Illness, and Care: Clinical Lessons From Anthropological and Cross-cultural Research." *Annual of International Medicine* 88 (1978): 251–58.

Knowles, J., ed. (1977): See Section A.

Knutson, A. *The Individual, Society, and Health Behavior.* New York: Russell Sage Foundation, 1965.

Kosa, J. et al. *Poverty and Health: A Sociological Analysis.* Cambridge, Mass.: Harvard University Press, 1969.

Kosa, J. and Coker, R. (1965): See Section G.

Kreps, G. "Health Communication and Aging: An Overview." Paper presented to the International Communication Association conference, Dallas, 1983.

Kreps, G. "Communication and Gerontology: Health Communication Education for Providers of Health Care to the Elderly." *Resources in Education* 17 (May 1982), ERIC # ED 209–702.

Kreps, G. "Humanizing Organizational Communication for Elderly Health Care Recipients." Paper presented to

the SCA conference, Louisville, Kentucky, 1982.

LaFargue, J. "Role of Prejudice in Rejection of Health Care." *Nursing Research* 21 (1972): 53–58.

Lambert, E. (1978): See Section A.

Langlois, P. "Helping Patients Cope With Hospitalization." *Nursing Outlook* 19 (1971): 334–36.

Larson, C. et al. "Staff-Resident Communication in Nursing Homes: A Factor Analysis of Staff Attitudes and Resident Evaluations of Staff." *Journal of Communication* 19 (1969): 308–16.

Lazare, A. et al. "The Customer Approach to Patienthood." *Archives of General Psychiatry* 32 (1975): 553–58.

Lederer, H. "How the Sick View Their World." *Journal of Social Issues* 8 (1952): 4–15.

Lennane, K. and Lennane, R. "Alleged Psychogenic Disorders In Women—A Possible Manifestation of Sexual Prejudice." *New England Journal of Medicine* 288 (1973): 288–92.

Lesser, M. (1974): See Section E.

Levine, C. "Doctor-Patient Communication With the Inner-City Adolescent." *The New England Journal of Medicine* 9 (1968): 494–95.

Levine, S. et al. "Community Interorganizational Problems In Providing Medical Care and Social Services." *American Journal of Public Health* 53 (1963): 1183–95.

Lewis, A. "Health As A Social Concept." *Journal of American Medical Association* 85 (1969): 109–24.

Long, A. and Atkins, J. (1974): See Section F.

Lynch, L., ed. *The Cross-Cultural Approach to Health Behavior.* Rutherford: N.J.: Fairleigh Dickinson University Press, 1969.

Magee, J. "The Pelvic Examination: A View from the Other End of the Table." *Annals of Internal Medicine* 83 (1975): 563–64.

Maiman, L. and Becker, M. "The Health Belief Model: Origins and Correlates in Psychological Theory." *Health Education Monographs* 2 (1974): 336–53.

Maltz, M. (1973): See Section B.

Martiney, C. "Community Mental Health and the Chicano Movement." *American Journal of Public Health* 43 (1973): 595–601.

Martiney, R. *Hispanic Culture and Health Care—Fact, Fiction and Folklore.* St. Louis: C. V. Mosby Co., 1978.

Maslow, A. *Motivation and Personality.* New York: Harper and Row, 1954.

Matarazzo, J. and Wiens, A. (1967): See Section B.

McClain, C. "Adaptation in Health Behavior: Modern and Traditional Medicine in a West Mexican Community." *Social Science and Medicine* 11 (1977): 341–47.

McIntosh, J. (1974): See Section A.

McKinley, J. "The Help-Seeking Behavior of the Poor." In J. Kosa and I. Zola, eds. *Poverty and Health—A Sociological Analysis.* Cambridge, Ma.: Harvard University Press, 1975.

McKinley, J. "Who is Really Ignorant—Physician or Patient? *Journal of Health and Social Behavior* 16 (1975): 3–11.

McLamb, J. and Huntley, R. "The Hazards of Hospitalization." *Southern Medical Journal* 60 (1967): 469–72.

Meador, C. "The Art and Science of Non-disease." *New England Journal of Medicine* 272 (1965): 92–95.

Mechanic, D. "The Influences of Mothers on the Children's Health Attitudes and Behavior." *Pediatrics* 33 (1964): 444.

Mechanic, D. *Medical Sociology.* New York: The Free Press, 1968.

Mechanic, D. *Public Expectations and Health Care: Essays on the Changing Organizations of Health Services.* New York: Wiley, 1972a.

Mechanic, D. (1966): See Section A.

Mechanic, D. "Social Psychologic Factors Affecting the Presentation of Bodily Complaints." *New England Journal of Medicine* 286 (1972B): 1132–36.

Mechanic, D. "The Sociology of Medicine: Viewpoints and Perspectives." *Journal of Health and Human Behavior* 7 (1966): 237–48.

Mechanic, D. and Volkhart, E. "Illness Behavior and Medical Diagnosis." *Journal of Health and Human Behavior* 1 (1960): 86–94.

Melzack, R. "The Perception of Pain." *Scientific American* 264 (1961): 41–49.

Mendelson, M. *Tender Loving Greed.* New York: Vintage Books, 1975.

Metsch, J. and Veney, J. "Consumer Participation and Social Accountability." *Medical Care* 14 (1976): 283–93.

Moore, B. (1974): See Section E.

Moss, G. *Illness, Immunity and Social Interaction.* New York: Wiley, 1973.

Mumford, E. and Skipper, J. *Sociology in Hospital Care.* New York: Harper & Row, 1967.

Myerhoff, B. and Larson, W. "The Doctor as Cultural Hero: The Routinization of Charisma." *Human Organization* 24 (1965): 188–91.

Nall, F. and Speilberg, J. "Social and Cultural Factors in the Response of Mexican-Americans to Medical Treatment." In R. Martney, ed. *Hispanic Culture and Health Care.* St. Louis: C. V. Mosby Co., 1978.

Nelson, B. (1973): See Section A.

Osfsky, H. "Some Socialpsychologic Issues in Improving Obstetric Care For the Poor." *Obstetrics and Gynecology* 31 (1968): 437–43.

Pederson, P. et al. (1976): See Section E.

Pegels, C. Health Care and the Elderly. Rockville Md.: Aspen Systems Corporation, 1980.

Pelletier, K. *Mind as Healer, Mind as Slayer: A Holistic Approach to Preventing Stress Disorders.* New York: Delacorte, 1977.

Peterson, J. (1973): See Section A.

Plaja, A. et al. "Communication Between Physicians and Patients in Outpatient Clinics: Social and Cultural Factors." *Milbank Memorial Fund Quarterly* 46 (1968): 161–213.

Pollack, S. "Changes in Attitudes of Medical Students Toward Psychological Aspects of the Doctor-Image and the Doctor-Patient Relationship." *Journal of Medical Education* 40 (1965): 1162–65.

Powers, L. et al. "Practice Pattern of

Women and Men Physicians." *Journal of Medical Education* 44 (1969): 481–91.

Pratt, H. (1965): See Section F.

Pratt, L. et al. (1957): See Section A.

Prior, J. "Some Aspects of the Clinical Communication of Pain." *Journal of American Medical Women's Association* 22 (1967): 725–31.

Quesada, G. and Heller, R. "Sociolcultural Barriers to Medical Care Among Mexican-Americans in Texas." *Medical Care* 15 (1977): 93–101.

Reading, A. "Illness and Disease." *Medical Clinics of North America* 61 (1977): 703–10.

Reeder, L. (1972): See Section A.

Rioch, D. (1963): See Section A.

Robinson, D. *The Process of Becoming Ill.* London: Routledge, 1971.

Roemer, M. and Elling, R. "Sociological Research on Medical Care." *Journal of Health and Human Behavior* 4 (1963): 49–68.

Rosen, R. "Occupational Role Innovators and Sex Role Attitudes." *Journal of Medical Education* 49 (1974): 554–61.

Rosenblatt, D. and Suchman, E. "Awareness of Physician's Social Status Within An Urban Community." *Journal of Health and Human Behavior* 7 (1966): 146–53.

Rosenstock, I. "The Health Belief Model and Preventive Health Behavior." *Health Education Monographs* 2 (1974): 354–85.

Rosenstock, I. "What Research in Motivation Suggests for Public Health." *American Journal of Public Health* 50 (1960): 295–302.

Roth, J. "Ritual and Magic in the Control of Contagion." *American Sociological Review* 23 (1957): 311–12.

Ruhly, S. *Orientation to Intercultural Communication.* Chicago: Science Research Associates, 1976.

Ruig, P. "Culture and Mental Health: A Hispanic Perspective." *Journal of Contemporary Psychotherapy* 9 (1977): 241–27.

Samovar, L. et al., *Understanding Intercultural Communication.* Belmot, Ca.: Wadsworth Publishing Co., 1981.

Scheifelbein, A. "The Female Patient: Heeded? Hustled? Healed?" *Saturday Review* (1980): 12–16.

Scott, C. "Health and Healing Practices Among Five Ethnic Groups in Miami, Florida." *Public Health Reports* 89 (1974): 524–32.

Scully, D. and Bart, P. "A Funny Thing Happened on the Way to the Orifice: Women in Gynecology Textbooks." *American Journal of Sociology* 78 (1973): 1045–1050.

Seagull, A. "Sociocultural Variation in Sick Role Behavioral Expectations." *Social Science and Medicine* 10 (1976): 47–51.

Seibold, D. and Roper, R. "Psychosocial Determinants of Health Care Intentions: Test of the Triandis and Fishbein Models." In D. Nimmo, ed., *Communication Yearbook 3.* New Brunswick, N.J.: Transaction-International Communication Association, 1979, 626–43.

Seward, J. (1969): See Section F.

Shader, R. and Levine, F. "Technical Reports: Staff–Patient Interaction Patterns and Opinions about Mental Illness." *Social Science and Medicine* 3 (1969): 101–03.

Simmons, L. and Wolff, H. *Social Science In Medicine.* New York: Russell Sage Foundation, 1954.

Simonton, O. and Matthews-Simonton, S. "Belief Systems and Management of the Emotional Aspects of Malignancy." *Journal of Transpersonal Psychology* 7 (1975): 29–47.

Sitaram, K. and Cogdell, R. *Foundations of Intercultural Communication.* Columbus, Oh.: Charles E. Merrill Publishing, 1976.

Skipper, J. and Leonard, R. (1968): See Section G.

Skipper, J. et al. "Some Barriers Between Patients and Hospital Functionaires." *Nursing Forum* 2 (1963): 14–23.

Skipper, J. et al. "Some Possible Consequences of Limited Communication Between Patients and Hospital Functionaries." *Journal of Health and Human Behavior* 5 (1964): 34–39.

Snow, F. "Folk Medical Beliefs and Their Implications for the Care of Patients." *Annals of Internal Medicine* 81 (1974): 82–91.

Spiegel, J. (1954): See Section E.

Stimson, G. (1974): See Section A.

Stratton, J. (1975): See Section E.

Sue, D. and Sue, D. "Barriers to Effective Cross-Cultural Counseling." *Journal of Counseling Psychology* 24 (1977): 420–29.

Tabery, J. et al. "Attitude Research for Intercultural Communication and Interaction." *Journal of Communication* 20 (1976): 180–200.

Tagliacozzo, D. and Mauksch, H. "The Patient's View of the Patient's Role." In E. Gartley Jaco, ed. *Patients, Physicians and Illness*, 2nd ed. New York: The Free Press, 1972.

Taylor, C. and Leslie, C. "Asian Medical Systems: A Symposium on the Role of Comparative Sociology in Improving Health Care." *Social Science and Medicine* 7 (1973) 307–18.

Twaddle, A. "The Concepts of the Sick Role and Illness Behavior." *Advances in Psychosomatic Medicine* 8 (1972): 162–79.

Welford, W. (1975): See Section A.

Wessen, A. (1958): See Section F.

White, E. "Health and the Black Person: An Annotated Bibliography." *American Journal of Nursing* 74 (1974): 1839–41.

Williams, J. et al. "The Teaching of Behavioral Sciences in the Family Medicine Residency Programs in Canada and in the U.S." *Social Science and Medicine* 8 (1974): 565–74.

Wilson, R. *The Sociology of Health.* New York: Random House, 1970.

Wolf, S. and Godell, H. *Behavioural Science in Clinical Medicine.* Springfield, Ill: Charles C. Thomas, 1976.

Zola, I. "Culture and Symptoms—An Analysis of Patients' Presenting Complaints." *American Sociological Review* 31 (1966): 615–30.

J. Communication In Health Care Organizations

Alpert, J. (1964): See Section A.

Ambuel, J. et al. (1964): See Section A.

Anderson, O. (1972): See Section H.

Anonymous. (1976): See Section A.

Apostle, D. and Oder, F. (1967): See Section H.

Bartlett, M. et al. "Access Library-Patient Information Service: An Experiment in Health Education." *New England Journal of Medicine* 288 (1973): 994.

Bates, E. and Moore, B. (1975): See Section G.

Beecher, H. (1961): See Section A.

Ben-David, J. "The Professional Role of the Physician in Bureaucratized Medicine: A Study In Role Conflict." *Human Relations* 11 (1958): 255–257.

Bloch, R. (1976): See Section F.

Bowers, W. (1960): See Section A.

Braunwald, E. (1972): See Section F.

Brunetto, E. and Birk, P. (1972): See Section F.

Burke, R. et al. (1976): See Section E.

Caplan, E. and Sassman, M. "Rank Order or Important Variables for Patient and Staff Satisfaction With Outpatient Service." *Journal of Health and Human Behavior* 7 (1966): 133–37.

Carlson, R. *The End of Medicine.* New York: Wiley Interscience, 1975.

Cartwright, A. (1964): See Section A.

Casella, C. *Training Exercises to Improve Interpersonal Relations In Health Care Organizations.* Greenvale, N.Y.: Panel Publishers, 1978.

Cavalier, R. "Ombudsman is Middle Man Between Clinic Patient and Hospital." *Modern Hospital* 116 (1970): 92–86.

Chamberlin, R. and Rodenbaugh, J. (1976): See Section H.

Charns, M. (1976): See Section F.

Chisani, F. et al. *The Consumers' Guide to Health Care.* Boston: Little, Brown and Company, 1976.

Churchill, S. and Glasser, P. (1974): See Section F.

Cohen, M. "Medication Error Reports." *Hospital Pharmacy* 10 (1975): 166.

Coleman, J. et al. *Medical Innovation: A Diffusion Study.* New York: Bobbs-Merrill, 1966.

Crosby, E. "Physician's Place in Health Care Administration." *Hospitals* 42 (1968): 47–49, 121.

Cruikshank, N. "The Public's Expectations in Changing Health Care Programs." *Journal of Medical Education* 42 (1972): 69–71.

Cumming, J. (1960): See Section A.

Cummins, A. and Dahl, R. (1972): See Section H.

Cunningham, R. *Hospitals, Doctors, and Dollars.* New York: F.W. Dodge Corp., 1960.

Falick, J. "Departments That Work Together Should Be Planned Together." *Modern Hospital* 116 (1970): 99–104.

Friedson, E. "The Development of Administrative Accountability in Health Services." *American Behavioral Scientist* 19 (1976): 286–98.

Fuchs, V. (1974): See Section A.

Georgopoulos, B., ed. *Organization Research on Health Institutions.* Ann Arbor, Mich.: Institute for Social Research, 1974.

Georgopoulos, B. *Hospital Organization Research: Review and Source Book.* Philadelphia: W.B. Saunders Company, 1975.

Georgopoulos, B. and Mann, F. *The Community General Hospital.* New York: MacMillan, 1962.

Goffman, E. (1961): See Section H.

Gordon, P. "The Top Management Triangle In Voluntary Hospitals, II." *Journal of the Academy of Management* 5 (1962): 66–75.

Goss, M. (1961): See Section A.

Goss, M. "Organizational Goal and Quality of Medical Care: Evidence from Comparative Research on Hospitals." *Journal of Health and Social Behavior* 11 (1970): 255–68.

Hall, B. (1964): See Section A.

Holland, T. "Organizational Structure and Institutional Care." *Journal of Health and Social Behavior* 14 (1973): 241–51.

Holloway, R. "Management Can Reverse Declining Employee Work Attitudes." *Hospitals* 50 (1976): 71–77.

House, R. (1970): See Section F.

Hsieh, R. "Evaluation of Formal Communications Systems In a Hospital." *Health Services Research* 1 (1966): 222–56.

Hunt, R. (1974): See Section E.

Illich, I. *Medical Nemesis.* New York: Random House, 1976.

Jaco, E. (1963): See Section H.

Jain, H. "Supervisory Communication Effectiveness and Performance in Two Urban Hospitals." *Personnel Journal* 50 (1971): 392–95.

Jelinek, R. et al. "Tell the Computer How Sick the Patients Are, And It Will Tell You How Many Nurses They Need." *Modern Hospital* 1, 119 (1973): 81–85.

Katz, E. et al. (1969): See Section A.

Knowles, J. "The Hospital." *Scientific American* 229 (1973): 128–37.

Kraegel, J. et al. *Patient Care Systems.* Philadelphia: J.B. Lippincott, 1974.

Kreps, G. "Organizational Reflexivity: Applying Interpretive Organizational Communication Research to Nurse Retention in an Urban Hospital," paper presented to the SCA/ICA Conference on Interpretive Approaches to Organizational Research, Alta, Utah, 1982.

Kreps, G. "Humanizing Organizational Communication for Elderly Health Care Recipients," paper presented to the Speech Communication Association Conference, Louisville, Kentucky, 1982.

Lambert, E. (1978): See Section A.

Lander, L. (1978): See Section A.

Langlois, P. (1971): See Section H.

Larson, C. et al. (1969): See Section H.

Levin, P. and Berne, E. (1972): See Section F.

Levine, S. et al. (1963): See Section H.

McLamb, J. and Huntley, R. (1967): See Section H.

McNamera, E (1976): See Section E.

Mechanic, E. *The Growth of Bureaucratic Medicine: An Inquiry Into the Dynamics of Patient Behavior and the Organization of Medical Care.* New York: Wiley, 1976.

Mechanic D. (1972): See Section H.

Mendelsohn, J. and Berklehamer, J. (1974): See Section G.

Mendelsohn, R. (1979): See Section A.

Metzagor, N. *Personnel Administration in the Health Services Industry.* New York:

Spectrum Publications, 1975.

Mitchell, W. "Communication and Organization." *Nursing Times* 72 (1976): 709–10.

Myers, R. "Organize the Medical Staff to Perform Functions, Not to Fill Committees." *Modern Hospital* (1969): 88–90.

Pellegrino, E. (1966): See Section A.

Perrow, C. "Hospitals, Technology, Structure and Goals." In J. March, ed. *Handbook of Organizations*. Chicago: Rand McNally, 1965.

Pfeffer, J. "Size, Composition and Function of Hospital Boards of Directors: A Study of Organization-Environment Linkage." *Administrative Science Quarterly* 18 (1973): 449–61.

Pfeffer, J. and Salancik, G. "Organizational Context and the Characteristics and Tenure of Hospital Administrators." *Academy of Management Journal* 20 (177): 74–88.

Plachy, R. "You Theory X, Me Theory Y!" *Modern Hospital* (1973): 73–78.

Portis, B. and Hunter, A. "In-Service Training By Mass Media." *Journal of Communication* 25 (1975): 167–70.

Quint, J. (1966): See Section A.

Quint, J. (1965): See Section B.

Ravich, R. et al. (1969): See Section G.

Reinhardt, V. "Proposed Changes in the Organization of Health Care Delivery: An Overview and Critique." *Milbank Memorial Fund Quarterly* 51 (1973): 169–222.

Revans, R. "Hospital Internal Communication." *Nursing Times* 64 (1966a): 41–44.

Revans, R. "Research Into Hospital Management and Organization." *Milbank Memorial Fund Quarterly* 44 (1966b): 207–48.

Revans, R. *Standards for Morale: Cause and Effect In Hospitals*. London: Oxford University Press, 1964.

Rosen, R. (1974): See Section H.

Rosen, S. and Tesser, A. "On Reluctance to Communicate Undesirable Information: The MUM Effect." *Sociometry* 33 (1970): 253–63.

Rosenblatt, D. and Suchman, E. (1966): See Section H.

Schaefer, J. (1974): See Section F.

Schimmel, E. (1964): See Section A.

Schlesinger, R. et al. (1962): See Section A.

Schulz, R. and Johnson, A. *Management of Hospitals*. New York: Council on Social Work Education, 1971.

Schultz, R. and Johnson, A. "Conflict in Hospitals." *Hospital Administration* 16 (1971): 36–50.

Schwartz, H. *The Case for American Medicine: A Realistic Look at Our Health Care System*. New York: McKay, 1972.

Seeman, M. and Evans, J. "Alienation and Learning in a Hospital Setting." *American Sociological Review* 27 (1962): 772–82.

Shenkin, B. and Warner, D. (1975): See Section A.

Skipper, J. and Ellison, M. "Personal Contact As a Technique for Increasing Questionnaire Returns From Hospitalized Patients After Discharge." *Journal of Health and Human Behavior* 7 (1966): 211–14.

Skipper, J. et al. (1963): See Section H.

Skipper, J. et al. (1964): See Section H.

Slocum, J. et al. (1972): See Section F.

Smith, R. "Bridging the Management-Employee Gap." *Health Care Management Review* 1 (1976): 7–11.

Spelman, M. et al. (1966): See Section A.

Stephens, L. (1967): See Section F.

Sterling, T. et al. "The Use of an Information System to 'Humanize' Procedures in Rehabilitation Hospital." *International Journal of Bio-Medical Computing* 5 (1973): 51–57.

Tannon, C. and Rogers, E. "Diffusion Research Methodology: Focus on Health Care Organizations." In G. Gordon and G. Fisher, eds. *The Diffusion of Medical Technology*. Cambridge, Mass: Ballinger Publishing Co., 1975, 51–73.

Tubesing, D. (1977): See Section A.

Valadez, A. and Anderson, E. (1972): See Section F.

Vernon, E. (1974): See Section A.

Weed, L. *Medical Records, Medical Education*

and Patient Care: The Problem-Oriented Record as a Basic Tool, 5th ed. Cleveland: The Press of Case Western Reserve University, 1971.

Weisbord, M. "Why Organization Development Hasn't Worked So Far In Medical Centers." *Health Care Management Review* 1 (1976): 17–28.

Wessen, A. (1958): See Section F.

Wilson, R. The Physician's Changing Hospital Role." *Human Organization* 18 (1959–1960): 177–183.

Wittenborn, J. et al. (1970): See Section A.

Yanda, R. (1977): See Section F.

Zaenglein, M. and Smith, C. "An Analysis of Individual Communication Patterns and Perceptions In Hospital Organizations." *Human Relations* 25 (1972): 493–504.

Zola, I. (1963): See Section A.

K. Communication With The Terminally Ill

Artiss, K. and Levine, A. (1973): See Section A.

Alvarez, W. "Care of the Dying." *Journal of the American Medical Association* 2 (1952): 86–91.

Barton, D. "The Need For Including Instruction on Death and Dying in the Medical Curriculum." *Journal of Medical Education* 47 (1972): 169–75.

Becker, E. *The Denial of Death*. New York: The Free Press, 1973.

Bloom, M. et al. (1971): See Section D.

Bowers, M. *Counseling the Dying*. New York: Thomas Nelson and Sons, 1964.

Brodlie, J. "Drug Abuse and Television Viewing Patterns." *Psychology* 9 (1972): 33–36.

Brody, M. "Compassion For Life and Death." *Medical Opinion and Review* 3 (1967): 108–13.

Bugen, L., ed. *Death and Dying*. Dubuque, Iowa: William C. Brown Company, 1979.

Bunch, B. and Zahra, D. "Dealing With Death: The Unlearned Role." *American Journal of Nursing 76* (1976): 1486–87.

Crane, D. *The Sanctity of Social Life: Physicians' Decisions to Treat Critically Ill Patients*. New York: Russell Sage, 1975.

Friedman, S. et al. "Behavior Observations on Parents Anticipating the Death of a Child." *Pediatrics* 32 (1963): 610–25.

Glaser, B. "The Physician and the Dying Patient." *Medical Opinion and Review* 1 (1965): 108–14.

Glaser, B. and Strauss, A. *Awareness of Dying*. Chicago: Aldine Publishing Company, 1965.

Goleman, D. "We Are Breaking the Silence About Death." *Psychology Today* 10 (1976): 44–48.

Kubler-Ross, E. *Death: The Final State of Growth*. Englewood Cliffs: N.J.: Prentice-Hall, Inc., 1975.

Kubler-Ross, E. *On Death and Dying*. New York: MacMillan, Inc., 1969.

Kubler-Ross, E. *Questions and Answers On Death and Dying* New York: MacMillan, Inc., 1974.

Kutscher, A. and Goldberg, M. eds. *Caring For the Dying Patient and His Family*. New York: Health Sciences Publishing Company, 1973.

Nelson, B. (1973): See Section A.

Rado, L. "Death Redefined: Social and Cultural Influences on Legislation." *Journal of Communication* 31 (1981): 41–47.

Rich, T. and Kalmanson, G. "Attitudes of Medical Residents Toward the Dying Patient In a General Hospital." *Postgraduate Medicine* 40 (1966): 127–30.

Ufema, J. "Dare to Care For the Dying." *American Journal of Nursing* 76 (1976): 88–90.

Verwoerdt, A. *Communication With the Fatally Ill*. Springfield, Ill: Charles C. Thomas Publishers, 1966.

Verwoerdt, A. and Wilson, R. "Communication With Fatally Ill Patients." *American Journal of Nursing* 67 (1967): 2307–09.

Westhoff, M. "Listening to Relieve the Fear of Death." *Supervisor Nurse* 3 (1972): 80–87.

White, J. "The Self-Image of the Physician and the Care of Dying Patients."

Annals of the New York Academy of Science 164 (1969): 822.

L. Media and Technology In Health Care

Adler, L. and Enelow, A. (1966): See Section D.

Adler, L. et al. (1970): See Section D.

Alger, I. and Hogan, P. (1969): See Section D.

Apostle, D. and Oder, F. (1967): See Section H.

Atkins, C. "Research Evidence On Mass Mediated Health Communication Campaigns." In D. Nimmo, ed. *Communication Yearbook 3*. New Brunswick, N.J: Transaction-International Communication Association, 1979, 655–88.

Atkins, C. "Effects of Drug Commercials on Young Viewers." *Journal of Communication* 28 (1978): 48–56.

Atkyns, R. et al. (1975): See Section H.

Baran, S. "TV Programing and Attitudes Toward Mental Retardation." *Journalism Quarterly* 54 (1977): 140–42.

Barnum, H. "Mass Media and Health Communications." *Journal of Medical Education* 50 (1975): 24–26.

Bartlett, M. et al. (1973): See Section J.

Batey, M. (1963): See Section A.

Bishop, R. (1974): See Section G.

Brenner, D. and Logan, R. "Some Considerations In the Diffusion of Medical Technologies: Medical Information Systems." In D. Nimmo, ed. *Communication Yearbook 4*. New Brunswick, N.J: Transaction-International Communication Association, 1980, 609–23.

Cannell, D. and MacDonald, J. "The Impact of Health News on Attitudes and Behaviors." *Journalism Quarterly* 35 (1956): 315–23.

Capalaces, R. and Starr, J. "The Negative Message of Anti-Drug Spots: Does It Get Across?" *Public Telecommunications* 1 (1973): 64–66.

Cassata, D. et al. (1977): See Section D.

Cassata, D. et al. (1976): See Section D.

Cassata, D. and Clements, P. (1978): See Section D.

Cassata, D. et al. "In Sickness and In Health." *Journal of Communication* 29 (1979): 73–80.

Coleman, J. et al. (1966): See Section J.

Day, S. (1975): See Section B.

Eisler, R. et al. (1973): See Section C.

Farquhar, J. and Maccoby, N. (1977): See Section H.

Feingold, P. and Knapp, M. "Anti-drug Abuse Commercials." *Journal of Communication* 27 (1977): 20–28.

Fejer, D. et al. (1971): See Section H.

Feldman, J. *The Dissemination of Health Information*. Chicago: Aldine, 1966.

Fritzen, R. and Mazer, G. (1975): See Section D.

Goldstein, H. "Guidelines For Drug Education Through Electronic Media." *Journal of Drug Education* 14 (1965): 157–71.

Greenberg, R. et al. "A Content Analytic Study of Daily Newspaper Coverage of Cancer." in D. Nimmo, ed. *Communication Yearbook 3*. New Brunswick, N.J.: Transaction-International Communication Association, 1979, 645–54.

Griffiths, W. and Knutson, A. "The Role of Mass Media in Public Health." *American Journal of Public Health* 50 (1960): 515–23.

Hanneman, G. (1973): See Section H.

Hawkins, et al. "Using Computer Programs to Provide Health Information To Adolescents: BARNY." Paper presented to the ICA conference, Boston, 1982.

Helfer, R. and Levin, S. (1967): See Section D.

Isguith, R. (1974): See Section H.

Janis, I. and Feshback, S. (1953): See Section A.

Kanter, D. "Research on the Effects of Over-The-Counter Drug Advertising." *Journal of Drug Issues* 4 (1974): 223–26.

Kaufman, L. "Prime-Time Nutrition." *Journal of Communication* 30 (1980): 37–46.

Kirscht, J. et al. (1975): See Section A.

Kobin, W. "Encouraging Better Health Through Television." *Journal of Medical Information* 50 (1975): 143–48.

Kreps, G. "The Youth Wellness Media Project: A Preliminary Report." Working paper Indiana University-Purdue University at Indianapolis, 1982.

Leventhal, H. "Fear Communications in the Acceptance of Preventive Health Practices." *Bulletin of the New York Academy of Medicine* 11 (1965): 1144–65.

Lindberg, D. *Growth of Medical Information Systems In the United States.* Lexington, Mass: Lexington Books, 1979.

Loeb, F. (1968): See Section C.

Maccoby, N. and Farquhar, J. "Communication for Health: Unselling Heart Disease." *Journal of Communication* 25 (1975): 114–26.

Mark, N. "How Television Tries to Close the Health Information Gap." *Today's Health* 54 (3), (1976): 31–33.

Maultsby, M. and Slack, W. "A Computer Based Psychiatry History System." *Archives of General Psychiatry* 25 (1971): 570.

McEwen, W. and Hanneman, G. "The Depiction of Drug Use in Television Programming." *Journal of Drug Education* 4 (1974): 281–93.

McLaughlin, J. "The Doctor Shows." *Journal of Communication* 25 (1975): 182–84.

Meadow, R. and Hewitt, C. (1972): See Section D.

Meyer, A. et al. "The Role of Opinion Leadership in a Cardiovascular Health Education Campaign." In B. Ruben, ed. *Communication Yearbook 1.* New Brunswick, N.J: Transaction-International Communication Association, (1977), 579–91.

Milausky, R. et al. "TV Drug Use Among Advertising and Proprietary and Illicit Drug Use Among Teenage Boys." *Public Opinion Quarterly* 39 (1975): 457–81.

O'Keefe, M. "The Anti-Smoking Commercials: A Study of Television's Impact on Behavior." *Public Opinion Quarterly* 35 (1971): 242–48.

Park, B. and Bashshur, R. "Some Implications of Telemedicine." *Journal of Communication* 25 (1975): 161–66.

Porterfield, J. "The Merchandising of Public Health." *New York Academy of Medicine Bulletin* 40 (1964).

Pratt, L. "How Do Patients Learn About Disease?" *Social Problems* 4 (1956): 29–40.

Puska, P. et al. "A Comprehensive Television Smoking Cessation Programme In Finland." *International Journal of Health Education* 22 (1979): 1–29.

Ray, M. and Ward, S. "Experimentation for Pretesting Public Health Programs: The Case of the Anti-Drug Abuse Campaigns." *Advances in Consumer Research* 3 (1976): 278–86.

Rosenblatt, D. and Kabasakalian, L. "Evaluation of Venereal Disease Information Campaign for Adolescents." *American Journal of Public Health* 56 (1966): 1104–13.

Schlegel, R. (1977–1978): See Section A.

Schlinger, M. "The Role of Mass Communications in Promoting Public Health." *Advances in Consumer Research* 3 (1976): 302–05.

Schmelling, D. and Wotring, C. "Agenda-Setting Effects of Drug Abuse Public Service Ads." *Journalism Quarterly.* 53 (1976): 743–46.

Scully, D. and Bart, P. (1973): See Section H.

Shaw, D. and Nevel, P. "The Informative Value of Medical Science News." *Journalism Quarterly* 44 (3) (1967): 548.

Simoni, J. and Ball, R. "Can We Learn From Medicine Hucksters?" *Journal of Communication* 25 (1975): 174–81.

Sinnett, E. et al. "Credibility of Sources of Information About Drugs." *Psychological Reports* 39 (1975): 299–309.

Slack, W. et al. "A Computer Based Medical History." *New England Journal of Medicine,* 274 (1966): 194–98.

Slack, W. et al. "Dietary Interviewing by Computer," *Journal of the American Diabetics Association.* 69 (1976): 514–17.

Smart, R. and Feger, D. "The Effects of High and Low Fear Messages About Drugs." *Journal of Drug Education* 4 (1974): 225–35.

Sobel, J. and Brown, J. "Public Health Agenda-Setting: Evaluation of a Cardiovascular Risk Reduction Campaign," paper presented at the ICA conference, Boston, 1982.

Stimson, G. "The Message of Psychotropic Drug Ads." *Journal of Communication* 25 (1975): 153–60.

Stoeckle, J. et al. "Learning Medicine by Videotaped Recordings." *Journal of Medical Education* 46 (1971): 518–24.

Swinehart, J. "Voluntary Exposure to Health Communication." *American Journal of Public Health* 58 (1968): 1265–75.

Tannon, C. and Rogers, E. (1975): See Section J.

Udry, J. "Can Mass Media Advertising Increase Contraceptive Use?" *Family Planning Perspectives* 4 (1972): 37–44.

Wade, S. and Schramm, W. "The Mass Media As Sources of Public Affairs, Science, and Health Knowledge." *Public Opinion Quarterly* 33 (1969): 197–209.

Wagner, H. "Videotape in the Teaching of Medical History Taking." *Journal of Medical Education* 42 (1967): 1055–58.

Winick, C. "A Content Analysis of Drug Related Network Entertainment Prime Time Programs." In *Social Responses to Drug Use, Commission of Marijuana and Drug Abuse*. Washington, D.C: Government Printing Office, 1973, 698–708.

Wright, W. "Mass Media as Sources of Medical Information." *Journal of Communication* 25 (1975): 171–73.

M. Ethical Aspects of Health Care

Alfidi, R. (1971): See Section D.

Alvarez, W. (1952): See Section K.

Bandman, E. and Bandman, B. *Bioethics and Human Rights: A Reader for Health Professionals*. Boston: Little Brown and Company, 1978.

Banks, S. and Vastyan, E. (1973): See Section A.

Barber, B. (1976): See Section A.

Barnlund, D. (1976): See Section A.

Barry, V. *Moral Aspects of Health Care*. Belmont, Ca.: Wadsworth Publishing Co., 1982.

Beauchamp, T. and Childress, J. *Principles of Biomedical Ethics*. New York: Oxford University Press, 1979.

Beauchamp, T. and Walters, L. *Contemporary Issues In Bioethics*. Encino: Ca.: Dickenson Publishing, 1978.

Beecher, H. (1961): See Section A.

Blaxter, M. (1978): See Section D.

Bok, S. *Lying: Moral Choice In Public and Private Life*. New York: Vintage Books, 1978.

Bok, S. "The Ethics In Giving Placebos." *Scientific American* 231 (1974): 17–23.

Campbell, A. *Moral Dilemmas In Medicine*, 2nd ed. London: Longman Press, 1975.

Campbell, A. (1976): See Section A.

Carlson, R. (1975): See Section J.

Casberg, M. "Toward Human Values in Medical Practice." *Medical Opinion and Review* 3 (1967): 22–25.

Collins, E. (1955): See Section D.

Corea, G. (1977): See Section H.

Cousins, N. (1979): See Section A.

Dangott, L. et al. "Communication and Pain." *Journal of Communication* 28 (1978): 30–35.

Davies, E. "The Patient's Right to Know the Truth." *Proceedings of the Royal Society of Medicine* 66 (1973): 533–36.

Dennert, J. (1976): See Section A

Dewitt, C. *Privileged Communications Between Physicians and Patients*. Springfield, Ill: Charles C. Thomas Publishers, 1958.

Diamond, B. and Weihofen, H. "Privileged Communication and the Clinical Psychologist." *Journal of Clinical Psychology* 9 (1953): 388–90.

Dlougy, A. et al. "What Patients Should Know About Their Diagnostic Tests." *Nursing Outlook* 11 (1963): 265–67.

Dodge, J. (1971): See Section H.

Duff, R. and Campbell, A. "Moral and Ethical Dilemmas in the Special Care Nursery." *New England Journal of Medicine* 289 (1973): 890–94.

Etziony, M. *The Physician's Creed: An Anthology of Medical Prayers, Oaths and Codes of Ethics*. Springfield, Ill: Charles C. Thomas, 1973.

Fenner, K. *Ethics and Law in Nursing: Profes-*

sional Perspectives. New York: Van Nostrand Press, 1980.

Fitts, W. and Fitts, B. "Ethical Standards in the Medical Profession." *Annals of the American Academy of Political and Social Science* 297 (1955): 25.

Fletcher, J. *Morals and Medicine.* Boston: Beacon Press, 1960.

Fox, R. "Ethical and Existential Developments in Contemporaneous American Medicine." *Milbank Memorial Fund Quarterly* 52 (1974): 445–83.

Fuchs, V. (1974): See Section A.

Gaylin, W. (1976): See Section E.

Gaylin, W. "Harvesting the Dead." *Harpers* 249 (1492), (1974): 23–29.

Gorovitz, S. and MacIntyre, A. (1976): See Section A.

Gorovitz, S. "Bioethics and Social Responsibility." *The Monist* 60 (1977): 3.

Horty, J. "Informed Consent: New Rule Puts Burden of Proof on Patient." *Modern Hospital* 116 (2), (1971): 54–55.

Illich, I. *Medical Nemesis.* New York: Random House, 1976.

Ingelfinger, F. "Informed (But Uneducated) Consent." *New England Journal of Medicine* 287 (1972): 465–66.

Ingelfinger, F. "Why Trust the Professional?" *New England Journal of Medicine* 286 (1972): 263–64.

Johnson, T. (1972): See Section F.

Kaiser, B. and Kaiser, I. (1974): See Section H.

Kalish, R. and Collier, K. *Exploring Human Values.* Monterey, Ca.: Brooks/Cole Publishing Co., 1981.

Kieffer, G. *Bioethics: A Testbook of Issues.* Menlo Park, Ca: Addison-Wesley Publishing Co., 1979.

Klemer, R. (1966): See Section D.

Ledermann, E. *Philosophy and Medicine,* Philadelphia: J. B. Lippincott, 1970.

Magee, J. (1975): See Section H.

Mappes, T. and Zembaty, J. *Biomedical Ethics.* New York: McGraw-Hill Co., 1981.

McFadden, C. *Medical Ethics.* Philadelphia: F. A. Davis, 1967.

Mendelsohn, R. (1979): See Section A.

Meyer, B. "Truth and the Physician."

Bulletin of the New York Academy of Medicine 45 (1969): 59–71.

Munson, R. *Intervention and Reflection: Basic Issues in Medical Ethics.* Belmont, Ca.: Wadsworth Publishing Co., 1979.

Purtilo, P. and Cassel, C. *Ethical Dimensions in the Health Professions.* Philadelphia: W. B. Saunders, 1981.

Presidents Commission for the Study of Ethical Problems in Medicine and Biomedical and Medical Research. *Making Health Care Decisions: A Report on the Ethical and Legal Implications of Informed Consent on the Patient-Practitioner Relationship.* Volume 1: Report, Washington, D.C.: U.S. Government Printing Office, 1982.

Ramsey, P. *Ethics at the End of Life.* New Haven, Conn.: Yale University Press, 1978.

Scannon, T. and Giacomo, J. *An Introduction to Bioethics* New York: Paulist Press, 1979.

Scheifelbein, S. (1980): See Section H.

Scully, D. and Bart, P. (1973): See Section H.

Silverman, M. and Lee, P. *Pills, Profits, and Politics.* Berkeley, Ca: University of California Press, 1974.

Standard, S. and Nathan, E., eds. *Should the Patient Know the Truth?* New York: Springer, 1955.

Steele, S. *Value Clarification in Nursing.* New York: Appleton-Century-Crofts, 1979.

Szasz, T. and Hollender, M. "A Contribution to the Philosophy of Medicine: The Basic Models of Doctor-Patient Relationship." *Archives of Internal Medicine* 97 (1956): 585–92.

Visscher, M. ed. *Humanistic Perspectives In Medical Ethics.* Buffalo, N.Y: Prometheus Books, 1972.

N. General Communication Literature

Anderson, K. and Clevenger, T. "A Summary of Experimental Research in Ethics." *Speech Monographs* 30 (1963): 59–73.

Anderson, W. "Bulletin Boards, Exhibits, Hotlines." In C. Ruess and D. Silvis, eds. *Inside Organizational Communication.* New York: Longman, Inc., 1981.

Bostrom, R. "Patterns of Communicative Interaction in Small Groups." *Communication Monographs* 37 (1970), 257–63.

Bradley, P. and Baird, J. *Communication for the Business and Professions.* Dubuque, Iowa: William C. Brown, 1980.

Burge, S. "Audiovisuals." In: *Inside Organizational Communication*, Reuss, C. and Silvis, D., eds., New York: Longman, 1981, 169–186.

Cohen, B. *The Press, the Public, and Foreign Policy.* Princeton, N.J.: Princeton University Press, 1963.

Deutsch, K. *Nationalism and Social Communication—An Inquiry Into the Foundations of Nationality.* Cambridge, Mass.: The M.I.T. Press, 1966.

Dewey, J. *How We Think.* Lexington, Mass.: Heath Publishing Co, 1933.

Elmore, G. "Integrating Video Technology and Organizational Communication." Paper presented to the Indiana Speech Association conference, Indianapolis, 1981.

Emery, E. et al. *Introduction to Mass Communications*, 2nd ed. New York: Dodd, Mead and Co., 1968.

Fayol, H. *General and Industrial Management.* London: Pitman, 1949.

Fisher, B. A. *Small Group Decision Making: Communication and Process.* New York: McGraw Hill, 1974.

Fisher, D. *Communication in Organizations.* St. Paul, Minn.: West Publishing Co., 1981.

French, J. and Raven, B. "The Basis of Social Power." In *Group Dynamics: Research and Theory*, 3rd edition, D. Cartwright and A. Zander, eds. New York: Harper and Row, 1968, 259–69.

Frost, J. and Wilmot, W. *Interpersonal Conflict.* Dubuque, Iowa: William C. Brown, 1978.

Giffin, K. "An Experimental Evaluation On the Trust Differential." Lawrence, K: The University of Kansas Communication Research Center, 1968.

Giffin, K. and Barnes, R. *Trusting Me,*

Trusting You. Columbus, Oh: Charles Merrill Co., 1976.

G. Goodman. *Winning By Telephone: Telephone Effectiveness for the Business and Professional Consumer.* Englewood Cliffs, N.J.: Prentice Hall, 1982.

Gouran, D. "Perspectives On the Study of Leadership: Its Present and Its Future." *Quarterly Journal of Speech* 60 (1974): 376–81.

Haakenson, R. "A Good Talk: C.O.D.: Content, Organization, and Delivery." In *Communication Probes*, B. Peterson et al., eds. Chicago: Science Research Associates, 1977.

Halpin, A. and Winer, B. *The Leadership Behavior of the Airplane Commander.* Columbus, Oh: State University Research Foundation, 1952.

House, R. "Role Conflict and Multiple Authority in Complex Organizations." *California Management Review* 12 (1970), 53–60.

Hyman, H. and Sheatsley, P. "Some Reasons Why Information Campaigns Fail." In W. Schramm and D. Roberts, eds. *Processes and Effects of Mass Communications.* Urbana, Ill.: University of Illinois Press, 1971.

Kreps, G. "A Field Experimental Test and Revaluation of Weick's Model of Organizing." In D. Nimmo, ed. *Communication Yearbook 4.* New Brunswick, N.J.: Transaction Press/International Communication Association, 1980, 389–98.

Mabry, E. and Barnes, R. *The Dynamics of Small Group Communication.* Englewood Cliffs, N.J.: Prentice-Hall, 1980.

Maccoby, N. et al. "Reducing the Risk of Cardiovascular Disease: Effects of a Community Based Campaign on Knowledge and Behavior." *Journal of Community Health* 3 (1977): 100–14.

McGregor, D. *The Human Side of Enterprise.* New York: McGraw Hill, 1960.

McLuhan, M. *Understanding Media: The Extensions of Man.* New York: McGraw Hill, 1964.

Taylor, F. *Scientific Management.* New York: Harper and Row, 1911.

Tortoriello, T. et al. *Communication in the Organization: An Applied Approach.* New York: McGraw Hill, 1978.

Vogel, A. and Krabbe, M. *Mass Communication.* Menlo Park, Ca.: Cummings, 1977.

Von Bertalanffy, L. *General Systems Theory.* New York: Braziler, 1969.

Weber, M. *The Theory of Social and Economic Organization.* Translated by A. Henderson and T. Parsons. New York: Oxford University Press, 1948.

Weick, K. *The Social Psychology of Organizing.* Reading, Mass.: Addison Wesley, 1969.

INDEX